T0336933

Veterinary Toxicology for Australia and New Zealand

Veterinary Toxicology for Australia and New Zealand

Rosalind Dalefield, BVSc PhD DABVT DABT
Masterton, New Zealand

Elsevier
Radarweg 29, PO Box 211, 1000 AE Amsterdam, Netherlands
The Boulevard, Langford Lane, Kidlington, Oxford OX5 1GB, United Kingdom
50 Hampshire Street, 5th Floor, Cambridge, MA 02139, United States

Notices
Knowledge and best practice in this field are constantly changing. As new research and experience broaden
our understanding, changes in research methods, professional practices, or medical treatment may become
necessary.

Practitioners and researchers must always rely on their own experience and knowledge in evaluating and
using any information, methods, compounds, or experiments described herein. In using such information or
methods they should be mindful of their own safety and the safety of others, including parties for whom they
have a professional responsibility.

To the fullest extent of the law, neither the Publisher nor the authors, contributors, or editors, assume any
liability for any injury and/or damage to persons or property as a matter of products liability, negligence or
otherwise, or from any use or operation of any methods, products, instructions, or ideas contained in the
material herein.

British Library Cataloging-in-Publication Data
A catalog record for this book is available from the British Library

Library of Congress Cataloging-in-Publication Data
A catalog record for this book is available from the Library of Congress

ISBN: 978-0-12-420227-6

For Information on all Elsevier publications visit our
website at https://www.elsevier.com/books-and-journals

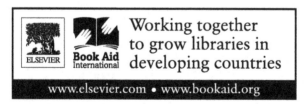

Working together
to grow libraries in
developing countries

www.elsevier.com • www.bookaid.org

Publisher: Sara Tenney
Acquisition Editor: Zoe Kruze
Editorial Project Manager: Molly McLaughlin
Production Project Manager: Chris Wortley
Designer: Greg Harris

Typeset by MPS Limited, Chennai, India

This book is dedicated to A.W.L., who would have found it interesting.

Contents

14. Metals

15. Metalloids

Rhian Cope

16. Site of First Contact Effects of Acids and Alkalis

Rhian Cope

17. Miscellaneous Inorganic Toxicants

Rhian Cope

22. Venomous and Poisonous Vertebrates

Part 1: Venomous and Poisonous Terrestrial Vertebrates
in Australia

Part 2: Venomous Aquatic Vertebrates

23. Venomous and Poisonous Invertebrates

Part 1: Aquatic Invertebrates

Part 3: Poisonous Native Plants of New Zealand

Foreword

Recent decades have seen the publication of a number of reference books on veterinary toxicology, but most of them have been produced in the United States of America, and concentrate on toxicants and venomous animals of importance to North America. The idea of this book, as originally conceived by Rosalind Dalefield and Rhian Cope, was to provide information more relevant to veterinary personnel in Australia and New Zealand. While it is hoped that the book will be interesting and informative to laypeople, it is not intended to replace a veterinary consultation, and it has been assumed that the reader has an education in veterinary medicine. It is further assumed that the reader is competent in general emergency medicine, including diagnostic procedures and techniques, and life support measures. Veterinary personnel seeking more information about emergency medicine are referred to appropriate reference books, notably Kirk & Bistner's *Handbook of Veterinary Procedures and Emergency Treatment*, also published by Elsevier.

In treating the poisoned animal, veterinary personnel should always bear in mind that the first rule of toxicology is *The Dose Makes The Poison* and the first rule of clinical toxicology is *Treat The Patient, Not The Poison*.

Chapter 1

Introduction and Definitions

INTRODUCTION

The purpose of this book is to present a convenient reference work on veterinary toxicology, that is applicable to Australia and New Zealand, for use by veterinary practitioners, veterinary nurses and practice staff, and related occupations.

With a few exceptions, the adverse side effects and effects of overdose of veterinary pharmaceuticals are not addressed in this book, because it is anticipated that veterinarians, veterinary nurses, and others who use veterinary pharmaceuticals will have appropriate training concerning those pharmaceuticals, and will also have access to package inserts and other sources of information.

Bacterial toxins that are synthesized by bacteria proliferating in the body of the affected animal are not addressed in this book, although botulism is covered because it is generally the result of ingestion of preformed toxin.

TOXICOLOGY: THE SCIENCE OF POISONS

A *poison* is any chemical that can interfere with cellular processes of the living organism.

The dictum of the Swiss-German physician and alchemist Paracelsus (1493−1541) is often quoted as the fundamental rule of toxicology: "Poison is in everything, and no thing is without poison. The dosage makes it either a poison or a remedy." While the fundamental principle that "the dose makes the poison" is correct, not all substances are poisonous. It would be more accurate to say that anything that can interact *chemically* with tissues is a poison at some dose. An insoluble polymer such as keratin or nylon is not poisonous, although ingestion of a large amount could cause a mechanical blockage of the gastrointestinal tract. Also, while all pharmacological agents are potentially poisonous if given in overdose, there are many poisons that have no therapeutic properties. The action of poisons is independent of temperature; liquid nitrogen and fire can have extremely adverse effects, but are not poisons.

The concept that all substances have a threshold below which they are not toxic is extremely important, but often overlooked.

Veterinary Toxicology for Australia and New Zealand
DOI: http://dx.doi.org/10.1016/B978-0-12-420227-6.00001-3

IMPORTANT DEFINITIONS AND CONCEPTS

Understanding and accurate use of the following terms and concepts is important in toxicology.

Acute toxicity	The effects of exposure lasting 24 hours or less; often used to describe toxicity from a single exposure
AUC	Area under the curve or total systemic exposure; see chapter on Toxicokinetics for more information
Chronic toxicity	Effects of repeated or continuous exposure lasting for 3 months or more
Dosage	The amount of poison per unit of the animal's bodyweight, e.g., mg/kg
Dose	The total amount of poison received by the animal
Dose−response curve	Graphical representation of the relationship between increasing dose on the x-axis and increasing severity of response on the y-axis. Typically sigmoid, and closest to linearity at the LD_{50} (see below)
Dose−response relationship	The relationship between increasing dose and increasing severity of response
Idiosyncratic response	An uncharacteristically severe response to a poison that occurs rarely and generally unpredictably in a population, because of individual metabolic or immune-mediated characteristics
Intoxication	The disease state caused by exposure to a poison. Synonymous with toxicosis. Not confined to the effects of ethanol in toxicology, although it is often used to refer only to effects of ethanol in common parlance
Latency or latent period	The delay between exposure to the poison and the onset of clinical signs. This is particularly relevant for protoxicants, i.e., when the poison is not toxic in itself, but is metabolized to a toxic metabolite
Lethal concentration	The lowest concentration of a poison in feed or in water that causes death. May be expressed in mg/kg feed or mg/L of water
Lethal dose, LD	The lowest dose that causes death. The lethal dose is often expressed as a percentage, and the most commonly used lethal dose is the lethal dose 50, or LD_{50}, which is the dose which will kill 50% of the population. The reason that LD_{50} is most often used is that the dose−response curve is closest to linear at LD_{50} and most reproducible
Median lethal dose	Synonymous with LD_{50}
Mycotoxin	A toxin synthesized by a fungus
Physiological adaptation (or subthreshold phase)	The part of the dose−response curve between a dose of zero and the threshold dose. In this part of the curve, the dose of the poison is increasing but the body is adapting and no toxic effects are manifested
Poison	A chemical that can interfere with processes required to maintain cellular viability in the living organism
Poisoning	The disease state caused by exposure to a poison. Synonymous with toxicosis

Prototoxicant (or protoxicant)	A substance that requires bioactivation by the exposed animal's body in order to produce toxic effects
Subacute toxicity	Effects of repeated or continuous exposure lasting for less than a month In practical terms, the duration varies but a subacute toxicity study is generally no longer than 2 weeks in duration
Subchronic toxicity	Effects of repeated or continuous exposure lasting for between 1 and 3 months
Threshold dose (or toxic threshold)	The dose at which detrimental effects on the organism first become manifested
Tolerance	An organism may adapt to a poison as a result of prolonged sublethal exposure, often by upregulation of metabolic enzymes that convert the poison to nontoxic metabolites
Toxic	An adjective that describes the adverse effects of a poison on an organism
Toxicant	A synonym for poison
Toxicosis	The disease state caused by exposure to a poison
Toxin	A poison synthesized by a living organism. The organism may belong to any of the taxonomic kingdoms, and organisms that synthesize toxins are found in all five kingdoms *Note*: Often but incorrectly used as a synonym for poison. All toxins are poisons, but most poisons encountered in veterinary practice are not toxins
Venom	A toxin produced or employed by an animal that exerts its effects when injected into another animal by means of a bite, sting, or similar active injection process *Note*: Toxins that are not injected, but affect those animals that mouth or ingest the animal producing the toxin, such as the poison of cane toads and their tadpoles, are not considered to be venoms
Venomous	An animal that uses venom in defense and/or predation
Xenobiotic	A substance that is foreign to the body. This is a useful term when referring to substances that may be harmless or therapeutic at intended dose but toxic in overdose
Zootoxin	A toxin synthesized by an organism from the Animal Kingdom

Chapter 2

Essentials of Toxicokinetics for Veterinary Practitioners

INTRODUCTION

To define *toxicokinetics*, it is helpful to revisit the definition of *pharmacokinetics*, which is the use of mathematical models to quantitate the time course of drug absorption and disposition in the body. Toxicokinetics differs from pharmacokinetics in two important aspects:

- The study of toxicokinetics is not confined to pharmaceuticals, but can be used to model all poisons.
- Toxicokinetics applies to the kinetics of poisons at doses at or above the dose at which metabolic pathways are saturated.

The toxicokinetics of a therapeutic drug often differs from the pharmacokinetics, and should never be assumed to be the same for any given drug. As an example, theophylline is excreted by *first-order kinetics* when given at therapeutic doses, which means that a fixed proportion of the total body burden is excreted per hour. However, when theophylline is given at toxic doses, it is excreted by *zero-order kinetics*, which means a fixed quantity is excreted per hour, regardless of the total body burden.

The biological aspects of toxicokinetics are *Absorption*, *Distribution*, *Metabolism*, and *Excretion*, often collectively referred to by the acronym *ADME*. These processes will be reviewed before the mathematical modeling of toxicokinetics is described. For the purpose of reviewing ADME processes, ingested substances that can lead to toxicity will be referred to as *xenobiotics*. This term also covers any substance that is "strange to the body" such as orally administered pharmaceutical substances as well as non-toxic substances. It is convenient to use this term because it also covers both those substances that are toxic as the parent compound and those that are metabolized to a substance that causes toxicity. The phenomenon whereby a parent compound of low or negligible toxicity is metabolized to the active toxicant is sometimes called *lethal synthesis*.

The intention of the following sections is to provide brief revision notes of the key points about ADME that are relevant to veterinary clinical toxicology. Comprehensive discussion of ADME is beyond the scope of this book.

Veterinary Toxicology for Australia and New Zealand
DOI: http://dx.doi.org/10.1016/B978-0-12-420227-6.00002-5

Absorption

Absorption is the movement of the poison from the site of administration into the circulating blood. The primary routes of absorption in toxicology are gastrointestinal, respiratory, and dermal.

The fraction of a xenobiotic that enters the body, relative to the total amount to which the animal is exposed, is termed the *bioavailability*, and is typically expressed as a percentage. The use of bioavailability data should always include the route of exposure. As an example, if the oral bioavailability of a xenobiotic is 50%, this means that 50% of the xenobiotic reaches the systemic circulation. This does not mean that the other 50% is passed out in the feces. It might be destroyed by stomach acid or intestinal flora, or metabolized by intestinal flora, intestinal mucosal cells (enterocytes), or on first pass through the liver or respiratory tract. For the purposes of toxicokinetics the gastrointestinal lumen, and the lumen of the respiratory tract, is treated as being "exterior" to the body.

Plasma concentration of a xenobiotic, drawn from a peripheral vein, is generally used as a representative default for determination of bioavailability of therapeutic drugs and other xenobiotics that are reasonably hydrophilic, although it can be misleading for lipophilic substances. Exposure to these can result a very low plasma concentration, suggesting that the xenobiotic has not been absorbed, when it has been absorbed but is dissolved hydrophobic compartments such as the Ito cells of the liver, adipose tissue and, if it can cross the blood—brain barrier, the central nervous system. For these substances, bioavailability may more accurately be determined by comparing excretion following intravenous administration to excretion following administration by the route of interest. Alternatively, total quantity measured in plasma over time following intravenous administration is compared to that quantity following administration by the route of interest. Bioavailability by intravenous bolus administration is by default 100%.

Gastrointestinal Absorption

To be absorbed by the gastrointestinal route, a xenobiotic must be soluble in gastric or intestinal fluids so that it can be transported across the mucosa, into submucosal capillaries and thus into the systemic circulation. In some cases the toxicant absorbed into the systemic circulation is not the parent xenobiotic but a metabolite produced by the action of gastric acid, intestinal fluids, or bacterial digestion in the rumen or large intestine.

For readily absorbed substances such as cyanide, or the nicotine in chewing tobacco, significant absorption may occur in the oral cavity. The oral mucosa is more permeable than skin, and buccal absorption bypasses the portal vein and escapes first-pass hepatic metabolism.

The epithelium of the esophagus and forestomachs, which include the reticulorumen of ruminants and the forestomach of rats, is keratinized (cornified), and absorption of xenobiotics across this barrier is generally low.

The gastric mucosa allows absorption, although the surface mucus may be a barrier to some xenobiotics. A more significant limiting factor to gastric absorption is the low pH of the stomach. Xenobiotics that are nonionized are most readily absorbed across bilipid membranes into cells. In the strongly acidic environment of the stomach, acidic xenobiotics are nonionized but basic xenobiotics are ionized, relatively hydrophilic, and unlikely to be absorbed. The stomach acid also destroys some substances completely. The transit time of xenobiotics in the stomach is generally short, which also limits absorption even of those xenobiotics that are nonionized. Ingestion of food delays gastric emptying and may promote gastric absorption. Although for most ingested xenobiotics the small intestine is the predominant site of absorption, for the reasons described in the next paragraph, it should not be assumed that absorption from the stomach does not occur.

The small intestine has evolved to facilitate the absorption of ingested substances. Characteristics that promote absorption include slightly basic pH, very well-perfused mucosa, the presence of pancreatic and bile secretions, the enormous surface area created by the microvilli and villi of the intestinal mucosa, and the enzymes expressed by the enterocytes.

Bile enhances the absorption of lipid-soluble xenobiotics by the formation of micelles with a hydrophilic surface and hydrophobic core, which deliver hydrophobic xenobiotics to the mucosal surface for diffusion across the lipid membranes of cells. Stimulation of bile release is another reason that ingestion of a poison with food may increase absorption, at least in carnivorous species that eat episodically. The proportion of fat in the food may significantly alter absorption of a lipophilic substance and is sometimes manipulated for this purpose.

Without the action of bile, extremely hydrophobic xenobiotics have limited absorption because they do not distribute well in gastrointestinal fluids and so access to enterocyte membranes is limited. On the other hand, extremely hydrophilic xenobiotics are unable to dissolve into bilipid membranes of cells. Xenobiotics that are most readily absorbed are those that are weak acids or weak bases.

The great majority of xenobiotics are absorbed by passive diffusion across, rather than between, enterocytes. However, enterocytes have specific active transport systems for absorption of some nutrients, and if a specific poison has a similar molecular configuration to such a nutrient, it may be absorbed by such a transport system. For example, some toxic minerals and metals are absorbed by mechanisms that have evolved to transport nutrient minerals. These transport systems tend to have very high capacity and are therefore unlikely to become saturated.

The role of the rumen in oral exposure to a xenobiotic is variable. In some cases it may protect against acute toxicosis by diluting the concentration of a xenobiotic and changing bolus ingestion to a more gradual release to the stomach and small intestine, while in other cases ruminal microbes may metabolize ingested xenobiotics to compounds of higher or lower toxicity.

Although the liver is commonly regarded as the primary site of metabolism of xenobiotics, the enterocytes, and/or intestinal flora, are capable of substantial metabolism of some xenobiotics. This is referred to as *prehepatic* or *presystemic metabolism.*

Dermal Absorption

The skin is generally a well-adapted barrier to xenobiotic absorption, with the result that systemic absorption following dermal exposure is almost always much lower than following oral or respiratory exposure. The primary barrier to absorption is the outermost layer of the epidermis, the stratum corneum. While most dermally applied toxicants have only local effects, if any, some have the chemical characteristics to reach the systemic circulation in toxic concentrations, particularly if the integrity of the skin barrier is reduced by circumstances such as abrasions, or prolonged soaking in water, or exposure to detergents or defatting agents.

There is no evidence for active transport of xenobiotics through the skin. Nonionized, lipid-soluble xenobiotics are largely absorbed by moving through the lipid layers between cells of the stratum corneum, rather than through the cells. Xenobiotics can also reach the dermis via hair follicles, sebaceous glands, and sweat glands, all of which penetrate to and are based in the dermis, although this route is believed to be significant only for very small and/or polar xenobiotics.

For those xenobiotics able to penetrate the epidermis, absorption from the dermis is facilitated by the highly vascular nature of this layer, and is increased when the dermal blood vessels are dilated.

Both Phase I and Phase II metabolic pathways have been identified in the skin, and resident bacteria on the skin may also metabolize xenobiotics.

Xenobiotics that can be absorbed through human skin should be assumed to be able to penetrate the skin of domestic animals, because as a generalization, human skin is at least as impermeable as the skin of cats and dogs, if not more so.

Respiratory Absorption

The same features that make pulmonary tissue ideally adapted for gas exchange also facilitate absorption of harmful gases. These are the great alveolar surface area, very thin epithelial membranes, and intimate association with abundant capillaries. Absorption into the systemic circulation by this route is the equivalent of intra-arterial administration, in that there is no opportunity for hepatic metabolism prior to systemic exposure (*first-pass hepatic metabolism*). However, nasal mucosal cells, as well as Clara cells and Type II pneumocytes in the lungs, have metabolic enzymes, and for some inhaled poisons these are significant sites of metabolism prior to absorption into the systemic circulation. As with any cell with metabolic capabilities, these cells are susceptible to injury from toxic metabolites of some inhaled xenobiotics.

Gases and vapors with high water solubility are primarily absorbed in the nasal passages and do not penetrate into the lower respiratory tract. For example, a highly water-soluble gas such as SO_2 is unlikely to penetrate beyond the upper respiratory tract unless adsorbed onto particles, whereas relatively water-insoluble gases such as ozone and NO_2 readily penetrate to the alveoli.

Irritant gases may induce upper respiratory inflammation, sneezing, tear production, and laryngospasm. Laryngospasm and bronchoconstriction are common acute responses to irritant gases, and can compromise respiratory function.

The rate of entry of a poisonous gas or vapor into the systemic circulation from the lower respiratory tract is determined by the solubility of the gas in blood, which determines how long it takes for a blood:gas equilibrium to be reached. The solubility of an inhaled gas in blood is expressed as the *blood: gas partition coefficient*. Gases and vapors that are highly soluble in blood have a high blood:gas partition coefficient whereas those that are poorly soluble in blood have a low blood:gas partition coefficient.

If a gas or vapor that reaches the alveoli is highly soluble in blood, it is very rapidly absorbed across the alveolar membrane and as blood passes continuously through the lungs, a large amount of the gas or vapor enters the body. In this situation the only way to increase the amount absorbed would be to increase the breathing rate and depth, so absorption of such gases and vapors is *ventilation-limited*. Equilibrium between the concentration of the xenobiotic in the air and the concentration of the xenobiotic in the blood takes longer to be achieved. Relative to a gas or vapor with poor solubility in blood, a gas or vapor with high solubility in blood takes longer to clear from the body by diffusion back into the alveoli from the blood, followed by exhalation, after exposure is halted.

For a gas or vapor that reaches the alveoli but has poor solubility in blood, the blood exposed to the xenobiotic rapidly becomes saturated, equilibrium between xenobiotic in the blood and xenobiotic in the alveoli is quickly reached, and unabsorbed xenobiotic remains in the alveoli and is exhaled. Systemic absorption can only be increased if the rate of blood flow through the lungs is increased, so absorption of such gases and vapors is *perfusion-limited*. Once exposure to such a gas or vapor is halted, the diffusion of the gas or vapor back into the alveoli, and subsequent removal from the body by exhalation, is relatively rapid. For this reason, poor solubility in blood is a desirable property in anesthetic agents, but anesthetic agents with this property are poor candidates for "gassing down" a patient and an induction agent such as a barbiturate is generally used to induce anesthesia, which is then maintained by the gas.

The factors affecting respiratory absorption of xenobiotics presented as aerosols or particulates are quite different, because the respiratory tract has a number of adaptations to prevent these reaching the alveoli. The upper respiratory tract presents numerous obstacles to particulates, such as the complexity of the nasal passageways, the presence of nasal mucus, and the sneeze and cough reflexes. On the other hand, some xenobiotics can be absorbed through the nasal mucosa and/or olfactory epithelium. Aerosol application to the olfactory epithelium is used in human beings as a method of delivering some pharmaceuticals directly to the central nervous system.

Protective features of the lower respiratory tract include the cough reflex, the mucociliary apparatus, and the changing directions of the branching bronchi and bronchioles. Particle sizes larger than 6 μm are unlikely to reach the alveolus. However, some xenobiotics can be absorbed through the mucous layer of the mucociliary apparatus and exert direct toxic effects on the underlying cells of the respiratory tract.

Particles and aerosols that are removed from the lower respiratory tract by the mucociliary apparatus are ultimately swallowed. Particles and aerosols caught on buccal mucus are swallowed, and most nasal mucus is also swallowed, the sneezing reflex notwithstanding. Thus, the body's exposure to inhaled particles and aerosols always includes some gastrointestinal exposure. For particles too large to reach the alveoli, and unable to penetrate the mucus of the mucociliary apparatus, the exposure will be gastrointestinal.

Insoluble particulate matter that does reach the alveoli is subject to phagocytosis by alveolar macrophages. However, insoluble particulates that are unable to reach the alveoli are not necessarily harmless. Chronic exposure to insoluble particulates as silica dust or coal dust can lead to severe pulmonary fibrosis in response to chronic irritant effects.

Distribution

To have a toxic effect, a xenobiotic must reach the target tissue at sufficient concentration, and for a sufficient period of time, to elicit its toxic effect. The xenobiotic must be in unbound, active form. A toxicant may be present in the systemic circulation but highly bound to components of the blood such as plasma proteins or erythrocyte membranes, and will not be able to exert a toxic effect on other components of the blood or vascular system, or move out of the vascular system to exert toxic effects on cells or tissues outside the vascular system. On the other hand, xenobiotic that is bound to plasma proteins is not available for renal excretion. A bound xenobiotic will be present in equilibrium with unbound xenobiotic, so as unbound xenobiotic is removed by metabolism and/or excretion, some bound xenobiotic will dissociate to maintain the equilibrium. Bound xenobiotic will also dissociate in the presence of a molecule for which it has a greater chemical affinity.

Tissues may also act as depots where a xenobiotic may be stored while having no toxic effect. Well-known examples are the storage of lead in bone, and the storage of chlorinated hydrocarbon pesticides in adipose tissue. This storage delays elimination, although equilibrium is maintained with plasma concentration such that, as the xenobiotic is removed from the plasma and ultimately from the body by metabolic and excretory processes, a proportion of the stored xenobiotic will be mobilized from the depot into the plasma. Storage in depots can lead to toxicity if the rate of absorption and storage exceeds the rate of elimination. For example, sheep are able to store copper in their livers but when the storage capacity is exceeded, the excess copper begins to damage the liver, precipitating a cascade of liver necrosis, free copper in the blood and hemolysis, which is usually fatal.

The perfusion of a given tissue and the affinity of the xenobiotic for that tissue, which in turn is determined by the physicochemical properties of the xenobiotic, affect the distribution of a xenobiotic to any given tissue. For most xenobiotics, movement from the blood into a tissue is by simple diffusion down a concentration gradient.

Some organs are relatively protected by barriers to xenobiotic penetration, such as the blood−brain barrier. The eyes, testes, and synovial joints are other examples. The placenta has some limited barrier functions, but should generally be regarded as a poor barrier.

The rate of metabolism of a xenobiotic has a major effect on the distribution. Metabolism generally results in a metabolite or metabolites that are more polar and more readily excreted, less able to cross cell membranes, and less likely to be stored in tissues.

Binding of xenobiotics in inactive form, storage of xenobiotics in depots, and rapid metabolism and excretion are among the reasons that a xenobiotic can have pharmaceutical or toxic effects on cells in cell culture but not toxic in the living organism. While studies in cultured cells can be extremely useful to elucidate mechanisms of toxic action, they cannot be used to replace toxicity studies in the living organism at present.

Metabolism

The liver is the major site of metabolism of most xenobiotics, and the most studied, although metabolic enzyme systems are widely distributed in the body. When the metabolic capacity of the liver for a given xenobiotic is saturated, systemic distribution of the xenobiotic to other metabolic sites is increased.

Metabolic enzyme systems in the body are numerous. Generally each enzyme pathway is capable of metabolizing numerous different substrates of similar physicochemical properties, although with different levels of activity. Metabolic processes have evolved to facilitate excretion of substances, including endogenous substances, from the body, rather than to make xenobiotics less toxic. Although it is common to refer to xenobiotics being "detoxified" by metabolism, a xenobiotic of low or moderate toxicity may be metabolized to a much more toxic metabolite or metabolites. Classic examples in veterinary toxicology include ethylene glycol and sodium fluoroacetate.

Metabolic processes are divided into Phase I and Phase II reactions, although these do not always happen sequentially as the names might suggest. Not all xenobiotics undergo metabolism, and of those that do, not all undergo both Phase I and Phase II reactions. Some xenobiotics are readily excreted unchanged, such as some gases that dissolve back across capillary and alveolar membranes into the alveolar spaces from the blood, and are exhaled unchanged. Some xenobiotics are rapidly excreted after Phase I metabolism and do not undergo Phase II metabolism. The substrates of Phase II metabolism may be metabolites produced by Phase I metabolism, or may be xenobiotics that do not first undergo Phase I metabolism. Both Phase I and Phase II metabolism may result in a metabolite that is more toxic than the parent compound.

The principal pathways included in Phase I metabolism are oxidation, reduction, hydrolysis, and hydration. Dethioacetylation and isomerization are also Phase I pathways. Phase II pathways include gluronidation, sulphation, methylation, acetylation, amino acid conjugation, glutathione conjugation, fatty acid conjugation, and condensation. Although metabolic pathways have generally evolved to facilitate excretion, sometimes metabolites are less readily excreted than the parent compound.

The Cytochrome P450 (*CytP450* or *P450*) mixed function oxidase system has been the most studied of metabolic systems, because many therapeutic drugs are metabolized by enzymes within this system, although not all metabolic enzyme pathways are part of this system. The CytP450 system is located in the endoplasmic reticulum of the liver. Hundreds of individual isoenzymes have been identified within this system. The level of activity of metabolic enzyme pathways, both within the CytP450 system and exclusive of it, often differs between species, and differences in metabolic enzyme activity may also be found based on age, sex, and breed. Furthermore, certain xenobiotics are known to induce increased activity of metabolic pathways, while others are known to inhibit them.

Excretion

The major routes of xenobiotic excretion are the renal and biliary routes, although volatile xenobiotics or metabolites may also be eliminated from the body by exhalation. Minor routes of xenobiotic elimination include sweat, semen, and keratinized structures including hair and hooves. Milk may be a significant pathway of excretion, and exposure of the offspring, in lactating animals.

Biliary Excretion

In addition to facilitating the absorption of dietary lipids, bile plays an important role in excretion. Biliary excretion is often the major route of excretion for xenobiotics or their metabolites with a molecular weight greater than 300 Da and a high degree of polarity. These substances enter bile by active transport processes, which are saturable and for which there may be competition. Passive diffusion into bile is negligible.

Xenobiotics and their metabolites excreted into bile may be subject to *enterohepatic circulation*, in which they are reabsorbed by the digestive tract and pass through the liver repeatedly, extending the duration of the xenobiotic or metabolite in the body. Enterohepatic circulation may include deconjugation of conjugated metabolites by intestinal flora. Intestinal flora may also degrade xenobiotics or metabolites that are excreted in the bile, confounding attempts to detect the substances in feces.

To reach the bile, xenobiotics must first be absorbed into hepatocytes. This principally occurs by passive diffusion but is generally a highly efficient process limited only by hepatic perfusion, because of the unique properties of the sinusoidal endothelium. Active transport mechanisms may be the principal or sole transport mechanism for highly polar molecules, and some xenobiotics are phagocytosed in protein-bound form by hepatocytes. Because many xenobiotics diffuse passively into hepatocytes but must then be transported into the bile by active transport processes, toxic xenobiotics or metabolites tend to accumulate in the liver. Consequently the liver is a common target organ of toxicity, and even when the hepatocytes are resistant to the toxic effects of the xenobiotic or metabolite, fresh liver is a recommended tissue for analytical detection of many poisons.

Xenobiotics and metabolites excreted in the bile do not always leave the body in the feces. It is common for the substances to be reabsorbed, with or without further metabolism by flora of the large intestine, and ultimately excreted in urine.

Biliary excretion varies between species. This is not only due to differences in metabolism but also due to differences in rate of bile flow and in composition of bile.

Urinary Excretion

Xenobiotics may enter the renal tubules as glomerular filtrate, by passive diffusion through tubule cells or by active tubular transport mechanisms. Xenobiotics may also be reabsorbed across tubule cells, so the total urinary excretion is the sum of glomerular filtration and secretion across tubule cells, less any reabsorption across tubule cells.

Only xenobiotics that are not protein-bound can enter the glomerular filtrate. Therefore the extent of glomerular filtration of a xenobiotic depends on both the degree of protein binding and the glomerular filtration rate. The glomerular filtration barrier possesses a net negative charge that limits the glomerular excretion of cationic xenobiotics or metabolites. Glomerular filtration is not saturable, so a constant fraction of the filterable xenobiotic presented to the glomeruli is filtered.

In contrast to glomerular filtration, active tubular pathways of excretion or reabsorption are saturable, and competition for the pathways may occur and alter excretion or reabsorption rate. Some xenobiotics can be actively transported into tubule cells but lack an equally efficient transport mechanism for transport out of the other side of the cell, with the result that the xenobiotic accumulates to toxic levels within the tubule cell.

There are two distinct excretory pathways for acids and bases through tubule cells. If two xenobiotics of similar ionic status are present in the circulation, they may compete for transport sites and affect each other's excretion. Many conjugated metabolites of Phase II metabolism are excreted by the acid excretion pathway.

Tubular reabsorption by passive back-diffusion may also occur. This process is affected by urine flow rate, lipid solubility of the xenobiotic, and urine pH. If urine production is low, excreted xenobiotic is likely to reach higher concentrations in the tubule lumen and there is greater time for back-diffusion to occur. Polar xenobiotics or metabolites are unlikely to diffuse back from the tubule lumen because they are unable to cross cell membranes, but nonionized, lipid-soluble xenobiotics or their metabolites may diffuse back into the circulation. Therefore the extent of back-diffusion is also influenced by the pK_a of the xenobiotic and the pH of the tubular fluid. Weak acids are most readily reabsorbed when the urinary pH is low while weak bases are most readily absorbed when the urinary pH is high. Carnivores tend to have acidic urine while herbivores tend to have slightly basic urine.

Some xenobiotics are known to be reabsorbed into tubules by pinocytosis, a low-capacity process that is readily saturated. Xenobiotics reabsorbed by this mechanism are generally broken down by lysosomes in the tubule cells, but for some xenobiotics such as aminoglycosides, this breakdown does not occur and the xenobiotic accumulates in the renal tubule cells.

Tubule cells have metabolic enzyme systems for both Type I and Type II metabolism, although there may be quantitative or qualitative differences in which isoenzymes are expressed. Some xenobiotics are metabolized in hepatocytes, some in renal tubule cells, and some in both. Of particular toxicological concern is relay metabolism such as when a metabolite that has been conjugated in the liver enters a tubule cell where the conjugate is cleaved off and free xenobiotic is released into the tubule cell.

As in the liver, lethal synthesis can occur in the kidney, with production of a toxic metabolite from a nontoxic xenobiotic.

MATHEMATICAL MODELING OF TOXICOKINETICS

The following is intended to be a brief review of critical terms and definitions that may be encountered in this book or in other textbooks of clinical veterinary toxicology. It is not intended to be a comprehensive explanation of toxicokinetic modeling, or to explore different types of compartmental modeling.

A semi-logarithmic plot of plasma concentration vs time, for a xenobiotic absorbed by a route other than intravenous injection, is shown in Fig. 2.1. This plot could represent the result of a single oral, dermal, or respiratory exposure, but not a bolus intravenous administration, for which the highest plasma concentration would be found at time 0, and therefore would lie on the y-axis.

The plot shows plasma concentration increasing to a peak as the xenobiotic is absorbed and then decreasing as metabolism and excretion clear the xenobiotic from the plasma.

Distribution into tissue depots may also clear the xenobiotic from the plasma and will prolong the final clearance of the xenobiotic from the body, because xenobiotic will be mobilized into plasma only as xenobiotic is cleared by excretion or metabolism, to maintain equilibrium between the plasma concentration and the tissue concentration.

The maximum plasma concentration, following exposure to a known amount of a xenobiotic, is abbreviated to the C_{max} or Cmax. This parameter is not referred to as much in clinical toxicology as the time from exposure to C_{max}, referred to as T_{max} or Tmax. T_{max} provides information on the rate of absorption or, when the toxic principle is a metabolite of the original xenobiotic, the rate at which the toxic metabolite is formed.

Of fundamental importance in clinical toxicology is whether the systemic absorption of the xenobiotic exceeds the *toxic threshold* above which it has

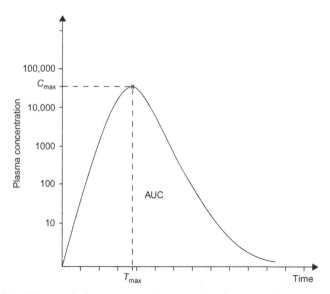

FIGURE 2.1 Diagram of plasma concentration over time, for routes of exposure other than intravenous.

detrimental effects on cells of the body. All poisons, without exception, have a toxic threshold below which the body is not harmed. The range of doses between zero and the toxic threshold is referred to as the range of *physiological adaptation*. It is sometimes asserted for a given xenobiotic that there is "no safe dose," e.g., "There is no safe dose of lead exposure in children" or "There is no safe dose of alcohol consumption in pregnancy." What these statements really mean is that the toxic threshold is unknown. It is incorrect to say that it does not exist.

Half-life or $T_{1/2}$ is an important but sometimes misused parameter in clinical toxicology, describing the time it takes for half of the xenobiotic in the body to be eliminated. This parameter gives information on the rapidity with which the xenobiotic can be metabolized and excreted. Half-life is the most easily measured parameter of the rate of removal from the body, because the downward curve is closest to linear at that point (see Fig. 2.1). However, the half-life in a toxic exposure is often assumed to be the same as the half-life in a pharmacological or other nontoxic exposure, and this is an unsafe assumption. At toxic levels, the pathways that dictate pharmacokinetics at nontoxic levels may be saturated, altering the kinetics of the xenobiotic. In addition, the toxic effects of the xenobiotic may affect metabolism or excretion. For example, a xenobiotic that causes liver necrosis may impair its own metabolism and/or biliary excretion, or a xenobiotic that lowers blood pressure and therefore reduces renal perfusion may impair its own renal excretion. It should never be assumed that half-life is the same in a toxic exposure as it is following a nontoxic exposure.

It should also be borne in mind that half-life is typically measured following an intravenous injection of the xenobiotic, a situation in which the curve shown in Fig. 2.1 is shifted to the left so that the C_{max} intersects with the y-axis.

The total plasma exposure to the xenobiotic is represented by the *area under the curve*, which is abbreviated to *AUC*. Decontamination techniques generally aim to reduce the total amount of xenobiotic absorbed in order to decrease the AUC. There are also methods for decreasing the AUC after absorption such as by increasing the rate of excretion or preventing metabolism of a xenobiotic. Techniques such as hemoperfusion, hemodialysis, or peritoneal dialysis aim to lower the AUC after absorption has taken place. Forced diuresis, with or without ion trapping, is intended to increase the rate of excretion of a xenobiotic.

Studies have shown that improvement in clinical outcome is unlikely to be achieved by decontamination methods unless the AUC is reduced by at least 50%. For this reason, many decontamination methods have been found to make no difference to clinical outcome and therefore they fail to meet the requirement for evidence-based medicine.

The plasma concentration of a xenobiotic immediately following intravenous injection of a known amount of a xenobiotic is used for the calculation of the *apparent volume of distribution* or V_D. This value can give information about the distribution and solubility of the xenobiotic. If the xenobiotic remains in the vascular system and does not readily move into extravascular spaces, the V_D will be similar to the total blood volume. If the xenobiotic is able to pass out of the blood vessels into interstitial spaces but is not readily distributed into cells or into adipose tissue, the V_D will be close to the total extracellular (blood plasma + interstitial fluid) fluid volume of the body. If the xenobiotic readily crosses cell membranes but is not readily distributed into adipose tissue, the V_D will be similar to the total fluid volume of the body. Some xenobiotics have a V_D significantly higher than the total volume of the whole body. This finding indicates that the xenobiotic is preferentially accumulating in a particular tissue or tissues. The most common examples in toxicology are lipid-soluble substances that accumulate in adipose tissue. Another example is iodine because it is actively scavenged from the plasma, against a concentration gradient, by thyroid tissue and also by lactating mammary gland. All extravascular concentrations of a xenobiotic exist in equilibrium with plasma concentrations, and xenobiotic molecules will move back into the plasma as the plasma concentration declines as a result of metabolism and excretion. However, this may be a very gradual process for substances sequestered in tissues with a slow metabolic rate, such as adipose tissue (e.g., chlorinated hydrocarbons and their metabolites) or bone (e.g., lead or fluoride).

The later part of the curve shown in Fig. 2.1 becomes asymptotic. That is, it approaches the *x*-axis but, in theory, never intersects with it. Although the point at which every last molecule of a xenobiotic is removed from the body is unknown, from the practical point of view the important parameter is when the level of xenobiotic in the body falls below a level at which it can cause toxic effects. For receptor-mediated toxicities, this is below the level at which receptor occupancy is sufficient to induce toxic effects. For xenobiotics that act by a mechanism that is not receptor-mediated, for example, corrosive substances that denature proteins indiscriminately, it is the level below which any damage is too slight to cause injury to the body.

Chapter 3

Emergency Care and Stabilization of the Poisoned Patient

Clinical poisoning cases represent a departure from the usual approach in veterinary clinical cases, which is that etiology should be determined before treatment is commenced. In the case of the poisoning emergency, stabilization and supportive treatment should be given priority over determining what poison the animal has been exposed to. Identifying the poison may be a slow process and the patient is likely to deteriorate or die in the interim. The majority of poisons do not have specific antidotes, and even for those that do, supportive symptomatic care is still critical. Most of the limited number of poisons that do have specific antidotes have distinctive toxidromes that make them readily diagnosable. The importance of giving priority to treatment of the patient rather than to identifying the toxic agent has led to the coining of the axiom of clinical toxicology.

TREAT THE PATIENT, NOT THE POISON

The first consideration in a poisoning case is to ensure that the situation does not pose a risk to the practitioner or support staff. However great the monetary or emotional value of the patient, the client, practitioner, or support staff should never put themselves at risk, such as by entering an environment in which there are deadly gases (e.g., hydrogen sulfide), handling an animal which has apparently toxic material on its coat (e.g., hydrogen fluoride or sulfuric acid) without appropriate protective clothing, or passing a gastric tube if the animal is likely to have toxic gas in the stomach (e.g., phosphine gas from ingestion of zinc phosphide rodenticide). This is not a merely theoretical risk. Fatalities have resulted from people trying to rescue workmates from environments in which there is toxic (e.g., chlorine or hydrogen sulfide) or asphyxiant (e.g., methane) gas. Veterinarians and support staff have been made ill as a result of inducing emesis, or passing a gastric tube, in canine cases of zinc phosphide poisoning.

Veterinary Toxicology for Australia and New Zealand
DOI: http://dx.doi.org/10.1016/B978-0-12-420227-6.00003-7

The priorities in stabilization are

- Ensuring oxygenation of tissues
- Maintaining cardiovascular function
- Controling central nervous function
- Maintaining body temperature within normal limits

Ensuring Oxygenation

In toxicology, this covers much more than the "Airway" of the traditional emergency "ABC." It cannot be assumed that a clear upper respiratory tract, larynx, and trachea are enough to ensure adequate oxygenation of hemoglobin if there is respiratory inhibition or arrest (strychnine, hydrogen sulfide poisoning, ethanol poisoning, ruminal tympany), bronchoconstriction (e.g., organophosphate poisoning), bronchiole obstruction (delayed effect of smoke inhalation) or pulmonary edema in the alveoli (chlorine gas poisoning). A clear airway and strong respiratory effort are of little value if the blood is unable to transport oxygen to the tissues due to cyanmethemoglobinemia (cyanide poisoning), methemoglobinemia (e.g., nitrite poisoning), or carboxyhemoglobinemia (carbon monoxide poisoning). Therefore the practitioner needs to consider all the steps from inhalation through to delivery of oxygenated blood to tissues, and recognize that if the animal is making respiratory efforts, this does not mean that the brain, heart, and other organs are getting sufficient oxygen for survival.

Maintaining Cardiovascular Function

Again, this covers much more than the "Bleeding" of the traditional emergency "ABC." Control of bleeding in hemorrhagic toxicoses such as anticoagulant poisoning is important, but it is also critical in the emergency situation to recognize and treat tachycardia, arrhythmia, and bradycardia. Correcting hypotension sufficiently to ensure adequate perfusion of all tissues, but particularly brain and kidneys, is also critical. Hypertension may also occur in clinical toxicology.

Controlling Central Nervous Function

Uncontrolled seizures can be rapidly fatal, and severe tremors alone can lead to exhaustion and cardiorespiratory failure. Central nervous depression is life-threatening if it is sufficient to paralyze the respiratory center (ethanol poisoning, barbiturate poisoning).

Maintaining Body Temperature

The potential of poisons to change body temperature should not be overlooked. Poisons may cause elevated body temperature (e.g., atropine, pentachlorophenol) or depressed body temperature (e.g., ethanol). Severe hyperthermia of small animals can be reversed by ice-water enema or, if an intravenous fluid line is in place, placing a loop of the tubing into a bowl of wet ice so that the fluid entering the body is chilled. Large animals, with the exception of sheep with more than minimal fleece, may be cooled by hosing or spraying, taking time to flatten the wet hair to the skin to remove the layer of dry air that would otherwise persist there. Shade and drinking water should be provided. Shearing will assist sheep, as well as long-haired goats or cattle, to cool. Warming of small animals can be promoted by hot water bottles, electric pads, or chemical hand-warmers. Large animals should be herded together to share body heat if possible. Woolen or reflective blankets help to conserve the animal's own body heat and will lead to gradual warming.

DECONTAMINATION

Decontamination has traditionally been described as "removing the animal from the poison and the poison from the animal" and is done to prevent further absorption, with the ultimate goal being to reduce the total systemic exposure or area under the curve (AUC). Removing the animal from the poison is fairly self-evident, although as noted previously, it should only be done if any risk of poisoning to those who would assist is controlled. The goal of removing the poison from the animal has been the goal of a number of practices, not all of which withstand the scrutiny of evidence-based medicine.

Gastrointestinal Decontamination

For ingested poisons, decontamination practices include:

- Inducing emesis
- Gastric lavage
- Rumenotomy and ruminal emptying
- Activated charcoal
  1. Single-dose activated charcoal (SDAC)
  2. Multiple-dose activated charcoal (MDAC)
- Catharsis
- Whole bowel irrigation (WBI)
- Enema
- Forced diuresis, with or without ion trapping
- Hemodialysis
- Hemoperfusion
- Peritoneal dialysis
- Intravenous lipid emulsion (ILE) also known as intravenous fat emulsion (IFE)

Inducing Emesis

Inducing emesis has been a standard part of treatment of poisoning in dogs and cats for many years, but does not withstand the scrutiny of evidence-based medicine and is very seldom justified. Extensive experimental studies in dogs and in human volunteers have shown that inducing emesis is rarely successful in removing more than half the stomach contents, even when the emetic is administered immediately after ingestion of the marker. Toxicokinetic studies have shown that prompt administration of an emetic makes little or no difference to the AUC as measured by plasma concentrations of the xenobiotic over time, and radiographic studies have shown that emesis is ineffective in removing radiodense pills or capsules from the stomach. Very large randomized prospective studies of human poisoning outcomes in multiple emergency rooms have shown that whether or not an emetic is administered makes no significant difference to morbidity, mortality, length of hospital stay, or long-term complications of poisoning. In short, there is no scientific evidence that inducing emesis improves clinical outcome in any poisoning in man or animals.

Absolute contraindications of inducing emesis are:

- Patient is a domestic animal other than a cat or dog.
- Ingestion of oil. This includes waxes that melt to oils at internal body temperature, such as the waxes used to formulate rodent baits.
- Ingestion of a corrosive substance.
- Ingestion of hydrocarbons or other volatile substances.
- Patient is exhibiting altered mental state (whether depressed or excited).
- Patient is at risk of seizures. Note that emesis itself can trigger seizures.
- Patient is at risk of stupor or coma.
- Patient has or is at risk of increased intracranial pressure or other risk factor(s) of cerebral hemorrhage, such as bleeding diathesis.

Disadvantages of administering an emetic are:

- It is highly unlikely to make any difference to clinical outcome in most poisonings, even if administered immediately after the poison was ingested.
- It causes discomfort and distress to the patient.
- Time spent administering an emetic and waiting for it to take effect means that commencement of effective measures is delayed.
- It has been shown that activated charcoal alone is more effective than activated charcoal after an emetic, possibly because activated charcoal administration is delayed.
- There is risk of aspiration of vomitus and resulting pneumonia.
- Clinical signs of nausea and abdominal discomfort, such as hypersalivation and abdominal muscle rigidity, may be confused with, or conceal, signs of poisoning.

- Emesis may be prolonged or severe, particularly if the toxicant is itself an emetic (e.g., chocolate, sodium fluoroacetate) and may lead to hypochloremia and dehydration.
- The dose of apomorphine that induces emesis also causes CNS and respiratory depression.
- Rare but reported complications of emesis include cerebral hemorrhage, esophageal tear or rupture, hiatal hernia, gastric rupture, pneumothorax, and pneumomediastinum.

The medical professions in the USA and the EU have nearly entirely abandoned the use of emesis since 1997, with no increase in morbidity, length of hospital stay, or mortality resulting.

The only situation in which emesis is indicated is when a deadly poison has been ingested in a delayed-release form. Good examples are ingestion of a puffer fish or a sea slug by a dog. These marine organisms are likely to carry the deadly bacterial toxin tetrodotoxin, but dogs often swallow puffer fish and sea slugs in largely intact form. If the puffer fish or sea slug can be recovered whole, then an emergency gastrotomy can be avoided.

Gastric Lavage

Gastric lavage is another technique that has largely failed to withstand the scrutiny of evidence-based medicine, and is likely to be useful only in rare circumstances.

Toxicokinetic and marker studies have demonstrated that gastric lavage results in at best only modest decreases in AUC, and then only if it is performed within 30 minutes of ingestion of the poison, which is rarely possible in clinical practice. The efficacy of the procedure declines rapidly with time since ingestion of the poison. High variability in effect on AUC between individual patients treated, and between practitioners, has been demonstrated. A beneficial effect on clinical outcome is generally unlikely unless the AUC is decreased by at least 50%, and this result is seldom achieved with gastric lavage, even when it is performed within 10−30 minutes after ingestion.

Gastric lavage is of no value in cases of poisoning with toxicants that are rapidly absorbed from the stomach, such as ethanol, isopropanol, xylitol, ethylene glycol, sodium chloride, and weak acids such as aspirin. Gastric lavage is also of no value when the poison acts as an emetic or promotes gastric emptying into the duodenum.

There is no clinical evidence that gastric lavage improves clinical outcome, and the progressive abandonment of the procedure in most situations by emergency medical personnel has not been associated with any increase in morbidity or mortality in human poisonings. On the contrary, human studies have shown that gastric lavage is correlated with worse outcomes, more complications and increased admissions into intensive care facilities.

The procedure is not innocuous, but is associated with significant risks. The risk of aspiration into the lungs is such that gastric lavage should never been performed unless the airway has been protected with a cuffed endotracheal tube.

Absolute contraindications of gastric lavage include:

- the airway is unprotected
- the ingested poison is an oil or hydrocarbon distillate
- the poison is corrosive
- there is potential for gastric perforation
- there is presence, or risk, of gastric hemorrhage

Recognized adverse effects of gastric lavage include

- aspiration and resultant pneumonia or respiratory tract damage
- conjunctival hemorrhages
- laryngospasm
- tension pneumothorax
- tachycardia and ectopic beats
- triggering or exacerbation of cardiac arrhythmias
- injury or perforation of the esophagus and/or stomach
- the use of saline or intravenous infusion fluids as lavaging fluid may lead to hypernatremia
- water intoxication, particularly in small patients
- hypothermia if lavaging fluid is not appropriately warmed

Gastric lavage should not be used routinely, if at all, in poisoning cases. Although the procedure may be useful for retrieving samples of stomach content for analysis, performing gastric lavage for this purpose is seldom justifiable. Gastric lavage is unlikely to be justified unless the following criteria are met:

- the ingested material is highly toxic
- the patient presents within 10–30 min of ingestion
- the poison is not effectively adsorbed by activated charcoal
- the poison is not rapidly absorbed from the stomach
- the poison is likely to be soluble in the lavaging fluid

For those poisons that are adsorbed by activated charcoal, the administration of activated charcoal is at least as effective as gastric lavage and is associated with significantly fewer risks.

Rumenotomy and Ruminal Emptying

Emptying of the rumen via a rumenotomy performed through an upper left flank incision may be indicated if a valuable ruminant has recently ingested a deadly poison that is believed to still be in the rumen, e.g., oleander, or has a structure in the rumen that is slowly releasing poison. The procedure may be performed with the sedated animal restrained standing or in sternal recumbency, and with a regional nerve block performed for anesthesia. If specialized rumenotomy equipment is not available, the rumen may be sutured to the edges of the incision through the abdominal wall prior to incision of the ruminal wall, in order to prevent spillage of ruminal contents into the peritoneal cavity. These sutures are removed after the ruminal incision is closed. If the ruminal contents are completely removed, it will be necessary to inoculate the rumen with ruminal fluid from a healthy animal of the same species to restore function.

A less invasive approach to decontamination of the rumen has been described, and involves perforating the rumen from the flank using a trochar and cannula, introducing fluid until the abdomen has expanded slightly, and then siphoning the fluid out using gravity. The effectiveness of this technique in significantly altering the contents of the rumen is unknown.

Enterogastric Lavage (Whole Bowel Irrigation)

Methods for WBI described in the veterinary literature include introducing an osmotically balanced solution of polyethylene glycol and electrolytes into the stomach by nasogastric tube, and irrigating until the solution is produced from the anus; using the same method but alternative lavage fluids; and introducing warm water or enema fluid *per rectum* to an animal that has a gastric tube in place, until the warm water flows from the gastric tube ("through and through enema").

There is very little information on the safety or efficacy of WBI available. WBI is very rarely indicated, and should not be performed routinely in poisoning cases. It is unlikely to be of any significant clinical benefit unless the total quantity of absorbed toxicant (AUC) is reduced by 50%, which is a rare situation. WBI may be of use if the toxicant is slowly released or in an extended-release formulation, the toxicant is not effectively bound by activated charcoal or too much time has elapsed since ingestion for activated charcoal to be useful, and the animal is presented while most of the material is still in the intestines. Examples of situations in which WBI has been found to be useful include ingestion of transdermal patches of fentanyl or clonidine, and extended-release formulations of potassium chloride.

The authors do not recommend WBI by methods other than the administration of an osmotically balanced solution of polyethylene glycol and electrolytes into the stomach by nasogastric tube. WBI is contraindicated if the gag reflex is compromised, or if there is cardiovascular or respiratory instability. Vomiting should be controlled before attempting WBI. Nasogastric tubes of rubber, silicone, or polyurethane tend to be superior to polyethylene which is inclined to kink, and a tube with a radiographic marker is highly desirable in order to verify correct placement of the tube. Chilling of the tube prior to placement, with a small kink near the end which is directed dorsally in the pharynx, assists in ensuring that the tube is directed into the esophagus. A small amount of local anesthetic is placed in the nostril prior to insertion of the tube. It is essential to ensure that the tube is in the esophagus rather than the trachea before commencing irrigation, because the irrigation volume is likely to be in the range of 2−3 L for an average-sized dog. If a tube with a radiodense marker is not available, measurement of the pH of aspirated fluid, or auscultation of the stomach while a small volume (e.g., 50 mL) of air is rapidly forced through the tube, may be used to confirm correct placement.

Irrigation is commenced gradually and may be increased to up to 400−500 mL/hour if no adverse effects are observed. Adverse effects which indicate that irrigation rate should be decreased include abdominal discomfort, bloating, and hemodynamic disturbances. Irrigation should be halted if defecation does not occur within an hour, if the procedure is causing adverse effects, or if no intestinal sounds can be auscultated.

Activated Charcoal

Activated charcoal is charcoal that has been treated with either a combination of heat and pressure, or with strong acid or base followed by carbonization, to make it highly porous, giving it a very large functional surface area for its volume.

There are a range of different activated charcoals, but only pharmaceutical grade powdered activated charcoal is suitable for use in clinical toxicology. Granular, extruded, or beaded activated charcoals are considerably less porous and are not suitable for use for adsorbing xenobiotics, and the same is true of activated charcoal biscuits, tablets, or capsules. The binding capacity of activated charcoal is usually expressed as iodine number, which is the number of milligrams of iodine bound by one gram of activated charcoal. Pharmaceutical grade activated charcoal has an iodine number in the range of 600−1100 mg/g.

There are a number of activated charcoal formulations marketed for veterinary use. Most are liquid formulations suitable for administration by nasogastric or gastric tube. Gel formulations are intended for oral administration.

Activated charcoal does not bind all xenobiotics. It is not effective for substances with a molecular or atomic weight < 100 Da, which means it is not effective for metals, other elemental poisons such as lithium or arsenic, or for small molecules such as metal salts, sodium chloride, ammonia, and cyanide. It is not effective for alcohols, including methanol, xylitol, and ethylene glycol. It is most effective for large nonpolar compounds and less effective for ionic compounds. However, poisons with a molecular weight in excess of 1000 Da, such as botulinum toxin, are poorly absorbed. The effectiveness of activated charcoal is poor for oily or viscous xenobiotics.

Activated charcoal is generally effective for binding plant toxins such as alkaloids, as well as many pharmaceuticals. Activated charcoal will bind oral antidotes such as *N*-acetyl-cysteine.

Activated charcoal should not be used if endoscopy is likely to be required, because it will coat surfaces and may conceal lesions. It is extremely irritating to the peritoneal cavity and for this reason should not be used if gastrointestinal surgery is likely to be required. It should not be used if there is any risk that the esophagus or stomach has been perforated by a corrosive toxicant. Activated charcoal is also contraindicated if the patient is dehydrated or hypernatremic.

Although activated charcoal itself is not emetic, it is extremely irritating to lung tissue if aspirated and should not be administered until vomiting has been controlled. Because of the inherent high risk of aspiration, activated charcoal should never be used if the poison is a hydrocarbon distillate. A cuffed endotracheal tube may be required if there is likelihood that the reflexes that protect against aspiration are not functioning normally. Some practitioners prefer to use a parenteral anti-emetic prior to administering activated charcoal.

There are some rare reports of complications including hypernatremia, hypokalemia, hypermagnesemia, metabolic acidosis, and intestinal obstruction by bezoars of activated charcoal in human beings.

Single-Dose Activated Charcoal

A number of human and animal studies have shown that administration of activated charcoal within 30 minutes of ingestion of a poison can lead to a significant decrease in absorption of the poison from the gastrointestinal tract. However, there is a lack of clear evidence that this decrease translates to an improved clinical outcome. On the other hand, activated charcoal is regarded as a low-risk therapy and remains popular.

To be effective, activated charcoal must come in contact with the toxicant and for this reason it should be administered as soon as possible after ingestion of the toxicant. The effectiveness of activated charcoal falls off rapidly as time from ingestion of the toxicant elapses, with the effectiveness of activated charcoal administered after 30 minutes generally only about half that of activated charcoal administered 5 minutes after administration of a xenobiotic. Unfortunately, presentation of a poisoned animal within 30 minutes of ingestion of the poison is rather uncommon in clinical practice. Administration after 60−120 minutes is unlikely to be beneficial unless the xenobiotic is in a delayed-release formulation, or there is inhibition of gastric emptying. Activated charcoal is unlikely to be of benefit if the xenobiotic is rapidly absorbed from the stomach (e.g., xylitol and aspirin).

If the activated charcoal is in a powder rather than a liquid formulation, it should be mixed to a slurry with 5−7 mL of water per gram of activated charcoal. A dust mask and safety glasses should be worn because activated charcoal is extremely irritant to the eyes and to the respiratory tract.

Activated charcoal may be placed in the stomach via nasogastric or gastric tube, or the gel may be syringed into the mouth, to deliver 1−3 g activated charcoal/kg bodyweight.

Multiple-Dose Activated Charcoal

MDAC is used with the objective of increasing elimination of toxicants that undergo enterohepatic cycling. Experimental data show that MDAC works best with agents that have a prolonged half-life ($t_{1/2}$) and an apparent volume of distribution (V_d) of <1 L/kg bodyweight, indicating that sequestration is not occurring. Among the toxicants for which MDAC has been shown to reduce total systemic exposure are:

carbamazepine	dapsone	digoxin and digitoxin
paracetamol	phenylbutazone	piroxicam
quinine		

However, the available data on clinical efficacy are mixed, and generally there is a lack of evidence that MDAC substantially reduces morbidity or mortality in poisoned patients. On the other hand, it is a relatively cheap therapy, and relatively safe.

The same limitations, contraindications, and adverse effects apply to MDAC as to the use of a single dose of activated charcoal.

Systemic Decontamination

Forced Diuresis With Ion Trapping

This method involves promoting diuresis by administration of intravenous fluid and at the same time adjusting the urinary pH so that the poison is not reabsorbed in the renal tubules. The theory behind this practice is that the rate of back-diffusion of a xenobiotic to the circulation from the renal tubular lumen is lowest when the xenobiotic is ionized and greatest when the xenobiotic is not ionized. For this reason, oral administration of ammonium chloride has been recommended to acidify the urine, in order to promote excretion of basic poisons, and intravenous sodium bicarbonate has been recommended to alkalinize the urine to promote excretion of acidic poisons.

Urinary alkalinization appears to be useful for enhancing the urinary clearance of a limited number of acidic poisons. It is endorsed for salicylate poisoning and may also be helpful in toxicosis due to fluoride salts or methotrexate. In combination with forced diuresis, it may also promote excretion of 2,4-D. Human cases of poisoning with cocaine or amphetamine have been treated with forced acid diuresis.

Forced diuresis, with or without ion trapping, should not be used indiscriminately to promote renal excretion of xenobiotics. Its use should be preceded by a literature search to determine whether there is good evidence that it is indicated for a particular poison, and that it makes a difference to clinical outcome. Renal function must be adequate to avoid complications such as pulmonary edema, and the patient must be monitored for derangements in systemic acid−base balance or electrolyte balances.

Hemoperfusion

Hemoperfusion consists of passing blood through a column that contains adsorbent particles, either activated charcoal or resin. Hemoperfusion was used in human clinical toxicology in the 1970s and 1980s but has been largely superseded by hemodialysis because the latter is simpler and has fewer complications. Hemoperfusion requires the use of anticoagulant such as heparin, or special treatment of the adsorbent particles, to overcome the problem of platelet aggregation. In the medical field hemoperfusion is usually performed using a machine that is expense beyond the reach of veterinary practice, but in an emergency situation hemoperfusion may be performed more simply using only tubing from an intravenous infusion set, the hemoperfusion cartridge and a peristaltic pump to move the blood along the tubing, through the cartridge and back to the body. Peristaltic pumps are relatively inexpensive and available from chemistry supply companies. Blood is usually drawn from an artery and returned to a vein, but venovenous transfer may be more feasible in most veterinary situations. An in-line filter is recommended to prevent embolism due to fragments of the adsorbent or to small thrombi.

Currently there appear to be no hemoperfusion cartridges commercially available that are small enough to be used with any domestic pets other than large breeds of dogs, which is unfortunate because although the procedure is relatively complex and carries a number of risks, such as embolism and thrombocytopenia, it does have the attraction that it has been shown to remove some highly toxic substances from circulation that otherwise carry a very poor prognosis. Such substances include paraquat, digoxin, amatoxins, phallotoxins, and sodium fluoroacetate. Charcoal hemoperfusion has been used to successfully treat sodium fluoroacetate poisoning in dogs and in humans in China. Hemoperfusion has also been used to remove methylxanthine alkaloids, tricyclic antidepressants, barbiturates, and salicylates.

Hemodialysis

Hemodialysis has largely replaced hemoperfusion in clinical toxicology for human patients, but because access to hemodialysis machines is extremely limited, even in the USA, the procedure will not be discussed further.

Peritoneal Dialysis

Because of the growing volume of medical literature showing that hemodialysis is effective in reducing the AUC for a number of poisons, there is interest in the veterinary field in using peritoneal dialysis as a practical alternative to hemodialysis.

This interest needs to be tempered with the recognition that peritoneal dialysis is significantly less effective (1/8 to 1/3 the efficacy) than hemodialysis in reducing plasma concentration of those poisons that can be removed by dialysis. Therefore it cannot be assumed that because hemodialysis is useful in a toxicosis in a human patient that peritoneal dialysis will be useful in a veterinary patient with the same toxicosis. It is important to bear in mind that an improvement in clinical outcome is unlikely unless the AUC is lowered by at least 50%. In other words, a small decrease in AUC is not a worthwhile goal of therapy.

Not all poisons are available to be removed by dialysis. To be removed by dialysis, a poison must have the following properties:

- relatively water-soluble (hydrophilic)
- not highly protein-bound
- low molecular weight
- small V_D
- slow intrinsic rate of clearance (i.e., long $t_{1/2}$)

Details on the method of performing peritoneal dialysis are beyond the scope of this book but can be found in publications in veterinary emergency medicine.

Case reports supporting a role for peritoneal dialysis exist for the following toxicoses:

barbiturates	borates	carbamazepine
ethanol	ethylene glycol	iron
lithium	methanol	salicylates
salt	theophylline	

It should be noted that if peritoneal dialysis is to be performed in ethylene glycol poisoning, it must be performed early in the toxicosis when the parent compound is the principal toxicant. If ethanol is used as an antidote in ethylene glycol toxicosis, this will also be removed by peritoneal dialysis.

The usefulness of peritoneal dialysis in caffeine poisoning and theobromine poisoning has not been explored, although the close chemical relationship between these methylxanthine alkaloids and theophylline suggests that peritoneal dialysis may be useful in these toxicoses.

The usefulness of peritoneal dialysis for paraquat poisoning has been explored, but current evidence suggests that diuresis is more effective, provided renal function is adequate.

Peritoneal dialysis should only be performed with purpose-made fluids and purpose-made catheters, and the fluid must be warmed to body temperature prior to introduction into the peritoneal cavity. The procedure is contraindicated in patients that have recently had abdominal surgery.

Complications and adverse effects of peritoneal dialysis may include:

- fluid and electrolyte imbalances
- perforation or laceration of viscera
- peritonitis with bacteria introduced from outside the body in the fluid or by technique
- peritonitis with bacteria from the gastrointestinal lumen, if visceral puncture
- adhesions
- hypothermia (if fluid has not been warmed appropriately)
- respiratory compromise/dyspnea

Peritonitis may be evident as cloudiness in the recovered dialysis fluid. If peritonitis occurs, the procedure must be abandoned and antibiotic therapy instituted. Peritoneal dialysis cannot be continued in conjunction with antibiotic therapy, because many antibiotics are removed by peritoneal dialysis and may therefore be reduced to below therapeutic concentration.

Intravenous Lipid Emulsion Also Known as Intravenous Fat Emulsion

ILEs were developed to provide energy and fatty acids to patients on parenteral nutritional support, but is gaining increasing popularity in human clinical toxicology for the trapping of lipophilic xenobiotics. By acting as a "lipid sink" or "lipid sponge," ILEs trap lipophilic substances and prevent their distribution into the intracellular compartment. The growing list of poisonings in which ILE has been used with apparent beneficial effect include bupropion, bupivacaine, verapamil, propranolol, clomiprazine, quetipine, sertraline, calcium-channel blockers, and beta-blockers. In the veterinary field, ILE has been used to successfully treat a puppy with moxidectin poisoning.

The use of ILE in clinical toxicology is a rapidly growing field that can be monitored through Pubmed or other online literature databases.

Dermal Decontamination

The skin has evolved as a barrier against xenobiotics, while the gastrointestinal tract or respiratory tract has essential roles in absorption into the body. As a generalization, bioavailability of a xenobiotic is much lower following dermal exposure than absorption of the same xenobiotic via the gastrointestinal or respiratory route, and for many xenobiotics, dermal absorption is negligible or nil.

When removing toxic xenobiotics from the skin, hair, or plumage, personnel should wear appropriate personal protective equipment that are likely to include gloves, long-sleeved garments, closed footwear, and safety glasses.

The skin should be flushed with copious water. Tepid water should be used, if possible, when flushing the skin of small dogs, cats, or small birds, to avoid hypothermia. However, water should not be warm enough to cause vasodilation, because this may lead to increased dermal absorption of xenobiotics. Water pressure should be controlled to ensure that damaged but viable tissue is not removed.

Neutralization of acids by application of bases, or bases by application of acids, should not be attempted. The reaction of acids with bases is exothermic and may lead to thermal injury. Instead, copious water should be used to remove the acid or base and correct the dermal pH by dilution. Powdered cement is acidic and should be removed with copious flushing with water for this reason.

A mild detergent such as dishwashing liquid for washing dishes by hand may be used. Strong detergents such as those intended for dishwashing machines or for laundry are corrosive and should not be used.

Solvents that are light petroleum distillates, such as turpentine, should not be used to decontaminate skin. These substances are dermal irritants and may increase dermal absorption by disrupting the barrier function of the skin. The solvents are themselves toxic and may be absorbed systemically through the skin or may be ingested or aspirated if the animal grooms them off its skin.

Although the animal's owner may be distressed by the presence of substances such as paints, adhesives, or tar on their animal's skin, the veterinarian should not be tempted to use solvents to remove such substances. It is preferable to leave adherent substances in place unless they are interfering with biological function. Attempts by the animal to remove adherent substances by grooming should be prevented by appropriate restraints such as an Elizabethan collar. If a substance is adhered directly to the skin and must be removed, it may be possible to soften and remove the substance by careful use of Tween 80, PEG 500, or cosmetic remover. Baby oil and vegetable oil have also been recommended by some authors. None of these proposed removers is sterile and all are potential media for bacterial growth.

Ocular exposure to toxicants should be treated with copious gentle flushing and referred for specialist care if there is any evidence of ocular injury.

Chapter 4

Antidotes

INTRODUCTION

There is no general accepted definition of the word "antidote." The Macquarie Dictionary defines an antidote as "a medicine or other remedy for counteracting the effects of poison, disease, etc.," which is very broad and would cover all therapeutic agents used to treat poisoning. The Oxford Dictionaries are somewhat more specific, defining an antidote as "A medicine taken or given to counteract a particular poison."

An antidote can act in a number of ways. Examples include:

- Limiting absorption
- Sequestering the poison
- Inhibiting metabolism to a toxic metabolite
- Promoting distribution from tissues
- Displacing the poison from a receptor or competing for the receptor
- Counteracting the toxic effect
- Enhancing detoxification

Because the term antidote is not clearly defined, there may be disagreement about whether a given therapeutic agent is an antidote or not. In this chapter, an agent is regarded as an antidote if it is specific for a certain poison or class of poisons.

Important facts to bear in mind about antidotes include the following:

- Administration of an antidote does not obviate the need for supportive and symptomatic treatment. On the contrary, supportive treatment may still mean the difference between survival and death.
- Poisonings for which there are antidotes are not necessarily less serious than those for which there is no antidote, and do not necessarily carry a better prognosis. If anything, the opposite is true; antidotes have been developed for some poisons because those poisons carry a particularly high mortality rate.
- A number of antidotes are toxic in their own right and may cause serious toxicosis if used when the animal is misdiagnosed, or if the antidote is given for too long a course. For example, atropine in the absence of anticholinesterase poisoning can cause life-threatening atropine poisoning,

Veterinary Toxicology for Australia and New Zealand
DOI: http://dx.doi.org/10.1016/B978-0-12-420227-6.00004-9

and the course of calcium disodium EDTA in lead poisoning must be limited because of the toxicity of the antidote.

Table 4.1 lists poisonings described in this book that have antidotes in alphabetical order, with their antidotes. Table 4.2 is a summary of antivenoms.

TABLE 4.1 Poisons for Which There Are Specific Antidotes

Poison	Antidote	Dose and Comments
Amitraz	Atipamezole OR Yohimbine	Dogs: intramuscular injection of 50 µg atipamezole/ kg bodyweight (BW) OR intravenous injection of 0.2 mg atipamezole/kg BW OR intravenous injection of yohimbine at 0.1 mg/kg BW
Anticholinergic drugs (atropine, hyoscamine, scopolamine, etc.)	Physostigmine	0.6 mg/kg IV
Anticoagulant rodenticides	Phytonadione	Small animals: 3−5 mg/kg/day PO, split into two doses/day, and followed by a fatty meal if possible Ruminants: 0.5−1.5 mg/kg phytonadione SC or IM, not more than 10 mL/site Pigs: 2−5 mg/kg phytonadione, SC or IM. Horses: as for ruminants but do not exceed 2 mg/kg/day
Arsenic	Dimercaptosuccinic acid (succimer), 2-3-dimercapto-1-propanesulfonate, or meso-2,3-dimercaptosuccinic acid OR Dimercaprol	Succimer: 10 mg/kg PO, three times daily for 10 days OR Dimercaprol: 3−6 mg/kg IM, 3 to 4 times daily, or 2−5 mg/ kg IM every 4 h for 2 days, then every 8 h for 1 day, and every 12 h thereafter
β-Sympathetic blocking agents	Insulin OR amrinone	Insulin IV OR amrinone as 4 mg/kg bolus

(Continued)

TABLE 4.1 (Continued)

Poison	Antidote	Dose and Comments
Benzodiazepines	Flumazenil	0.1 mg/kg IV
Calcium channel blocking agents	Calcium	IV calcium gluconate or calcium chloride, 10% solution in saline
Carbamate insecticides	Atropine OR glycopyrrolate	Atropine 0.25 to 0.5 mg/kg BW. Give 1/4 of dose immediately, IV if possible. Remainder is administered IM or SC if a response is seen to the IV bolus OR Glycopyrrolate 0.5 mg/kg IM or SC
Carbon monoxide	Oxygen (pure or with not more than 5% CO_2)	By mask
Cholecalciferol	Pamidronate sodium (or other bisphosphonate as available)	Pamidronate sodium: slow (2–4 h) intravenous infusion in saline, at 1.3–2 mg pamidronate sodium/kg BW
Copper	Ammonium tetrathiomolybdate OR D-Penicillamine	Ammonium tetrathiomolybdate, 1.7–3.4 mg/day IV or SC, for three treatments on alternate days OR D-Penicillamine, 50 mg/kg orally for up to 6 days
Cyanide, HCN orally or by inhalation	Sodium nitrite followed by sodium thiosulfate OR Hydroxocobalamin Sodium thiosulfate may be used alone in mild toxicosis	Sodium nitrite IV, 16–22 mg/kg, as a 3% solution followed by IV sodium thiosulfate, 1.65 mL of a 25% solution. Treatment may be repeated at half the initial doses after 30 min OR Hydroxocobalamin: Human dose is one 2.5 g ampoule with 100 mL of 0.9% saline, administered IV over 15 min, followed by a second ampoule in the same volume over the same time. This is sufficient to bind 100 mg of cyanide. The recommended dose rate in acute cyanide poisoning in dogs is 79 mg/kg

(Continued)

TABLE 4.1 (Continued)

Poison	Antidote	Dose and Comments
Cyanogenic glycosides	Sodium nitrite + sodium thiosulfate OR Methylene blue	10–20 mg/kg sodium nitrite administered IV as 20% solution, up to 600 mg/kg of sodium thiosulfate as 20% solution Methylene blue, IV, at 9–22 mg/kg. Do not use both sodium nitrite and methylene blue Methylene blue is a cost-effective treatment of cyanogenic glycoside poisoning in large herbivores
Digitalis and analogs	Digibind	Digibind (digoxin-specific antibody)
Ethylene glycol	Ethanol OR 4-Methylpyrazole (never use together)	Ethanol—dogs: 5.5 mL/kg BW every 4 h for five treatments then every 6 h for four treatments Ethanol—cats: 5 mL/kg BW every 6 h for five treatments followed by four treatments at 8 h intervals OR 1.3 mL/kg of a 30% ethanol solution as an IV bolus, followed by 0.42 mL/kg/h for 48 h 4-Methylpyrazole (dogs only) 20 mg/kg BW initially, followed by 15 mg/kg at 12 and 24 h, and 5 mg/kg at 36 h
Fluoride (acute) and hydrofluoric acid	Calcium borogluconate	IV, titrate while monitoring cardiac function
Heparin	Protamine sulfate	1% protamine sulfate by slow IV push. This drug will antagonize heparin at a 1:1 ratio by mass
Iron	Deferoxamine	Deferoxamine IV at 15 mg/kg/h, or at 40 mg/kg every 4–6 h
Lead	Calcium disodium EDTA OR Calcium disodium EDTA + dimercaprol OR Meso-2,3-dimercaptosuccinic acid (Succimer) OR D-Penicillamine	Ca disodium EDTA: details by species are beyond the scope of this table. See entry for lead WITH/WITHOUT Dimercaprol: 3–6 mg/kg IM, 3 to 4 times daily, or 2–5 mg/kg IM every 4 h for 2 days, then every 8 h for one day, and every 12 h thereafter

(Continued)

TABLE 4.1 (Continued)

Poison	Antidote	Dose and Comments
		OR Succimer: 10 mg/kg PO, three times daily for 10 days OR D-Penicillamine—dogs: 30–110 mg/kg/days PO, divided into four doses. Treatment should be suspended after 5–7 days and then resumed after a further 5–7 days. D-Penicillamine and Ca-EDTA can be cycled Cats: D-penicillamine PO 125 mg/cat every 12 h for 5 days Cage birds: D-penicillamine 55 mg/kg PO every 12 h, for up to 2 weeks before giving a 5 day rest
Mercury	D-Penicillamine OR Succimer	See entry for lead, above
Molybdenum	Copper glycinate	Copper glycinate SC; 120 mg/adult cow; 60 mg/calf
Nitrates	Methylene blue	1%, administered IV at 4–15 mg/kg
Nonprotein nitrogen (urea, ammonia)	5% acetic acid (vinegar)	Cattle is 2–8 L; sheep or goats, 0.5–2 L
Opioids	Naloxone	0.01–0.02 mg/kg IV, IM or SC
Organophosphate insecticides	Atropine OR glycopyrrolate AND Pralidoxime (2-PAM) chloride	Atropine or glycopyrrolate, see carbamate toxicity, above 2-PAM chloride 20 mg/kg IM, twice daily
Para-aminopropiophenone	Methylene blue	Dogs: 4–22 mg/kg as a 1% solution, by slow IV infusion Cats: use with caution, starting at 4 mg/kg, administer as for dogs
Paracetamol	N-acetylcysteine	Orally or intravenously at a dose of 140 mg/kg, followed by doses of 70 mg/kg every 6 h for five to seven treatments. N-acetylcysteine should be

(Continued)

TABLE 4.1 (Continued)

Poison	Antidote	Dose and Comments
		If N-acetyl cysteine is not available, administer S-adenosylmethionine. The suggested treatment regime for dogs is 40 mg/kg orally, followed by 20 mg/kg every 24 h for 9 days, while a tentative regime for cats is 180 mg orally, every 12 h for 3 days, followed by 90 mg orally every 12 h for 14 days. Another treatment regime is sodium sulfate at 50 mg/kg IV, every 4 h for six treatments, in a 1.6% solution
Parasympathomimetic drugs, e.g., physostigmine, pilocarpine		Atropine, as for organophosphate insecticides (see above) 2-PAM is only useful for echothiophate
Quinidine	Sodium bicarbonate	IV sodium bicarbonate
Selective serotonin reuptake inhibitors	Cyproheptadine	Cyproheptadine, orally or per rectum, divided into three or four doses/24 h, 1.1 mg/kg for dogs or a total dose of 2–4 mg to a cat
Sodium nitrite	Methylene blue	Dogs: 4–22 mg/kg as a 1% solution, by slow IV infusion Cats: use with caution, starting at 4 mg/kg, administer as for dogs
Tropane alkaloids	Physostigmine	0.6 mg/kg IV
Zinc	Ca-EDTA OR D-Penicillamine	See entry for lead

TABLE 4.2 Antivenoms

Organism	Antivenom
Australian paralysis tick, *Ixodes holocyclus*	APVA-approved tick antivenom
Black snakes, *Pseudoechis* spp.	CSL Black snake antivenom
Broad-headed snakes, *Hoplocephalus* spp.	CSL Tiger snake antivenom
Brown snakes, *Pseudonaja* spp.	CSL Brown snake antivenom
Copperheads, *Austrelaps* spp.	CSL Tiger snake antivenom
Curl snake, *Suta suta*	CSL Polyvalent antivenom
Death adders, *Acanthophis* spp.	CSL Death Adder antivenom
Gray snake, *Hemiaspis daemeli*	CSL Polyvalent antivenom
Katipo, *Latrodectus katipo*	*Lactrodectus hasselti* antivenom
Major box jelly, *Chironex fleckeri*	*Chironex fleckeri* antivenom?
Redback spider, *Lactrodectus hasselti*	*Lactrodectus hasselti* antivenom
Rough-scaled snake, *Tropidechis carinatus*	CSL Tiger snake antivenom
Sea snakes, *Elapidae*	CSL Sea snake antivenom? Or CSL Tiger snake antivenom?
Small-eyed snake, *Rhinoplocephalus nigrescens*	CSL Tiger snake antivenom
Stonefish, scorpionfish, lionfish Order Scorpaeniformes	Stonefish antivenom (not effective for bullrout stings)
Tasmanian paralysis tick, *Ixodes cornuatus*	APVA-approved tick antivenom
Taipans, *Oxyuranus* spp.	CSL Taipan antivenom
Tiger snakes, *Notechis* spp.	CSL Tiger snake antivenom

Chapter 5

Vulnerable Patients

Some patients are particularly vulnerable to the toxic effects of xenobiotics. Some preexisting diseases may alter absorption, distribution, metabolism, or excretion of xenobiotics. For example, a xenobiotic may be more readily absorbed through broken, inflamed skin, less efficiently metabolized if there is preexisting liver disease, or less efficiently excreted if there is preexisting renal disease. In addition certain stages of life may make an animal particularly sensitive to toxicosis. These include:

- Neonatal and juvenile patients
- Breeding stud males
- Cycling and pregnant animals and more particularly their embryos or fetuses
- Animals suckling a lactating dam
- Geriatric animals

In addition some breeds of animal are recognized to have particular susceptibilities to xenobiotics due to inherited characteristics of xenobiotic metabolism. Some of the better-known examples are briefly reviewed in this chapter.

Finally, animals may have hypersensitivity reactions to xenobiotics. Although some breeds are more likely to develop hypersensitivity reactions than others, whether or not a particular animal will develop hypersensitivity is not predictable. The types of hypersensitivity reaction are briefly reviewed at the end of this chapter.

NEONATAL AND JUVENILE PATIENTS

Relatively little is known about pediatric differences in Absorption, Distribution, Metabolism, and Excretion (ADME) in domestic animals, although it is clear from studies of experimental animals, particularly the rat, and from studies of human beings that substantial changes in all these aspects of toxicokinetics exist between the neonate, the juvenile, and the adult.

It is very difficult to generalize because of differences in maturity at birth, and developmental rate, between species, not to mention the great diversity of chemical characteristics of potentially toxic xenobiotics. However, physiological differences to be considered include the following:

- Newborns have a near-neutral gastric pH.
- Gastric emptying rate is lower in neonates.
- If the animal is not weaned, milk may bind some xenobiotics.
- Preruminant juveniles lack the diluting effect of the ruminal volume that is often protective in adult ruminants. Absorption rate may be greatly increased if the ruminal bypass mechanism is triggered. On the other hand, xenobiotics that are activated to a toxic form by ruminal microbes will not be activated in the preruminant.
- The biliary system may not be fully functional and therefore fat-soluble xenobiotics may be less readily absorbed from the gastrointestinal tract.
- The balance of large intestinal microbial flora may be different, leading to differences in extrahepatic metabolism and/or enterohepatic cycling.
- Thermoregulation may be poor in neonates, reducing dermal absorption but increasing risk if exposed to toxicants that cause hypothermia.
- However, skin hydration is highest in neonates, and this is directly correlated with rate of percutaneous absorption of xenobiotics.
- Neonates and juveniles have a higher minute volume and are therefore more sensitive to inhaled gases.
- Juveniles may have lower levels of plasma proteins, resulting in a greater proportion of the absorbed xenobiotic circulating in unbound, active form.
- Neonates and juveniles tend to have less body fat than adults. Therefore a greater proportion of a lipid-soluble xenobiotic will be circulating in the plasma. This may increase the risk of toxic levels being reached, but also means that the half-life is likely to be shorter.
- A larger proportion of the juvenile body is water, compared to the adult body, and a greater proportion of the total body water is in the extracellular compartment.
- A greater proportion of the cardiac output is directed to the brain and heart in juveniles.
- The brain—blood barrier is more permeable in the neonate, compared to the adult.
- The blood—testis barrier is also more permeable in immature animals. This is relevant if the animal is intended as a future stud.
- Hepatic and renal excretion are often lower in neonates and juveniles than in adults.
- The profile of activity of Phase 1 and Phase II enzymes can be very different in neonates and/or juveniles, as compared to adults. This may result in reduced detoxification, but it can be protective, in the case of xenobiotics that undergo metabolic activation to the toxic form (lethal synthesis) in the liver.
- Expression of cytochrome P450 enzymes may be less inducible in juveniles.

- Renal excretion tends to be slower in neonates, particularly those born in a particularly immature, helpless state, such as puppies and kittens.

THE STUD MALE

The testes of the adult male animal are partially protected from circulating xenobiotics by the blood—testis barrier. This barrier is formed by myoid cells and by tight junctions between Sertoli cells. Leydig cells are outside this barrier and may be harmed by xenobiotics that do not reach the seminiferous tubules.

Deleterious effects on male reproduction are not confined to those that act directly on the testes, but include those that interfere with normal male endocrinology, such as exposure to estrogenic compounds, and those that affect the physical ability to mate, such as skeletal effects of fluorosis in cattle or hypervitaminosis A in the cat.

Any xenobiotic that causes pyrexia (e.g., phenoxy herbicides) or which interferes with cellular replication (e.g., chemotherapeutics) may cause a decline in spermatogenesis. This may be reversible once the xenobiotic has been largely metabolized and/or excreted, provided the spermatogonia are not harmed.

The length of the spermatogenic process varies between species, and this should be borne in mind when choosing the time to test the sperm count of a stud male to determine if recovery from toxic effects of a xenobiotic has occurred. The estimated length of the spermatogenic cycle for the common domestic species is summarized in Table 5.1.

Veterinary therapeutics known to have deleterious effects on male reproductive function are listed in Table 5.2. Some environmental xenobiotics that are known to have deleterious effects on male reproductive function are listed in Table 5.3. These lists are not exhaustive, and if there is any question

TABLE 5.1 Estimated Duration of the Spermatogenic Process in Males of the Common Domestic Species

Species	Duration (days)
Horse	57
Bull	56—63
Ram	46—49
Goat	48
Boar	36—40
Dog	62
Cat	47

TABLE 5.2 Veterinary Therapeutics Known to Have Deleterious Effects on Male Reproductive Function of Mammals

Type or Use of Xenobiotic	Xenobiotic	Effect/s
Hormones	Testosterone	Doses in excess of physiological levels cause decreased sperm count, testicular degeneration
	Anabolic steroids (including zeranol)	Decreased sperm count and motility, morphological changes in sperm
	Estrogens	Decreased sperm count, feminization of behavior
	Progestins	Decreased sperm count and quality
	Prolactin	Decreased sperm count, testicular degeneration
	Trenbolone	Decreased sperm quality
Antibiotics	Metronidazole	Decreased sperm count, morphological changes in sperm
	Nitrofurantoin	Decreased sperm count
	Tetracycline	Decreased sperm count, testicular degeneration
	Trimethoprim	Decreased sperm count
Antifungal	Ketoconazole	Decreased testosterone levels and libido
		Decreased sperm count and motility
Chemotherapeutics	Adriamycin	Testicular degeneration
	Cisplatin	Decreased sperm count
	Cyclophosphamide	Decreased sperm count
	Cytarabine	Decreased sperm count
	Vincristine	Decreased sperm count (may be persistent)
Antiparasitic	Bunamidine	Interference with spermatogenesis
Diuretic	Acetazolamide	Decreased libido, impotence
Behavioral modification	Buspirone	Decreased libido, impotence
	Benzodiazepines	Decreased libido, impotence
	Phenothiazines	Priapism, impotence
	Tricyclic antidepressants	Decreased libido, impotence

(Continued)

TABLE 5.2 (Continued)

Type or Use of Xenobiotic	Xenobiotic	Effect/s
Antacid	Cimetidine	Decreased prostaglandins in semen
Antiemetic	Metaclopramide	Impotence
Nonsteroidal antiinflammatories	Sulfasalazine	Decreased sperm count and motility
Glucocorticoids	Prednisone	Decreased sperm count and motility, decreased testosterone levels
Anesthetics	Thiamylal	Decreased testosterone levels

TABLE 5.3 Some Environmental Xenobiotics Known to Have Deleterious Effects on Male Reproductive Function of Mammals

Type or Use of Xenobiotic	Xenobiotic	Effect/s
Metals	Cadmium	Ischemic necrosis of the testis
	Lead	Decreased sperm count and testosterone levels
	Chromium	Decreased sperm count and quality; decreased testosterone levels
	Mercury	Decreased sperm quality
Insecticides	Carbamates	Decreased sperm quality
	Pyrethrins	Competitively bind to androgen receptors; in vivo impact unclear
Herbicides	Dichlorophenoxyacetic acid	Decreased sperm quality, testicular degeneration
Fungicides	Vinclozolin	Androgen receptor antagonist
Nematocides	Dibromochloropropane	Decreased sperm count
Antifreeze	Ethylene glycol	Decreased sperm count and motility
Recreational drugs	Marijuana	Decreased sperm count and testosterone levels
	Tobacco	Decreased sperm count
Food additives	Cyclamate	A metabolite, cyclohexylamine, is toxic to the testes
	Phytoestrogens	Soy phytoestrogens may act as estrogens in stud cats

of the safety of a chemical to the reproductive abilities of a stud animal, further information should be sought from a pharmacopeia, *Materials Safety Data Sheet*, or chemical databank, as appropriate.

DEVELOPMENTAL AND REPRODUCTIVE TOXICITY

Reproductive Inhibition

Fertility of breeding females may be adversely affected by xenobiotics with estrogenic activity. Sources of such xenobiotics to livestock include subterranean clover (*Trifolium subterraneum* in Australian or *Trifolium repens* in New Zealand; q.v.), and the mycotoxin zearalenone (q.v.). *Medicago sativa* (lucerne or alfalfa) produces coumestrol, which has a weak estrogenic effect, and is suspected of causing infertility in livestock.

Abortifacient Agents

Consumption of *Cupressus macrocarpa* ("Macrocarpa"; q.v.) is well-recognized cause of bovine abortions in both Australia and New Zealand. Other abortifacients to which domestic animals may be exposed include ergot alkaloids (q.v.).

Teratogenic and Fetotoxic Agents

Many xenobiotics cross the placenta, and some may cause developmental abnormalities in the embryo or fetus. As a generalization, if a xenobiotic has shown to be teratogenic or fetotoxic in one species, it is considered likely to cause deleterious effects in the embryos or fetuses of other species, although the target organ/s may not be the same, and the window of sensitivity is likely to differ.

There are relatively few teratogens known to affect the common domestic species. Dietary teratogens and fetotoxic xenobiotics relevant to Australia and New Zealand are presented in Table 5.4. This list should not be regarded as exhaustive.

Pharmaceutical agents that cross the placenta and that may cause teratogenic or fetotoxic effects are presented in Table 5.5. This list should not be regarded as exhaustive, and the manufacturer's information or a pharmacopeia should be consulted for xenobiotics not listed here.

Synthetic prostaglandins and corticosteroids should be avoided during pregnancy, unless induction of labor is intended, as they are likely to be abortifacient. Ketamine may also induce premature labor.

Most anesthetic agents, with the exception of nitrous oxide, cause neonatal respiratory depression but in the cases of the following agents, this may be readily reversed with naloxone, which is well tolerated by neonates:

pethidine	morphine	oxymorphone
butorphanol	codeine	Fentanyl

TABLE 5.4 Dietary Teratogens and Fetotoxicants of Domestic Animals in Australia and/or New Zealand

Teratogen or Fetotoxin	Source	Effects	Species Affected
Coniine	*Conium maculatum* Poison Hemlock	Joint contracture, sometimes cleft palate	Cattle, goats, sheep, and pigs
Ergovaline and other ergot alkaloids	*Festuca arundinacea* (Tall Fescue) pasture or hay infected with the endophyte *Neotyphodium coenophialum*	Weak, dysmature foals	Horses
Iodine	Kelp or other seaweed used as fodder or feed supplement	Congenital hypothyroidism	Horses
Unknown	Sudan grass (*Sorghum* spp.)	Joint contracture	Horses
		Arthrogryposis	Cattle
Nitrates	Water, annual ryegrass, and other plants	Congenital hypothyroidism	
Pyrrolizidine alkaloids	Numerous plant genera including *Senecio, Echium, Heliotropium,* and others	Congenital liver failure	Observed in a human patient
Mycotoxins: Aflatoxin (confirmed), Ochratoxin A (confirmed), Ergot alkaloids (suspected)		Various teratogenic effects	Effects observed in laboratory animals but theoretically possible in domestic animals

TABLE 5.5 Toxic and Teratogenic Effects of Antimicrobials and other Pharmaceuticals

Drug	Effects
Antibacterials	
Amikacin	Toxic to the eighth cranial nerve and to kidneys
Chloramphenicol	May decrease protein synthesis, particularly in bone marrow
Ciprofloxacin	Toxic to developing articular cartilage
Doxycycline	Staining of developing bones and teeth
Gentamicin	Toxic to the eighth cranial nerve and to kidneys
Kanamycin	Toxic to the eighth cranial nerve and to kidneys
Metronidazole	Teratogenic in laboratory animals
Oxytetracycline	Staining of developing bones and teeth
Streptomycin	Toxic to the eighth cranial nerve and to kidneys
Sulphonamides	Teratogenic in laboratory animals
Tetracycline	Staining of developing bones and teeth
Tobramycin	Toxic to the eighth cranial nerve and to kidneys
Antifungals	
Griseofulvin	Skeletal and brain malformations in cats
Ketoconazole	Fetal deaths in dogs
Cancer Therapeutics	
Azathioprine	Teratogenic in laboratory animals but has been used in pregnant women without adverse outcomes. Probably the chemotherapeutic of choice if a pregnant animal must be treated
Doxorubicin	Teratogenic and embryotoxic
Chlorambucil	Teratogenic and embryotoxic
Cisplatin	Teratogenic and embryotoxic
Cyclophosphamide	Teratogenic and embryotoxic
Methotrexate	Teratogenic and embryotoxic
Vincristine	Teratogenic and embryotoxic
Analgesics	
Aspirin	Teratogenic effects observed in laboratory animals but not in other species
Aurothioglucose	Teratogenic in laboratory animals

(Continued)

TABLE 5.5 (Continued)

Drug	Effects
Anesthetic and Preanesthetic Drugs	
Atropine	Causes fetal tachycardia; safe for short-term use
Halothane	May be neurotoxic to the embryo or fetus
Pentobarbital	Associated with high neonatal mortality; thiobarbiturates should be used instead
Cardiovascular Drugs	
Atropine	Causes fetal tachycardia; safe for short-term use
Isoproterenol	May cause fetal tachycardia, may inhibit uterine contractions
Lidocaine	May cause fetal bradycardia
Procainamide	May cause fetal bradycardia
Propanolol	May cause neonatal cardiac and respiratory depression and hypoglycemia. Do not use near term
Quinidine	May cause fetal bradycardia
Thiazide diuretics	Possible cause of perinatal mortality
Warfarin	Teratogenic and embryotoxic
Anticonvulsants	
Diazepam	Teratogenic in human beings and laboratory animals
Phenobarbital	Possibly teratogenic, may cause hemorrhagic diathesis
Phenytoin	Teratogenic in human beings and laboratory animals
Primidone	Possibly teratogenic, may cause hemorrhagic diathesis
Valproic acid	Teratogenic
Endocrine Drugs	
Corticosteroids	Teratogenic and abortifacient
Estradiolcypionate	Malformation of reproductive tracts of embryos of both genders, bone marrow suppression
Testosterone	Causes masculinization of the female fetus in a number of species
Miscellaneous	
Dimethylsulfoxide	Teratogenic in laboratory animals

Agalactia in the dam may be caused by ingestion of ergot alkaloids (q.v.) or *F. arundinacea* (Tall Fescue; q.v.)

SUCKLING (PREWEANED) ANIMALS AND TOXICITY VIA LACTATION

A large variety of xenobiotics are transferred into milk, although relay toxicosis from the dam to the suckling young is generally rare.

Xenobiotics may enter the alveolar lumen by passive diffusion or by active transport. Most xenobiotics enter milk by passive diffusion, and the concentration in the milk will be directly proportional to the concentration of free xenobiotic in the maternal plasma. The protein-bound fraction of a xenobiotic in the plasma will not diffuse into milk and therefore suckling animals will be at least partially protected from toxicosis from xenobiotics that are highly protein-bound in the plasma. Other physicochemical characteristics that govern the level of a xenobiotic in milk include atomic or molecular mass, lipophilicity, and ionization. Xenobiotics with an atomic or molecular weight less than approximately 200 kDa readily move into milk through intercellular pores in the alveolar membrane, whereas larger molecules must pass across cells, including dissolving in the basal and apical lipid membranes of the cell. Water-soluble xenobiotics can only enter milk through the intercellular pores, whereas lipid-soluble xenobiotics can dissolve in the cell membranes of the alveolar cells. As a generalization, lipid-soluble xenobiotics pass into milk in greater quantities and at a more rapid rate than water-soluble xenobiotics. Milk is slightly more acidic than plasma, so weak bases like antihistamines tend to pass into milk more readily than weak acids like barbiturates.

Xenobiotics that pass into milk may be protein-bound there, but on the whole, milk proteins do not bind xenobiotics strongly.

Retrograde diffusion from the milk into plasma can occur and has been demonstrated using intramammary medications in cows.

Metals and minerals are of small enough atomic mass to pass readily into milk, but on the other hand most are largely protein-bound in the plasma and this is probably the reason that they are usually present at lower concentrations in milk than in the maternal plasma. An exception is iodine, which is scavenged by the lactating mammary gland with greater avidity than that of the thyroid gland. Toxicosis due to excessive iodine may occur in the suckling young of a dam that is not showing any signs of toxicosis. Lead, which accumulates in the bones of growing animals, enters the milk of lactating animals if they are exposed to it.

A wide range of plant toxins that have been found in milk include pyrrolizidine alkaloids, piperidine alkaloids, quinolizidine alkaloids, sesquiterpene lactones, and glucosinolates. Goiters have been observed in the young of lactating dams that were grazing plants of the genus *Brassica*.

Mycotoxins may also enter milk, but generally only at trace amounts relative to the maternal exposure. Transfer into milk has been demonstrated for aflatoxins, trichothecenes, zearalenone, and fumonisin.

Many pharmaceuticals enter the milk of a lactating animal, although reports of toxicosis in the offspring are rare. Pharmacopeias may provide the milk to plasma ratio (M:P ratio) for pharmaceuticals. Usually the concentration of the pharmaceutical in the milk is lower than that in the maternal plasma, and the M:P ratio is therefore <1. However, some pharmaceuticals have an M:P ratio >1. Examples include fentanyl and morphine.

Organophosphates, carbamates, pyrethroids, phenoxy herbicides, and dipyridyl herbicides are excreted into milk in trace amounts relative to maternal exposure, and relay toxicosis by this route is highly unlikely. A toxic level of metaldehyde was relayed from a cow, that itself was showing clinical signs of toxicosis, to a kitten that drank its milk. Anticoagulant rodenticides are transferred in milk, and oral administration of Vitamin E to any suckling puppies or kittens is a prudent measure if the dam develops anticoagulant rodenticide toxicosis. Cholecalciferol is also transferred into milk, but on the other hand, sodium fluoroacetate and zinc phosphide have not been found in the milk of exposed dams. It is not clear whether 4-aminopyridine, alphachloralose, or para-aminopropiophenone can pass into milk.

GERIATRIC ANIMALS

As with neonatal and juvenile patients, geriatric patients have age-related characteristics that may affect ADME of xenobiotics. The effect may be protective or detrimental, depending on the ADME of the particular xenobiotic. As a generalization, farmed ruminants seldom reach old age, and the geriatric patient is most often encountered in companion animal practice. Physiological and pathological changes to be considered include the following:

- Preexisting chronic disease may be present. In particular, hepatic and renal reserve may be compromised.
- Decreased cardiac output, with increased circulatory transit time, may alter toxicokinetics in a favorable or unfavorable manner.
- Decreased liver size and hepatocyte numbers, and decreased protein synthesis. Hepatic metabolism may be altered.
- Decreased renal glomerular filtration rate and tubular absorption. Perfusion of the kidneys is also decreased.
- Decreased lean body mass, increased proportion of body fat, and decreased proportion of body water.
- Decreased plasma volume, and decreased plasma albumin.
- Decreased hydrochloric acid production in the stomach, leading to increased gastric pH.
- Decreased rate of gastric emptying.
- Decreased active transport in intestinal absorption.

- Decreased tissue perfusion.
- Increased vascular wall thickness with decreased elasticity, and increased systolic blood pressure.
- Decreased residual lung volume.

GENETIC SUSCEPTIBILITIES

Ivermectin in Some Breeds of Dogs

In veterinary medicine, this is perhaps the best-known genetic susceptibility to toxicosis. It has been reported in a variety of dog breeds, principally but not solely herding breeds, including Border Collies, Old English Sheepdogs, Shetland Sheepdogs, Australian Shepherds, German Shepherds, Collies (rough and smooth-coated), Skye Terriers, long-haired Whippets, and merle Pomeranians. Not all individuals within any of these breeds will be affected.

Although the susceptibility to ivermectin is the best-known effect, the genetic defect is in the multidrug resistance gene (MDR1) that codes for P-glycoprotein. P-glycoprotein is an ATP-dependent drug transporter that transports a wide range of substrates over cellular barriers in the body, and plays a major role in maintenance of the blood—brain barrier by excluding those substrates from the brain. The genetic defect renders P-glycoprotein effectively nonfunctional, and affected dogs will also be particularly susceptible to toxic effects of all xenobiotics that are substrates of P-glycoprotein. Not only ivermectin, but all the macrocyclic lactones are P-glycoprotein substrates. Macrocyclic lactones used in veterinary medicine include milbemycin, milbemycin oxime, moxidectin, selamectin, and doramectin. Other P-glycoprotein substrates to which dogs may be exposed include loperamide, domperidon, erythromycin, grepafloxacin, cyclosporin A, tacrolimus, dexamethasone, hydrocortisone, quinidine, digoxin, vincristine, vinblastine, and doxorubicin.

The mutated version of the normal MDR1 is termed mdr1-1Δ. Homozygotes may be fatally affected by doses that are in the therapeutic range for normal dogs. In the USA, it is estimated that approximately 35% of Collies are homozygous for mdr1-1Δ, and most Collies are heterozygous for it.

Dogs without the genetic mutation may also exhibit hypersensitivity to toxic effects of P-glycoprotein substrates if they have suffered head trauma or meningitis, or if they are puppies. Ivermectin toxicosis has also been reported in cats when significantly overdosed.

Clinical signs often develop within 12 hours of exposure in severe toxicosis, but may be delayed for up to 96 hours in milder cases. Clinical signs include miosis, depression, hypersalivation, emesis, anorexia, disorientation, tremors, weakness, recumbency, bradycardia, bradypnoea, hyperesthesia, seizures, stupor, or coma. Transient improvement in response to physostigmine is supportive, but not confirmatory, of the diagnosis.

Activated charcoal should be administered if exposure was oral and recent, and may be repeated if not contraindicated, because ivermectin undergoes enterohepatic cycling. There have been a small number of recent case reports of the use of intravenous lipid emulsion (ILE) for systemic decontamination in the treatment of ivermectin toxicosis in dogs and cats. ILE was well tolerated and appeared to significantly reduce the clinical course from the expected duration. Because this is currently an emerging therapy, the reader is advised to search for the most recent case reports for further details.

There is no antidote for ivermectin toxicosis and beyond the decontamination measures described in the previous paragraph, treatment is largely supportive. Seizures and persistent tremors must be controlled, preferably by barbiturates or propofol. It has been suggested that diazepam should not be used to control seizures, on the grounds that it may potentiate toxicosis by stimulating GABA receptors, but this has not been confirmed.

An intravenous fluid line should be established and, in the comatose dog, urinary catheterization. Body temperature should be monitored and kept within normal limits as required. Mechanical ventilation may be required. The dog may be recumbent in stupor or coma for a prolonged period, so it should be provided with a soft bed and turned regularly to prevent decubitus ulcers. Lubrication of the eyes, intravenous feeding, and/or intravenous electrolyte supplementation may be required. Physostigmine may provide transient improvement in the critically ill patient. Generally, it is considered that if the dog survives the first 24 hours, then prognosis is favorable, although recovery may be protracted.

Barbiturates in Sighthounds

The sensitivity of sighthounds, such as Greyhounds, Afghan hounds, Borzois, deerhounds, wolfhounds, whippets, and Salukis, to barbiturates has long been recognized. It is attributable in part to their low proportion of adipose tissue, which is an important "sink" in the distribution of barbiturates, and in part to lower expression of the hepatic enzymes responsible for barbiturate metabolism than in other breeds of dog. The use of barbiturates as anesthetic induction agents in sighthounds should be avoided. Alternative induction methods that are well tolerated by sighthounds include propofol, medetomidine/atipamezole, ketamine/diazepam, and oxymorphone/diazepam. Alternatively, anesthesia may be induced by administering isoflurane by mask, without using an induction agent. If the use of a barbiturate cannot be avoided, the sighthound should be administered one-third of the dose that would be administered to a dog of the same bodyweight that is not a sighthound.

Acetylpromazine in Some Dog Breeds and in Stallions

Acetylpromazine is generally a well-tolerated preanesthetic agent with a long history of safe use, but it has been noted that dogs of giant breeds, and greyhounds, may be particularly sensitive to the adverse effects of acetylpromazine, including bradycardia and hypothermia, while Boxers appear to have a susceptibility to vasovagal syncope when administered acetylpromazine. Alternative preanesthetics, such as butorphanol, should be used in these breeds.

Acetylpromazine causes paralysis of the retractor penis muscle, and in an extremely small number of male horses worldwide, this paralysis has been permanent. The risk of this outcome is remote, but it is generally recommended that acetylpromazine should not be used in breeding stallions.

Halothane in Pigs, Quarter Horses, and Dogs

Malignant Hyperthermia in response to exposure to halothane, similar to anesthetic gases and some other triggers has been detected in some breeds of pigs, Quarter horses, and dogs, most commonly Labrador retrievers. These individuals share with some human beings the genetic defect in the ryanodine receptor gene (*RYR1*) that causes Malignant Hyperthermia. Animals or people with this genetic defect are susceptible to developing Malignant Hyperthermia if administered halothane or other triggering xenobiotics, characterized by severe pyrexia, as well as tachycardia, tachypnea, miosis, acidosis, seizures, muscle rigidity, and rhabdomyolysis. Affected individuals are also particularly susceptible to the adverse effects of caffeine, and are also thought to be particularly intolerant of high ambient temperatures or vigorous exercise. Malignant Hyperthermia is inherited as an autosomal dominant trait in human beings and Quarter horses, but as an autosomal recessive trait in pigs and dogs. Pig breeds in which this genetic defect tend to be lean, heavily muscled breeds and include Pietrain, Poland China, Landrace, Duroc, and Large White.

The ryanodine receptor is located in the sarcoplasmic reticulum of skeletal muscle and controls the release of Ca^{2+}. In affected animals, the defective receptor floods the myoplasm with an excessive and prolonged release of Ca^{2+}. This leads to a hypermetabolic state in the muscle with contraction, ATP depletion, and excessive production of lactic acid and CO_2. Core body temperature escalates rapidly. The condition is self-amplifying in that the increased temperature, acidosis, and ATP depletion lead to rhabdomyolysis, and this releases more Ca^{2+}, leading to more contraction and energy consumption. Death in an acute episode is likely to be due to hyperkalemic cardiac failure, whereas if the animal survives the acute episode, it may die of renal failure secondary to myoglobinuria.

Although isoflurane has largely replaced halothane in veterinary medicine, this is not cause for complacency, because isoflurane, as well as desflurane and sevoflurane, can also trigger Malignant Hyperthermia, although onset may be delayed relative to the onset in response to halothane. In addition, severe reactions to caffeine, severe behavioral stress, vigorous exercise, or excessive ambient temperature remain risks to animals with this genetic defect. The treatment for Malignant Hyperthermia is dantrolene sodium

4–5 mg/kg IV, which should be administered as soon as possible. Dantrolene therapy may be repeated as necessary. In addition, vigorous efforts to cool the animal, by measures such as ice-water enemas, chilled IV fluids, and packing ice or snow around the patient, must be made. If the animal is being administered an anesthetic gas, the gas should be stopped immediately, the anesthetic administration system flushed, and oxygen flow increased. Urinary output should be promoted by intravenous fluid therapy, and the animal monitored for renal failure. Fluid therapy should also be directed toward correcting acidosis.

Successful surgery under halothane has been performed in patients pre-treated with dantrolene sodium, but it is more prudent to avoid the use of triggering anesthetic agents altogether.

There is evidence that in dogs with this genetic defect, an episode of Malignant Hyperthermia may be precipitated by low blood glucose, and it is therefore recommended that such dogs should be fed small quantities at frequent intervals, rather than a single large meal each day.

Genetic testing for the defect can be performed at some centers, and in addition there are protocols for sensitivity testing using limited exposure to halothane, caffeine, or ryanodine.

Copper Storage Hepatopathy in Dogs

The genetic predisposition to pathogenic storage of copper is best known in Bedlington Terriers, although it has also been found in West Highland White Terriers, Skye Terriers, Doberman Pinschers, and Labrador Retrievers. The inheritance in the Bedlington Terrier is autosomal recessive, and the defect has been shown to be due to the absence of a specific gene (COMMD1) that codes for a liver protein involved in the biliary excretion of copper in the bile. The prevalence of this genetic defect in Bedlington Terriers has been greatly reduced in recent years by genetic testing and selective breeding. The prevalence of chronic hepatitis due to excess copper storage is believed to be 4%–6% in Doberman Pinschers.

Copper storage hepatopathy usually presents as a chronic condition, and is usually first diagnosed in dogs between 2 and 6 years of age. In chronic presentation, clinical signs are polydipsia and polyuria, depression, anorexia, weight loss, emesis, diarrhea, ascites, icterus, melena, and hemorrhagic diathesis. Hepatic encephalopathy may develop if the disease is not treated promptly. Rarely, a dog with copper storage hepatopathy may present acutely with clinical signs that include depression, anorexia, emesis, icterus, anemia, bilirubinuria, and, rarely, hemolytic crisis and hematuria. Acute presentations, while rare overall, are more likely to be seen in younger dogs.

Serum chemistry reveals elevated ALT, AP, AST, and bilirubin, but serum copper and plasma ceruloplasmin levels are typically within normal range. On the ultrasound examination the liver may be enlarged or abnormally small, depending on the stage of the disease. Liver biopsy is diagnostic, with copper levels in the biopsy sample in excess of 2000 ppm dry weight in an affected dog. If the biopsy sample is of sufficient size to perform histopathology as well, lesions are those of chronic active hepatitis and cirrhosis, and rubeanic acid stain reveals copper accumulation in hepatocytes. However, if the biopsy sample is limited, determination of copper content should be given priority.

Dogs with a genetic propensity to copper storage may require oral D-penicillamine therapy, 10−15 mg/kg twice daily, for weeks, months, or years. Oral ascorbic acid (Vitamin C) at 500−1000 mg/day may be helpful to enhance copper excretion. Corticosteroids may be helpful. The dog should be placed on a diet that minimizes copper intake and also minimizes the metabolic burden on the liver. Dogs that carry this genetic defect should be avoided as breeding stock, and people who are interested in buying a Bedlington Terrier or a dog of one of the other potentially affected breeds should be given advice on how to avoid buying a dog that will develop or perpetuate this problem.

Sporidesmin in Most British Isles Sheep

Genetic predispositions in response to xenobiotics are not always adverse. Merinos enjoy much greater resistance to sporidesmin toxicosis when compared with breeds originating from the British Isles. Unfortunately, Merinos, which come from the dry climates of Spain, are substantially more susceptible to footrot and therefore are unsuited to the North Island areas where sporidesmin toxicosis is a significant problem. Among the breeds of British Isles origin the Wiltshire, a meat breed with the atavistic trait of shedding its fleece in the spring, is reputed to be much less susceptible to sporidesmin toxicosis than the other breeds. Efforts to select for tolerance to sporidesmin are being made for some other breeds.

HYPERSENSITIVITY REACTIONS

Allergic and other hypersensitivity reactions fall within the realm of toxicology, but are unusual and unpredictable, in that they affect only some individuals in a population.

Four types of immune hypersensitivity reaction are recognized.

Type I Hypersensitivity

Type I hypersensitivity is also known as immediate or anaphylactic hypersensitivity. Milder manifestations are referred to as an allergy. Clinical signs of Type I hypersensitivity may include an eczematous reaction of the skin, conjunctivitis, rhinorrhea or rhinitis, asthma, and/or gastroenteritis. The reaction is usually evident within 15—30 minutes of exposure to the antigen, although sometimes it may be delayed up to 12 hours.

Immediate hypersensitivity is mediated by IgE. The primary cellular component in this hypersensitivity is the mast cell or basophil, with amplification or modification of the reaction by platelets, neutrophils, and eosinophils. Biopsy of the reaction site reveals infiltration by mast cells and eosinophils.

The antigen in Type I hypersensitivity is often called an allergen.

The mediators of the Type 1 reaction, and their effects, are:

Preexisting Mediators in Cell Granules

histamine	bronchoconstriction, mucus secretion, vasodilatation, vascular permeability
tryptase	proteolysis
kininogenase	kinins and vasodilatation, vascular permeability, edema
eosinophil chemotactic factor of anaphylaxis (ECF-A) (tetrapeptides)	attract eosinophil and neutrophils

Mediators Synthesized During the Reaction

leukotriene B4	basophil attractant
leukotriene C4, D4	same as histamine, but much more potent
prostaglandins D2	edema and pain
platelet activation factor	platelet aggregation and heparin release, formation of microthrombi

Cyclic nucleotides appear to play a significant role in the modulation of Type I hypersensitivity reaction, although their exact function is not understood. However, substances which increase intracellular cAMP significantly relieve clinical signs.

Diagnostic tests for immediate hypersensitivity include skin (prick and intradermal) tests, measurement of total IgE and specific IgE antibodies against the suspected allergens. Increased IgE levels may indicate an atopic condition, although IgE may be elevated in some nonatopic diseases including parasitic infection.

Symptomatic treatment is achieved with antihistamines that block histamine receptors. The leukotriene-mediated bronchoconstriction seen in some Type I cases may respond to leukotriene receptor blockers or inhibitors of the cyclooxygenase pathway. Inhaled bronchodilators such as isoproterenol derivatives offer short-term relief. Theophylline elevates cAMP and is also used to relieve bronchoconstriction. Some allergies in human beings are treated with IgG antibodies against the Fc portions of IgE that binds to mast cells, in order to block mast cell sensitization.

Hyposensitization (immunotherapy or desensitization) is another treatment modality which is successful in a number of allergies, and is successful for some allergic problems encountered in veterinary practice, such as some cases of flea allergy. The mechanism is not clear, but there is a correlation between appearance of IgG (blocking) antibodies and relief from symptoms. Suppressor T cells that specifically inhibit IgE antibodies may also play a role.

Type II Hypersensitivity

Type II hypersensitivity is also known as cytotoxic hypersensitivity. The antigens may be endogenous, but xenobiotics can also lead to Type II hypersensitivity, if they act as haptens by binding with cell membranes. Examples of xenobiotics causing Type II hypersensitivity are drug-induced hemolytic anemia, granulocytopenia, and thrombocytopenia. The reaction time following exposure may be minutes to hours. Type II hypersensitivity is primarily mediated by antibodies of the IgM or IgG classes and complement, although phagocytes and K cells may also play a role.

Histologically, the lesion contains antibody, complement, and neutrophils. Diagnostic tests include detection of circulating antibody against the tissues involved and the presence of antibody and complement in the lesion (biopsy) by immunofluorescence.

Treatment involves antiinflammatory and immunosuppressive agents.

Type III Hypersensitivity

Type III hypersensitivity is also known as immune complex hypersensitivity. The reaction may be a general systemic response, such as serum sickness, or may involve individual organs.

The reaction may take several hours to develop after exposure to the antigen, and is mediated by soluble immune complexes, mostly of the IgG class, although IgM may also be involved. Exogenous antigens include chronic bacterial, viral or parasitic infections, or endogenous as in systemic lupus erythematosus. The antigen is not attached to the organ involved. Primary components are soluble immune complexes and complement, but the damage is caused by platelets and neutrophils. Histologically, the lesion contains primarily neutrophils and deposits of immune complexes and complement, although macrophages may be present in later stages. Diagnosis procedures include examination of tissue biopsies for deposits of immunoglobulin and complement by immunofluorescence microscopy, detection of immune complexes in serum, and depletion in the level of complement. Treatment includes antiinflammatory agents.

Type IV Hypersensitivity

Type IV hypersensitivity is also known as cell mediated or delayed type hypersensitivity. The classical example of this hypersensitivity is the tuberculin (Mantoux) reaction, which peaks 48 hours after the injection of antigen. The lesion is characterized by induration and erythema.

Type IV reactions are divided into three further types: contact, tuberculin, and granuloma. A number of xenobiotics cause Type IV contact hypersensitivity, which is dermal. These include organic chemicals and poison ivy. The clinical appearance is that of eczema, usually developing after 48—72 hours. Histologically there is edema with infiltration of lymphocytes, later followed by macrophages.

The tuberculin reaction arises over the same time range and is that of local induration at the site of intradermal injection of the antigen. Histologically, cellular infiltrates are those of lymphocytes, monocytes, and macrophages. The granuloma reaction takes 3—4 weeks to develop and features macrophages, epithelioid and giant cells, and fibrosis. It is triggered by persistent antigens such as occur in tuberculosis or leprosy, or by the presence of a foreign body.

Mechanisms of damage in delayed hypersensitivity include T lymphocytes and monocytes and/or macrophages. Cytotoxic T cells (Tc) cause direct damage whereas helper T (TH1) cells secrete cytokines which activate cytotoxic Tc and recruit and activate monocytes and macrophages, which cause most of the damage. Major lymphokines involved in delayed hypersensitivity reaction include monocyte chemotactic factor, interleukin-2, interferon-gamma, TNF alpha/beta, etc.

Diagnostic tests in vivo may include delayed cutaneous reaction such as the Mantoux test, or a patch test for contact dermatitis. In vitro tests for delayed hypersensitivity include mitogenic response, lympho-cytotoxicity, and IL-2 production.

Corticosteroids and other immunosuppressive agents are used in treatment.

Chapter 6

Sample Collection, Handling, and Submission in Toxicology

INTRODUCTION

For the purpose of reaching or confirming a diagnosis in clinical toxicology, laboratory testing may include testing of a variety of pre- or postmortem tissue samples for xenobiotics or their metabolites. In addition, testing of feed or drinking water may be desirable, as well as identification of plants, chemicals, organisms, or objects of uncertain composition.

Relatively few poisons create distinctive, let alone pathognomonic, lesions on histopathology, but histopathology of biopsy or necropsy samples still has a place, not least in eliminating possible differential diagnoses. However, even the most skilled pathologist cannot extract useful information out of improperly fixed, poorly handled, or absent tissues.

Collection of fresh samples is more important in toxicology than some other clinical disciplines and again, it is critical to collect the correct samples and to ensure that they reach the laboratory while still in condition suitable for analysis.

The most common mistake made by practitioners, in this author's experience, is to fail to collect samples, leaving the pathologist and/or analytical toxicologist saying regretfully "If only we had a sample of..." Therefore a good rule is *If in doubt, collect it. You can always throw it out later.*

Communication with the pathology/analytical laboratory is valuable, and the practitioner should not be reluctant to call the laboratory and ask what samples they find most useful. In analytical toxicology, there are no stupid presubmission questions, but there are many inadequate submissions.

SAMPLES FROM THE LIVING ANIMAL

Veterinary practitioners are generally familiar with the principles of appropriate collection and handling of samples of blood, serum, and urine, and they will not be reiterated here. Sample sizes should be as generous as feasible. Vacuum collection tubes with sodium citrate anticoagulant for determination of clotting factors, in particular, should be filled. Whenever possible, the volume serum or blood should be 5–10 mL, and that of urine at least 50 mL.

Veterinary Toxicology for Australia and New Zealand
DOI: http://dx.doi.org/10.1016/B978-0-12-420227-6.00006-2

If facilities exist and serum rather than whole blood is specified, the serum should be separated from the clot prior to shipment.

Changes in hematology and/or clinical chemistry in response to the toxic mechanism of the xenobiotic (e.g., anemia, hypoproteinemia) are discussed in the description of each toxicosis.

The samples of blood, urine, or other substances, which may be collected from the live animal, for analytical detection of poisons or their metabolites, are covered in Table 6.1. The list of poisons is not intended to be exhaustive. Biotoxins and plant toxins are not included in this table, because in all these cases, submission of the suspected source material is much more likely to be useful than attempts to isolate the toxin or its metabolites in clinical samples.

POSTMORTEM SAMPLES

Both fresh and fixed samples may be collected at necropsy to determine whether the cause of death was poisoning.

Note: A postmortem examination of an animal other than a human being is a necropsy. The term autopsy, which literally means "examination of self" applies only to human postmortem examination, and should not be used for the postmortem examination of any other species.

Fresh Samples

As a generalization, if the cause of death is not determined by the gross necropsy findings and poisoning is a possibility, generous samples of *liver* and *kidney* should be collected as fresh (unfixed) tissue. If submission to the laboratory is anticipated within 24–48 hours, these samples may be stored in a refrigerator. Otherwise, they should be frozen, sealed in plastic bags against freezer burn. Samples should be shipped chilled or on ice. Other samples the practitioner may consider for collection if the cause of death is unknown at the end of the gross necropsy, all of which may be stored frozen for possible future testing, are, *ruminal/gastrointestinal content*, *bile*, *adipose* tissue, and *urine* aspirated from the bladder.

Brain should be removed if nervous signs were present prior to death or the cause of death is undetermined at the end of the gross necropsy. If poisoning is suspected, the brain should be bisected longitudinally and one side fixed while the other is retained as fresh tissue. Brain is particularly important for the postmortem diagnosis of organophosphate poisoning.

Samples for toxicological analysis should be generous, 200 g if possible. For small animals, after removing a slice for fixation, retain all the rest of the kidney tissue as fresh specimen. For very small animals (e.g., kitten or small puppy) the same should be done with liver. Rumen content volume should be 500 g, and stomach/abomasum content 500 g if possible.

TABLE 6.1 Samples for Analytical Detection of Xenobiotics or Their Metabolites in the Live Animal

Poison	Samples	Comments
Metals and Minerals		
Arsenic	Urine, feces, hair	Hair in chronic poisoning
Cadmium	Urine	
Copper	Serum or whole blood	
Fluoride	Penultimate caudal vertebra from the tail in the cow	The last palpable vertebra in the bovine tail is generally not ossified and is not useful. The penultimate vertebra can be readily extruded as a biopsy sample
Iron	Serum	
Lead	Blood	Lead poisoning should not be diagnosed on blood lead levels alone because these correlate poorly to clinical signs
Mercury	Blood or urine	
Molybdenum	Blood	Also measure blood copper
Selenium	Blood, hair, hooves	Hair or hoof in chronic poisoning
Thallium	urine	
Zinc	Serum, urine	It is critical that the serum sample does not come in contact with rubber, including the rubber bung of a vacuum collection tube or the rubber grommet of a syringe. A vacuum collection tube with a plastic rather than a rubber stopper should be used
Insecticides, Repellents, Molluscicides, Fungicides, Herbicides, and Vertebrate Pesticides		
3-Chloro-*p*-toluidine HCl		
Amitraz	Blood, urine	
Anticoagulant rodenticides	Blood, urine	

(Continued)

TABLE 6.1 (Continued)

Poison	Samples	Comments
Anticholinesterase insecticides	Whole blood from most species; plasma from cats	Depression of AChE indicates exposure but correlates poorly with clinical signs. AChE depression from organophosphates is long-lasting but from carbamates are transient, so a false-negative result may be obtained if the agent is a carbamate
Boric acid	urine	
Chlorinated hydrocarbons	Blood, milk, adipose biopsy	Blood in acute exposure. Milk or biopsy of adipose tissue in chronic exposure
N,N-diethyl-m-toluamide (DEET)	Blood, urine	
Dipyridyl herbicides (paraquat and diquat)	Urine	
Fipronil	Hair or skin biopsy	Only confirms exposure, not toxicosis
Imidacloprid	Urine. Hair or skin biopsy	Only confirms exposure, not toxicosis
Methoprene	Hair or skin biopsy	Only confirms exposure, not toxicosis
Metaldehyde	Serum, urine	Detection is difficult and interpretation is uncertain
Phenoxy herbicides	Urine	Interpretation is uncertain
Pyrethrins/pyrethroids		Detection is difficult and interpretation of any agents or their metabolites is uncertain
Sodium fluoroacetate		Detection is difficult and interpretation is uncertain
Pharmaceuticals and Recreational Drugs		
Amphetamines	Serum, urine	
Aspirin	Serum	Detection of salicylates only confirm exposure
Barbiturates	Serum, urine	
Benzodiazepines	Serum, urine	
Cocaine	Urine	

(Continued)

TABLE 6.1 (Continued)

Poison	Samples	Comments
Ethanol	Blood	
Ketamine	Urine	Rapidly excreted with short half-life
Lysergic acid diethylamide	Serum, urine	
Marijuana	Serum, urine	
Metronidazole	Blood	
Nicotine	Urine, blood	
NSAIDs, other than aspirin	Urine	May confirm exposure
Opioids	Serum, urine	
Paracetamol	Serum, urine	
Phencyclidine (PCP)	Urine	
Tricyclic antidepressants	Serum, urine	
Household, Farm, and Industrial Poisons		
Ethylene glycol	Blood or urine	
Macrolide parasiticides (e.g., ivermectin)	Serum	Only confirms absorption
Methanol	Blood	
Methylxanthine alkaloids (caffeine, theobromine, theophylline)	Serum or urine	
Phenol-based antiseptics	Urine	
Strychnine	Serum, urine	

Fixed Samples

Fixed samples to collect routinely from any necropsy, regardless of suspected cause of death, are *liver*, *kidney*, *lung*, and *lesions*.

- *Liver*. Although it is tempting to snip a sample from the edge of the liver, this area may have been poorly perfused if the animal was in shock prior to death. Effects of some hepatotoxic poisons, such as sporidesmin, are typically less severe in the edges of the liver than in more central regions, suggesting that the edges are less exposed to xenobiotics even in animals that are not in shock. If there are no obvious lesions on the liver, cut a slice not more than 8 mm thick from the greater curvature, near the thickest part of the liver. If a biliary toxicant is suspected, a further section from the lesser curvature, including major biliary ducts leading into the gallbladder (when present) may be collected in addition.

- *Kidney.* Although from the point of view of gross necropsy, opening the kidney longitudinally may give the greatest visibility, from the point of view of histopathology, a transverse cut through the kidney has the advantage that the renal papilla is better preserved for examination, and the contents of the renal pelvis may be held in place by the surrounding connective tissue. With a longitudinal cut, the renal papilla is often cut sagitally with little tissue on one side, and the pelvic epithelium and any pelvic contents are easily lost. If a longitudinal cut has been made, examine the two sides and fix a slice of the side on which there is more renal papilla remaining. When sampling the bovine kidney, cut a sample that includes a renal papilla, and the perihilar tissue beyond it to protect it from damage in transit.
- *Lung.* As for liver, although it may seem tempting to snip a sample from an edge, the most useful lung tissue for histopathology is perihilar, because peripheral lung may not be effectively perfused in the moribund animal, and because a perihilar sample enables the pathologist to examine bronchioles of various sizes and may also include major vessels. Even in the healthy animal, the peripheral lung undergoes little inflation when the animal is at rest.
- *Lesions.* If lesions are focal, try to cut a sample that includes both the gross lesion and the apparently normal tissue around it. Do not be reluctant to submit multiple samples if lesions are multifocal or are diffuse but vary in apparent severity across the organ.

Use buffered formalin whenever possible, to avoid the formation of formalin pigment. Although the presence of formalin pigment does not usually preclude diagnosis, it can make it impossible to find a field of photographic quality, and if a case is particularly interesting or unusual, the practitioner should be able to expect coauthorship, if not lead authorship, on a publication. If the case leads to legal action, good quality photographs may be important.

When using formalin, with the exception of brain, always ensure that the section is no thicker than 8 mm from cut edge to cut edge, to ensure proper fixation. To ensure penetration of formalin, hollow tissues should be opened and tissue capsules incised, unless the subject is a rodent or no larger than a rat (e.g., neonatal puppy or young kitten) in which case incision of capsules is unlikely to be required.

In a suspected poisoning with central nervous signs, half the *brain* should be kept fresh and the other half fixed in formalin, with a small number of transverse cuts to the outside, that do not completely separate the brain into pieces, to allow fixation. As a guide, one such cut that penetrates as far as the lateral ventricles is adequate for the brain of a dog or sheep, but two or three may be required for the brain of a horse or cow. When handling brain, avoid applying pressure as much as possible, because this may result in artefactual changes to neurons. For very small animals such as kittens and puppies, consider fixing the brain in situ after removing the calvarium, to avoid damage associated with prising it out of the skull.

Formalin is suitable for most tissues but if the termination of the animal is elective and it is intended to take samples of *eye* or *testis*, contact the pathology laboratory in advance to determine whether they prefer to have those tissues fixed in Bouin's fixative or some other fixative, and if so, whether they can supply that fixative. Many pathologists prefer fixatives other than formalin for eye and testis.

The volume of fixative should always be at least 10 times the total volume of the tissue/s fixed. If the total tissue volume is large, as in the case of multiple tissues from one large animal in the same container, the tissues can be moved to a smaller volume of formalin for shipping purposes after a few days' fixation.

If sections of *spinal cord* are collected, notch the distal end with a small longitudinal cut to enable the pathologist which end is proximal and which is distal; and fix cervical, thoracic, and lumbar spinal cord samples separately in marked containers if the spinal cord has not been removed as one piece. Cutting a small distal notch can also be done for other longitudinal organs of large animals, e.g., *peripheral nerves*, *ureters*, or *oviducts*. For small animals, if these longitudinal organs are too small to allow the use of a distal notch, the organ may be laid over a piece of cardboard and the ends secured in small slits cut in either side of the cardboard. The cardboard is then marked with a pencil to indicate which end is proximal and which is distal. This information can be important in diagnosis, for example, in a "dying-back" axonopathy. For very small animals such as kittens, if a peripheral nerve sample is indicated, consider taking the biceps femoris and sciatic nerve as one piece of tissue, using the biceps femoris as a means of securing and identifying the sciatic nerve. This is an effective routine practice for laboratory rodents, and minimizes trauma to the nerve associated with handling.

Do not wash tissues in water if they are intended for histopathology, because this is likely to render the exposed surfaces of the tissue refractory to stains. Likewise, do not wipe mucosal surfaces, or scrape them with a knife, if they are intended for histopathology. If there is copious content of the viscus (e.g., stomach, intestine), the content may be shaken off a sample of tissue, or the sample tissue may be agitated in the formalin container, to dislodge the content and improve formalin penetration of the tissue, but wiping or scraping the content off manually often damages the mucosa beyond diagnostic quality. Pieces of *intestine* should always be opened longitudinally, preferably by a cut sagittal to the mesenteric attachment, prior to fixation. Do not attempt to strip off the mesenteric attachment.

Table 6.2 provides recommendations of tissues to fix from necropsy for various poisonings, *in addition to liver, kidney, lung,* and *lesions* which should be routinely fixed from all necropsies, as described above. These core tissues are *not* reiterated in Table 6.2, even if they are the primary site of lesions (e.g., liver in aflatoxicosis, kidney in ochratoxicosis, lung in dipyridyl herbicide toxicosis) because they should be collected routinely in any case.

Table 6.2 is not intended to be comprehensive, and for further details the section on the particular poisoning should be referred to. If there is sufficient time to do so, it is also advisable to call the laboratory and ask to talk to a pathologist about what tissues they consider useful.

Note that if tissues listed in Table 6.2 are submitted and no lesions are found in them, this does not necessarily preclude poisoning by that agent, unless so determined by a pathologist or toxicologist.

In the event of postmortem investigation of the fetus, samples to be fixed for histopathology are *fetal liver, kidney, lung,* and *placenta.* In the event that a deformed fetus is delivered and a teratogen is suspected, it is highly unlikely that the teratogen will be present in the fetus or fetal membranes.

FEED AND WATER SAMPLES

At least 2 kg of feed should be provided, if possible, and at least 500 mL of water. If volatile toxicants such as cyanide or ammonia are suspected, the sample should be frozen as soon as possible. For most analyses, samples can be stored frozen until a suitable analytical laboratory is located, and shipped on ice, without having a deleterious effect on the analytical results. The volume of ice should be at least four times the volume of submitted material.

Dry feeds containing <15% moisture can be shipped as is, but wet feed such as silage or pasture should be either dried or refrigerated to prevent growth of mold.

PLANT SAMPLES

For plant identification, high-quality photographs or pressed specimens may be of more use than plant material that has been allowed to wilt. If a laboratory with plant identification capability is close enough to permit shipping of fresh material, the material should be sent in paper or cloth bags rather than in plastic bags, which promote rotting. As many parts of the plant as possible should be submitted, including mature leaves, new shoots flowers, fruits or seeds, stems, bark and, for small plants, root system.

For analysis of plant material for plant toxins, at least 2 kg of material should be either dried, or frozen and shipped on ice.

TABLE 6.2 Tissues to Fix *in Addition to Liver, Kidney, Lung,* and *Lesions*

Poison	Tissues to Fix *in Addition to Liver, Kidney, Lung,* and *Lesions*
Metals and Minerals	
Arsenic	Gastric/abomasal and intestinal mucosa
	For organic arsenicals, brain and spinal cord, peripheral nerve
Copper	Abomasum/stomach in acute toxicosis
Fluoride	Bone; sites most likely to show lesions are metacarpal, metatarsal, rib, mandible
Iodine	Thyroid, trachea, skin
Iron	Abomasum/stomach and intestine in oral toxicosis. Injection site and regional lymph node if toxicosis follows iron injection
Lead	Brain including cerebellum. Peripheral nerve in horses. Myocardium and gizzard (proventriculus) in birds
Mercury	Gastrointestinal tract. Brain, including cerebellum, in the case of alkyl mercurials or organomercurials. Heart of cattle. Peripheral nerve in swine.
Molybdenum	Periosteum, epiphyseal growth plate in young animals
Selenium	Gastrointestinal tract, heart. Pancreas of sheep. Brain and spinal cord of swine
Sodium	Brain. Skeletal and cardiac muscle
Sulfur	Brain
Zinc	Pancreas. Spleen. Abomasum in ruminants. Humerus (ends) in swine. Fetlock joints of horses; epiphyseal plates of young horses. Gizzard (proventriculus) including lining in birds
Insecticides, Repellents, Molluscicides, Fungicides, Herbicides, and Vertebrate Pesticides	
3-Chloro-*p*-toluidine HCl	Brain
Amitraz	Adrenal gland
Anticholinesterase insecticides	Pancreas
Boric acid	Brain. Skin and/or gastrointestinal tract if affected
Bromethalin	Brain, spinal cord
Chlorinated hydrocarbons	Adrenal gland

(Continued)

TABLE 6.2 (Continued)

Poison	Tissues to Fix *in Addition to Liver, Kidney, Lung,* and *Lesions*
Cholecalciferol	Heart, gastrointestinal tract, skeletal muscle, tendons, and ligaments. Note that mineralization can be widespread and any palpably mineralized soft tissue should be submitted
DEET	Skin. Testes
Dipyridyl herbicides (paraquat and diquat)	Skin and/or gastrointestinal tract if affected by caustic properties
	Brain if pulmonary toxicosis leads to functionally decerebrate state prior to death
Fipronil	Dermal application site if lesions
Imidacloprid	Dermal application site if lesions
Metaldehyde	Gastrointestinal tract. Heart. Medulla of brain
Naphthalene	Gastrointestinal tract
Pyrethrins/pyrethroids	Skeletal muscle
Sodium fluoroacetate	Heart. Brain. Intestinal tract
Zinc phosphide	Heart. Gastrointestinal tract
Biotoxins (Bacterial Toxins, Algal Toxins, Mycotoxins, and Poisonous Fungi)	
Aflatoxin	Heart. Skeletal muscle
Cyanobacterial ("blue-green algal") toxins	No specific lesions, other than the hepatic lesions caused by microcystin
Corynetoxins (annual ryegrass toxicity)	Brain
Ochratoxin/citrinin	Lymphoid tissues including spleen, tonsils, lymph nodes, thymus if present, Bursa of Fabricius in birds. Proventriculus and bone marrow of birds
Ergot alkaloids	Brain. Gastrointestinal tract. Placenta and fetal lung in fescue toxicosis of the pregnant/parturient mare
Fumonisin	Brain (horses)
Phomopsins	Heart. Skeletal muscle
Sporidesmin	Skin lesions
Stachybotryotoxins	Oral/gastrointestinal lesions, dermatitis if present. Lymphoid tissues, including gut-associated lymphoid tissues (includes Peyer's patches that are most readily found in the terminal ileum). Bone marrow. Myocardium of birds
Tremorgenic mycotoxins	Brain (cerebellum)

(Continued)

TABLE 6.2 (Continued)

Poison	Tissues to Fix *in Addition to Liver, Kidney, Lung,* and *Lesions*
Plant Toxins	
Cardiac glycosides (e.g., oleander, lily-of-the-valley)	Heart
Cyanogenic glycosides	Heart
Cycasin (e.g., cycad palm)	Gastrointestinal tract
	Brain if hepatic encephalopathy is suspected
Diterpene esters (*Euphorbia* species)	Oral mucosa, gastrointestinal tract
Glucosinolates/thiocyanates/isocyanates (e.g., rape, kale)	Reticulum and rumen
Lectins (e.g., castor oil plant)	Gastrointestinal tract. Spleen. Heart. Skeletal muscle
Oxalates, insoluble	Oral cavity, pharynx
Oxalates, soluble	Gastrointestinal tract, heart
Persin (Avocado)	Heart
Phytoestrogens	Gonads. Female reproductive tract
Piperidine alkaloids (e.g., poison hemlock)	Skeletal muscle
Propyl disulfide (e.g., onion, garlic)	Spleen
Protoanemonins	Oral cavity, gastrointestinal tract
Ptaquiloside	Bone marrow
Tannins (e.g., oak)	Gastrointestinal tract
Household, Farm, and Industrial Poisons	
Carbon monoxide	Heart, brain
Ethylene glycol	Gastrointestinal tract in cats. Terminal colon, uterus, and heart in swine. Brain of birds
Ionophores	Heart. Skeletal muscle. Spleen in horses. Peripheral nerves in cat and dog, and eye in dog

OTHER SAMPLES

Insects or arachnids suspected of envenomation may be useful for identification if they can be captured without risk of further injury. Attempting to capture snakes or sea jellies for identification is not recommended.

Household, industrial, or farm chemicals suspected of causing toxicosis should be saved and full details from the label included in any laboratory submission of samples from the affected animal.

If in doubt about how to preserve or submit any specimen, or whether the laboratory can use it for analysis, contact the laboratory in advance. Retrieving a specimen that has been submitted to an inappropriate laboratory can be difficult and frustrating. With the exception of fixing slices of tissue in formalin for histopathology, never add any preservative to samples unless advised to do so by the laboratory.

Full history and clinical details should be provided with any submission.

CHAIN OF CUSTODY AND LEGAL CONSIDERATIONS

The chain of custody may be important if there are likely to be legal matters arising from the case, including insurance claims. Submitted samples should be packed carefully in numbered boxes in the style "Box 1 of 2," "Box 2 of 2." A full inventory of submitted samples should be included. The boxes should be sealed with tape and indelible ink used to cross-hatch the tape, or draw waving lines on it, so that the ink markings repeatedly go beyond the tape onto the adjacent box wall. This makes it extremely difficult to move the tape and replace it undetected, because of the difficulty in matching up all the points at which the markings cross from tape to box wall or from box wall to tape. Submission documents should be placed in a sealed envelope that is taped to the outside of the first box.

Prior to submission, the laboratory should be contacted and the name of a person responsible for receipt obtained. The box or boxes should be addressed for the specific attention of this person. The person responsible for receipt should be informed in advance that the case may have legal implications, and all boxes should be clearly marked "EVIDENCE."

Full history and clinical details should be included in the submission. Suspicions concerning insurance fraud or malicious poisoning should be communicated with great discretion, and in particular the person or company suspected of being responsible should not be named in any discoverable documents.

Chapter 7

Poisons by Toxic Action

INTRODUCTION

This chapter is intended for quick memory prompts, and to assist in navigating the rest of the book. Not all the poisons included in the book are listed in this chapter, because some substances that are extremely rare, are of very low toxicity, or are of very poorly characterized toxicity, that are described in other chapters are not included in these lists. Furthermore, prescription pharmaceuticals, introduced plants, and indigenous Australian plants are not included because they are already listed by target organ or system in their respective chapters.

Most poisons are listed only by the most important target organ or system, although some poisons that act on multiple organs are listed in several categories (e.g., cholecalciferol). A sound understanding of pathogenesis, with the ability to recognize or predict secondary effects of the primary toxic insult (to use a tired old cliché, "first principles"), is assumed.

Categories in this chapter are as follows:

- Neurotoxic poisons
- Hepatotoxic poisons
- Nephrotoxic poisons
- Cardiotoxic poisons
- Poisons with effects on the blood
- Poisons with effects on the gastrointestinal tract
- Poisons with effects on the respiratory system
- Poisons with effects on skin
- Poisons with effects on muscle
- Poisons with effects on the skeleton
- Poisons with effects on reproduction
- Poisons with effects on the endocrine system
- Poisons with effects on the immune system

Important: Also see chapters on prescription pharmaceuticals, indigenous Australian plants and introduced plants, if a pharmaceutical or plant poisoning is possible.

Veterinary Toxicology for Australia and New Zealand
DOI: http://dx.doi.org/10.1016/B978-0-12-420227-6.00007-4

Within each category, poisons are listed under the chapter in which they are described, and in the order in which they appear in that chapter (usually alphabetical), rather than in order of likelihood, or in order of toxicity.

NEUROTOXIC POISONS

Autonomic Nervous System

Insecticides and Acaricides
  Carbamates
  Organophosphates
Over the Counter (OTC) Pharmaceuticals
  Antihistamines
  Decongestants
Alternative Medicines
  Ephedra
Mycotoxins and Mushrooms
  Slaframine
Aquatic Invertebrates
  Cyanobacteria
Australian Terrestrial Invertebrates
  Redback spiders, *Latrodectus hasselti*
New Zealand Terrestrial Invertebrates
  Katipo, *Latrodectus katipo*
  Australian redback spider *L. hasseltii*
Indigenous New Zealand Poisonous Plants
  Kowhai   *Sophora* species
  Ongaonga   *Urtica ferox*
  Poroporo   *Solanum aviculare, Solanum laciniatum*

Central Nervous System

Insecticides and Acaricides
  Amitraz
  Chlorinated hydrocarbons
  Pyrethroids
  Rotenone
Molluscicides
  Metaldehyde
Vertebrate Pesticides
  Cyanide
  Phosphides
  Phosphorus
  Sodium fluoroacetate

Strychnine
Alphachloralose
Herbicides and Fungicides
Phenoxy herbicides
OTC Pharmaceuticals
Antihistamines
Loperamide
Cough suppressants
Alternative Medicines
5-Hydroxytryptophan (*Griffonia* extract)
Artemisia absinthium (Absinthe; wormwood)
Aconite
Camphor oil
Citrus oils
Guarana
Kava kava
Melaleuca oil
Recreational Drugs
Amphetamines
Barbiturates
Benzodiazepines
Cocaine
Ethanol
Ketamine
LSD
Marijuana
Phencyclidine
Psilocybin
Household Foods and Products
Pine oil disinfectants
Methylxanthine alkaloids (coffee, tea, and chocolate)
Salt (sodium chloride)
Turpentine
Xylitol
Metals
Lead
Mercury
Molybdenum
Metalloids
Boron and borates
Organic arsenicals
Miscellaneous Inorganic Substances
Bromides
Selenium

Industrial Toxicants
Petroleum hydrocarbons
Agricultural and Feed-Related Toxicants
4-Methylimidazole poisoning
Botulism
Nonprotein nitrogen
Raw soybeans
Sulfur
Smoke and Other Inhaled Toxicants
Smoke
Carbon dioxide
Carbon monoxide
Hydrogen cyanide
Hydrogen sulfide
Methane
Mycotoxins and Mushrooms
Corallocytostroma ornicopreoides toxin
Ergot alkaloids
Fumonisin
Penitrem A
Roquefortine
Swainsonine
Lolitrems, paspalinine, and paspalitrems
Agaricus spp.
Amanita spp.
Psilocybe and related spp.
Australian Terrestrial Vertebrates
Venomous terrestrial Australian snakes
Aquatic Vertebrates
Sea snakes
Aquatic Invertebrates
Ciguatoxin and related toxins
Dinoflagellate/shellfish poisonings
Tetrodotoxin
Cnidaria (sea jellies)
Australian Terrestrial Invertebrates
Australian paralysis tick, *Ixodes holocyclus*
Australian tarantulas (*Selenotholus, Selenotypus, Coremiocnemis, Phlogius* spp.)
Redback spiders, *L. hasselti*
Tasmanian Paralysis tick *Ixodes cornuatus*
New Zealand Terrestrial Invertebrates
Katipo, *L. katipo*
Australian redback spider *L. hasseltii*

Indigenous New Zealand Poisonous Plants
Karaka   *Corynocarpus laevigatus*
Ongaonga   *U. ferox*
Poroporo   *S. aviculare, Solanum laciniatum*
Pukatea   *Laurelia novae-zelandiae*
Rangiora   *Brachyglottis repanda*
Rarauhe   *Pteridium esculentum*
Tutu   *Coriaria* species

Peripheral Nervous System

Metalloids
Arsenic
Australian Terrestrial Vertebrates
Platypus, *Ornithorhynchus anatinus*
Aquatic Vertebrates
Eeltail catfish, *Tandanus tandanus*
Old Wife, *Enoplosus armatus*
Rabbitfishes, *Siganus* species, and Scat (family Scatophagidae)
Fish of the Order Scorpaeniformes (stonefish, scorpionfish, waspfish, soldierfish, bullrout, etc.)
Stingrays
Aquatic Invertebrates
Cyanobacteria
Ciguatoxin and related toxins
Conotoxins
Dinoflagellate/shellfish poisonings
Tetrodotoxin
Cnidaria (sea jellies)
Fire corals, genus *Millipora*
Sponges, phylum *Porifera*
Sea urchins, class *Echinoidea*
Australian Terrestrial Invertebrates
Redback spiders, *L. hasselti*
Hymenoptera
New Zealand Terrestrial Invertebrates
Katipo, *L. katipo*
Australian redback spider *L. hasseltii*
Hymenoptera
Indigenous New Zealand Poisonous Plants
Kakariki   *Cheilanthes sieberi*
Ongaonga   *U. ferox*

HEPATOTOXIC POISONS

Vertebrate Pesticides
Phosphides
Phosphorus
OTC Pharmaceuticals
Antifungals
Aspirin
Paracetamol
NSAIDs
Alternative Medicines
Camphor oil
Comfrey
Oil of wintergreen
Pennyroyal oil
Household Foods and Products
Clay pigeons
Pine oil disinfectants
Mothballs
Xylitol
Metals
Copper
Iron
Zinc
Mycotoxins and Mushrooms
Aflatoxins
Phomopsins
Sporidesmin
Amanita phalloides
Phallus spp.
Aquatic Invertebrates
Cyanobacteria
Australian Terrestrial Invertebrates
Sawflies, *Lophyrotoma interrupta*
Indigenous New Zealand Poisonous Plants
Ngaio   *Myoporum laetum*
Rangiora   *B. repanda*

NEPHROTOXIC POISONS

Vertebrate Pesticides
Cholecalciferol
Phosphorus

CARDIOTOXIC POISONS

Australian Terrestrial Vertebrates
Cane toads, *Rhinella marinus*
Aquatic Invertebrates
Ciguatoxin and related toxins
Cnidaria (sea jellies)
Australian Terrestrial Invertebrates
Australian tarantulas (*Selenotholus, Selenotypus, Coremiocnemis, Phlogius* spp.)

POISONS WITH EFFECTS ON THE BLOOD

Vertebrate Pesticides
Anticoagulant rodenticides
Para-aminopropiophenone
Sodium nitrite
Starlicide
OTC Pharmaceuticals
Aspirin
Paracetamol
NSAIDs
Alternative Medicines
Garlic
Household Foods and Products
Garlic
Onion
Phenol disinfectants
Fertilizer
Mothballs
Metals
Copper
Iron
Lead
Molybdenum
Zinc
Industrial Toxicants
Petroleum hydrocarbons
Mycotoxins and Mushrooms
Ergot alkaloids
Stachybotryotoxins
Trichothecenes
Australian Terrestrial Vertebrates
Notechis spp.—Tiger snakes
Oxyuranus spp.—Taipans
Pseudoechis spp.—Black snakes

Pseudonaja spp.—Brown snakes
Indigenous New Zealand Poisonous Plants
Rarauhe *P. esculentum*

POISONS WITH EFFECTS ON THE GASTROINTESTINAL TRACT

Vertebrate Pesticides
Chloropicrin
Cholecalciferol
Phosphorus
Herbicides and Fungicides
Phenoxy herbicides
OTC Pharmaceuticals
Antifungals
Aspirin
NSAIDs
Alternative Medicines
Aloe
Oil of wintergreen
Household Foods and Products
Batteries
Bleaches
Detergents
Phenol disinfectants
Pine oil disinfectants
Fertilizer
Food waste
Turpentine
Metals
Iron
Molybdenum
Metalloids
Antimony
Boron and borates
Arsenic
Miscellaneous Inorganic Substances
Selenium
Agricultural and Feed-Related Toxicants
Nonprotein nitrogen
Raw soybeans
Smoke and Other Inhaled Toxicants
Mycotoxins and Mushrooms
Stachybotryotoxins
Trichothecenes

Agaricus spp.
Aseroërubra
Chlorophyllum molybdites
Phallus spp.

Aquatic Invertebrates
Ciguatoxin and related toxins
Dinoflagellate/shellfish poisonings

Indigenous New Zealand Poisonous Plants
Karaka   *C. laevigatus*
Pinatoro   *Pimelea prostrata*
Waoriki   *Ranunculus amphitrichus*

POISONS WITH EFFECTS ON THE RESPIRATORY SYSTEM

Vertebrate Pesticides
Chloropicrin
Cholecalciferol

Herbicides and Fungicides
Dipyridyl herbicides (paraquat and diquat)

Household Foods and Products
Bleaches
Pine oil disinfectants
Teflon (Polytetrafluoroethylene; PTFE)
Turpentine

Miscellaneous Inorganic Substances
Iodine
Selenium

Industrial Toxicants
Petroleum hydrocarbons
Asbestos
Formaldehyde

Smoke and Other Inhaled Toxicants
Smoke
Ammonia
Hydrogen sulfide
Methane
Nitrogen dioxide
Teflon/PTFE

Mycotoxins and Mushrooms
Fumonisin

Aquatic Invertebrates
Cnidaria (sea jellies)

POISONS WITH EFFECTS ON SKIN

Insecticides and Acaricides
DEET
Vertebrate Pesticides
Chloropicrin
Household Foods and Products
Bleaches
Metalloids
Antimony
Boron and borates
Acids and Alkalis
Acids, alkalis, bases
Miscellaneous Inorganic Substances
Selenium
Industrial Toxicants
Petroleum hydrocarbons
Mycotoxins and Mushrooms
Stachybotryotoxins
Aquatic Invertebrates
Cnidaria (sea jellies)
Fire corals, genus *Millipora*
Sponges, phylum *Porifera*
Sea urchins, class *Echinoidea*
Australian Terrestrial Invertebrates
Ants of the genus *Myrmecia*
Ants of the genus *Solenopsis*
Ants: *Rhytidoponera metallica, Anoplolepis gracilipes, Oecophylla smaragdina*
Caterpillars of Australian *Lepidoptera*
Funnel-web spiders (*Atrax, Hadronyche, Illawarra* spp.)
Scorpions, centipedes, and millipedes
Hymenoptera
New Zealand Terrestrial Invertebrates
Hymenoptera
Indigenous New Zealand Poisonous Plants
Ongaonga *U. ferox*

POISONS WITH EFFECTS ON MUSCLE

Skeletal Muscle

Agricultural and Feed-Related Toxicants
Ionophores

Australian Terrestrial Vertebrates
  Oxyuranus spp.—Taipans
  Rhinoplocephalus nigrescens—Small-eyed snake
Aquatic Vertebrates
  Sea snakes
Indigenous New Zealand Poisonous Plants

Smooth Muscle

Insecticides and Acaricides
  Amitraz
Mycotoxins and Mushrooms
  Ergot alkaloids

POISONS WITH EFFECTS ON THE SKELETON

Metals
  Lead
  Molybdenum
  Zinc
Miscellaneous Inorganic Substances
  Fluoride

POISONS WITH EFFECTS ON REPRODUCTION

OTC Pharmaceuticals
  Antifungals
Metals
  Molybdenum
Agricultural and Feed-Related Toxicants
  Gossypol
Mycotoxins and Mushrooms
  Zearalenone
Australian Terrestrial Invertebrates
  Caterpillars of *Ochrogaster lunifer*

POISONS WITH EFFECTS ON THE ENDOCRINE SYSTEM

OTC Pharmaceuticals
  Antifungals
Miscellaneous Inorganic Substances
  Iodine
Mycotoxins and Mushrooms
  Zearalenone

POISONS WITH EFFECTS ON THE IMMUNE SYSTEM

Mycotoxins and Mushrooms
    Stachybotryotoxins
    Trichothecenes
Australian Terrestrial Invertebrates
    Hymenoptera
New Zealand Terrestrial Invertebrates
    Hymenoptera
Indigenous New Zealand Poisonous Plants
    Ongaonga   *U. ferox*

Chapter 8

Insecticides and Acaricides

INTRODUCTION

There are a very large number of insecticides and acaricides on the market in both Australia and New Zealand, although many fall within a limited number of chemical classes: organophosphates (OPs), carbamates, and pyrethroids.

An insect repellent (diethyltoluamide, DEET) and two insect growth regulators (cyromazine and methoprene) are also briefly covered in this chapter. Citrus oils are covered in the chapter on alternative medicines, and that section is applicable to citronella oil, often used as an insect repellent.

Agents covered in this chapter are as follows:

- Amitraz
- Anticholinesterase insecticides: organophosphates and carbamates
- Chlorinated hydrocarbon insecticides
- Cyromazine
- DEET
- Fipronil
- Hydramethylnon
- Imidacloprid
- Methoprene
- Pyrethrins and pyrethroids
- Rotenone
- Spinosad

AMITRAZ

Amitraz is an acaricide used in the control of ticks, mites, and lice on domestic animals; for the control of Varroa mite in beehives; and for control of some plant pathogens such as aphids and leaf rollers.

Amitraz should not be used on horses.

Toxicokinetics

Amitraz is readily absorbed orally. Dermal absorption is low. T_{max} is approximately 3 hours in the dog. Amitraz is rapidly metabolized to a number of metabolites. Excretion is primarily (65%–84%) by the renal route, and most amitraz is excreted within 24 hours of exposure. Excretion is practically complete after 72 hours.

Mode(s) of Action

Clinical signs of amitraz toxicosis are largely attributable to central α_2-adrenergic agonist activity, leading to sedation, with some peripheral α-adrenergic effects of diminished sympathetic tone, resulting in decreased heart rate. At high doses, amitraz inhibits monoamine oxidase. Amitraz suppresses insulin secretion in the dog, may induce moderate methemoglobinemia, and may inhibit platelet aggregation.

The acute oral LD_{50} of amitraz in the dog is 100 mg/kg bw. In the laboratory setting, dogs survived 0.25 mg/kg/day for 90 days, with mild clinical signs. Dogs developed some tolerance of amitraz after the first few days.

Amitraz inhibits contraction of intestinal smooth muscles. It has been associated with fatal ileus in horses, apparently due to inhibition of blood flow to the colon.

Amitraz disrupts LH secretion in laboratory rats.

Amitraz is often formulated with xylene which may contribute to CNS depression.

Clinical Signs

Clinical signs in domestic pets most often include depression, ataxia, vomiting, polyuria, hypothermia, and bradycardia. Blood pressure may be increased or decreased. In severe poisoning, there may be coma or seizures.

In ruminants, clinical signs may include hypersalivation, depression, anorexia, ataxia, tremors, and decreased milk production.

Horses may exhibit CNS depression and may also exhibit severe colic due to ileus.

Clinical signs most often develop within 4 hours of exposure, although delayed onset has been reported.

Diagnostic Aids

Hyperglycemia may be present.

Urine may be collected if analysis for the principal urinary metabolite, 4-amino-3-methylbenzoic acid, is available.

Treatment

Antidotes for amitraz toxicosis are atipamezole or yohimbine. Of these, atipamezole is better tolerated by dogs, while yohimbine induces significant tachycardia and tachypnea. Successful treatment regimes in the dog have included:

- intramuscular injection of 50 μg atipamezole/kg bw;
- intravenous injection of 0.2 mg atipamezole/kg bw;
- intravenous injection of yohimbine at 0.1 mg/kg bw.

Seizures should be treated with diazepam.

In the case of dermal exposure, bathing may be helpful once the patient is stabilized, but the likelihood of hypothermia should be borne in mind.

Amitraz is adsorbed by activated charcoal, but may be released later in the course of delayed intestinal transit time. Activated charcoal should not be administered if emesis has not been controlled. It should also be borne in mind that activated charcoal in the intestinal tract is highly undesirable if surgery is needed, e.g., to remove pieces of a tick collar.

Prognosis

Amitraz poisoning is usually mild and often requires no treatment. Prognosis is good in most species, particularly if an antidote is administered. Prognosis is guarded to poor in horses that develop colic.

Necropsy

In most domestic species there are no specific findings. Horses may have large intestinal impaction.

ANTICHOLINESTERASE INSECTICIDES

The anticholinesterase insecticides are a very large class of insecticides, divided into the organophosphates (OPs) and the carbamates. They are widely used in numerous insect control applications.

Toxicokinetics

Both OPs and carbamates are readily absorbed through the skin, gastrointestinal tract, and respiratory surfaces. They are widely distributed in the body but, unlike chlorinated hydrocarbons, do not sequester in adipose tissues. Phase I metabolism by mixed-function oxidases (MFOs) increases toxicity, but hydrolysis of the ester linkage decreases toxicity. Both OPs and carbamates are rapidly excreted, although chlorinated OPs such as chlorpyrifos are somewhat more persistent. Excretion is usually as products of hydrolysis in the urine. OPs and carbamates may be excreted in the milk.

The range of toxicity of these insecticides is very wide.

Mode(s) of Action

OPs and carbamates inhibit cholinesterases. Clinically the most significant inhibition is that of acetylcholinesterase (AChE). When AChE is inhibited, acetylcholine accumulates, causing excessive activity at the sites at which it is the neurotransmitter: muscarinic cholinergic synapses of the parasympathetic autonomic nervous system and of the CNS, and at the nicotinic cholinergic sites of the neuromuscular junctions in smooth muscle, cardiac muscle, and exocrine glands. Clinical signs therefore include *muscarinic* signs, *nicotinic* signs, and *CNS* signs.

The important distinction between OPs and carbamates is that the OP insecticides bound to AChE undergo "aging" such that the bond becomes unbreakable. Once this happens, the AChE will not be functional again and must be replaced by the body. However, the binding of carbamates to AChE is reversible, with a half-life of 30—40 min. This is long enough for clinical signs and even death to occur in the untreated patient, but makes a difference to treatment (q.v.).

Clinical Signs

Clinical signs often develop rapidly after oral exposure, and generally within 6 hours at the most. Clinical signs may be more delayed in the event of dermal exposure.

In large doses or with the most toxic members of the class, there may be sudden collapse and death from respiratory failure, with terminal signs of asphyxiation.

Muscarinic clinical signs include copious salivation, as well as lacrimation, urination, defecation followed by diarrhea, vomiting (often foamy due to swallowed saliva), miosis, coughing, dyspnea due to bronchoconstriction and overproduction of fluids in the lungs, bradycardia, abdominal pain due to hypermotility of the intestines, and cyanosis. Abdominal discomfort is often pronounced. Large animals may stamp, kick at the abdomen, and adopt unusual "tucked" posture. Dogs will often seek to lie in sternal recumbency with the ventral abdomen in contact with the ground, particularly if the ground is a cold surface such as concrete.

Various mnemonics have been suggested for the muscarinic toxidrome, which may be useful to veterinary students but are generally rendered superfluous by experience with a single clinical case of OP poisoning:

SLUD (salivation, lacrimation, urination, defecation).

SLUDGE (salivation, lacrimation, urination, diarrhea, GI upset, emesis).

SLUDGEM (salivation, lacrimation, urination, defecation, gastrointestinal motility, emesis, miosis).

DUMBELS (diarrhea, urination, miosis, bronchospasm, bradycardia, emesis, lacrimation, salivation).

DUMBBELLS (diarrhea, urination, miosis, bradycardia, bronchorrhea, emesis, lacrimation, salivation).

MUDDLES (miosis, urination, diarrhea, diaphoresis, lacrimation, emesis, salivation).

Nicotinic signs include muscle tremors that start at the head and neck and then progress to affect the whole body, muscle stiffness, and weakness progressing to paresis and paralysis.

CNS signs may include anxiety, restlessness, depression, seizures, depressed respiration, and coma. Seizures are more common in small animals than large animals and are most likely to reflect cerebral hypoxia. CNS signs are relatively rare.

Death in acute anticholinesterase poisoning is usually due to respiratory insufficiency, which is a result of the combination of bronchoconstriction and excessive fluid production in the lungs.

Intermediate syndrome has been described in dogs, cats, swine, and human beings. It may occur following an acute toxicosis or by itself following prolonged exposure. Intermediate syndrome primarily involves nicotinic signs and in domestic pets it includes anorexia, weakness, muscle tremors, abnormal positions, cervical ventroflexion, depression, and death. Animals may have convulsions. Animals may or may not exhibit miosis. Intermediate syndrome is most often associated with the most lipid-soluble OPs such as chlorpyrifos, fenthion, dimethoate, and phosmet, although it has been reported in association with carbaryl in swine.

Diagnostic Aids

Anticholinesterase insecticide toxicosis is confirmed by measurement of cholinesterase activity in heparinized whole blood. This assay measures the activities of AChE and pseudocholinesterase. The normal cholinesterase level differs between species and between diagnostic laboratories. Cholinesterase activity in the blood < 50% of normal for that species is considered to be indicative of exposure, while cholinesterase activity 25% or less than normal is considered confirmatory of poisoning.

It should be noted that in the case of carbamate toxicosis, dissociation of the carbamate from the cholinesterase may occur after the blood is collected. This will result in a "false negative" result.

Clinical pathology findings in anticholinesterase poisoning may include elevations in plasma amylase, lipase, glucose, potassium, CK, and AST. There may be leucocytosis and acidosis.

Treatment

The first line of treatment is atropine, which blocks muscarinic signs but not nicotinic signs. The dose is 0.25−0.5 mg/kg bw, of which one quarter of the dose should be administered immediately IV if possible. The rest of the dose should be administered IM or SC if a response is seen to the IV bolus.

It should be noted that atropinization of an animal that does not have anticholinesterase poisoning is hazardous and may result in death from atropine poisoning. When the diagnosis is uncertain, the animal may be treated with a preanesthetic dose of atropine, i.e., 01−0.2 mg/kg IV. If the animal shows mydriasis, tachycardia, and/or dry mouth, the animal does not have anticholinesterase poisoning and no more atropine should be given. Atropine poisoning is a serious condition that can be hard to reverse.

Atropine may be repeated after 2−6 hours if muscarinic signs return, but becomes progressively less effective with each readministration. Atropine is the specific physiological antidote for both OP and carbamate toxicosis.

No more than a total dose of 65 g atropine should be administered to a horse, since horses are particularly susceptible to ileus if given excessive atropine.

If atropine is not available, or the patient is refractory to atropine, an alternative is glycopyrrolate, which appears to be equally effective although it takes longer to reach full effect if given IM or SC. A dose of 0.5 mg/kg has been suggested for the treatment of OP poisoning in dogs. Glycopyrrolate is rapidly eliminated, with only minimal serum levels detectable 3 hours after IV administration.

For OP poisoning, oximes such as pralidoxime chloride (2-PAM) accelerate the hydrolysis of phosphorylated AChE, but cannot reverse phosphorylated enzmes that have "aged." Therefore early treatment is essential. For small animals the recommended dose rate of 2-PAM is 20 mg/kg IM, twice daily. Oximes relieve muscarinic, nicotinic, and CNS signs. 2-PAM can be given by very slow IV (over 5−10 min), but IV administration can lead to musculoskeletal paralysis and respiratory arrest.

The decision of whether to use an oxime when the toxicant is unknown has been debated, because there is evidence that 2-PAM is contraindicated in carbaryl poisoning. However, there is a lack of evidence that 2-PAM is contraindicated for other carbamate poisonings, although it may not have much therapeutic effect either. Carbaryl poisoning is unlikely, because carbaryl is an older carbamate with relatively low toxicity, and therefore the use of 2-PAM when it is not clear whether the toxicant is an OP or a carbamate is probably safe.

Diphenhydramine, 4 mg/kg PO, three times daily, may be helpful for refractory nicotinic signs, but should not be used in conjunction with atropine.

Diazepam may be beneficial to treat CNS effects and bradycardia. There is some evidence from experimental animals that diazepam improves the prognosis.

Morphine, physostigmine, phenothiazine tranquillizers, pyridostigmine, neostigmine, succinylcholine, local anesthetics, aminoglycoside antibiotics, clindamycin, lincomycin, and theophylline are *contraindicated* because they interfere with cholinesterase activity.

When exposure is dermal, bath with hand dishwashing liquid or a gentle shampoo once the animal is stabilized. Appropriate personal protective equipment should be used to protect owners and veterinary staff from exposure to the poison.

OPs and carbamates are generally well absorbed by activated charcoal but it should not be administered unless vomiting has been controlled. Activated charcoal is particularly useful in ruminants.

Treatment is otherwise symptomatic and supportive. Cats in particular may have prolonged anorexia and may need parenteral nutrition, and B vitamins to promote appetite.

Intermediate syndrome requires intense symptomatic care, and may involve weeks of convalescence. Repeat doses of 2-PAM, 20 mg/kg IM or SC every 12 hours, may save some animals.

Prognosis

Prognosis is guarded, because mortality rate with OP or carbamate poisoning is high, but prognosis improves with early, aggressive treatment.

Further exposure to OPs or carbamates should be avoided for at least 6 weeks, because cholinesterase levels recover to normal levels only slowly.

There is a significant risk of acute pancreatitis as a complication of OP poisoning in dogs, as in human beings. Pancreatitis is hemorrhagic and necrotizing.

Necropsy

Pulmonary edema may be present. The intestinal tract may contain excessive fluid, and the stomach may contain abundant fluid (saliva). Stomach and rectum are typically empty. Gross and microscopic findings are otherwise nonspecific.

The postmortem sample of choice for analysis of cholinesterase activity is brain. Postmortem samples for analysis for pesticide include stomach/rumen contents if exposure was oral, hair or skin if exposure was dermal, and urine that may contain metabolites of the toxicant. However, analysis is often not rewarding.

CHLORINATED HYDROCARBON INSECTICIDES

These insecticides have been phased out in Australia and New Zealand due to their persistent and bioaccumulative nature, and because some have been shown to be carcinogenic. However, they are included here because residues may persist in old dump sites or in lake sediments. It is also possible that containers of chlorinated hydrocarbon insecticide may still exist on farms or in garden sheds.

Examples of chlorinated hydrocarbon insecticides include:

- Diphenyl aliphatics including DDT, methoxychlor, perthane, and dicofol;
- Aryl hydrocarbons such as lindane, mirex, kepone, and paradichlorobenzene;
- Cyclodiene insecticides such as aldrin, dieldrin, endrin, chlordane, hepta-chlor, and toxaphene.

Toxicokinetics

Chlorinated hydrocarbon insecticides are highly lipid-soluble and are readily absorbed through the skin and across mucous membranes, although they are not particularly volatile and therefore inhalation is not an important route of exposure.

They rapidly distribute to liver, kidney, and brain, and accumulate and persist in adipose tissues, with the result that the half-life in the body is typically protracted and may be measured in months or even years.

Diphenyl aliphatics and cyclodienes are metabolized by mixed function oxidases (MFOs), and metabolites may be more toxic than the parent compound. Agents that upregulate MFO activity, including repeated exposures to the chlorinated hydrocarbons themselves, may increase toxicity of chlorinated hydrocarbon insecticides. Metabolism of aryl hydrocarbons includes glucuronidation and sulfation. Metabolism generally does not facilitate excretion significantly.

Excretion is primarily via bile, and enterohepatic recycling occurs and contributes to the long half-life. Chlorinated hydrocarbons are also excreted in milk.

Mode(s) of Action

The toxic mechanisms of most chlorinated hydrocarbon insecticides in mammals are incompletely understood. However, they all cause central nervous hyperexcitability.

DDT is known to interfere with sodium channels in nerve membranes, enhancing sodium influx and inhibiting potassium efflux. This enhances the initiation of action potentials and increases the risk of seizures.

In addition, some metabolites of DDT cause selective necrosis of the zone fasciculata and the zona reticularis. Mitotane, used for the treatment of hyperadrenocorticoidism, is such a metabolite.

The mechanism of action of cyclodiene insecticides is unclear, but they cause nervous system excitability. Chlorinated hydrocarbons in the cyclodiene group are the most toxic. They appear to enhance neurotransmitter release at cholinergic synapses, and may impair glutamine synthesis, leading to an increase in ammonia in the brain.

Some chlorinated hydrocarbon insecticides, including lindane, heptachlor, and mirex, have been shown to inhibit the postsynaptic binding of GABA.

LD_{50s} in dogs generally range from 15 to 65 mg/kg bw. Cats are the most sensitive domestic species.

Clinical Signs

Early clinical signs in animals are those of apprehension, tremors, incoordination, and hyperexcitability. Animals may become aggressive. Cattle may walk backward or exhibit abnormal chewing or licking activity. Clinical signs may occur within a very few minutes of exposure, or may be delayed for up to 2 days.

As toxicosis progresses, animals develop muscle fasciculations that are usually first seen in muscles of the head and neck, and then develop intermittent seizures which typically progress cranial to caudal, and include opisthotonus, paddling, and champing of the jaws. Animals may be normal or depressed between seizures. Hyperthermia commonly develops. Seizure activity may persist for 3 days.

Nervous signs in birds include depression, abnormal postures, disorientation, and apparent blindness, or the birds may be found dead.

Diagnostic Aids

The presence of pesticide in the blood or milk can confirm exposure, if diagnostic testing is available. Specimens should be packaged so that contact with plastic is prevented, because a number of plasticizers interfere with analytical testing.

Treatment

In the event of dermal exposure, animals should be bathed, using mild shampoo or hand dishwashing detergent, but personnel should wear appropriate personal protective equipment to prevent dermal contact.

Chlorinated hydrocarbon insecticides are adsorbed by activated charcoal, which should be used if oral exposure is recent and emesis has been controlled. Cholestyramine or mineral oil are alternative decontaminants.

Seizures must be controlled with diazepam or barbiturates, body temperature controlled and trauma prevented. Intravenous dextrose and electrolytes will help the animal restore homeostasis after seizure activity.

Phenothiazine tranquilizers, epinephrine, and other adrenergic amines are contraindicated.

Livestock that have been exposed to chlorinated hydrocarbon insecticides should not be used for production of milk or meat. Excretion may be improved by repeated administration of activated charcoal to inhibit enterohepatic cycling, and clearance of residues from adipose tissue may be enhanced by inducing the animal to lose weight under a gradual, controlled regime. There are anecdotal reports of severely contaminated animals developing clinical signs as a result of severe abrupt weight loss. Lactation enhances excretion of chlorinated hydrocarbon insecticides, but environmental authorities should be consulted on the safe disposal of the milk.

Prognosis

Prognosis in acute toxicosis is guarded to favorable, depending on dose, and on timeliness and aggressiveness of treatment. Protracted coma (several hours) signifies a poor prognosis.

Necropsy

Gross lesions are generally nonspecific consequences of trauma or seizures. In dogs, there may be liver necrosis and/or hemorrhagic necrosis in the adrenal cortex. At doses below those causing liver necrosis, enzyme induction may cause enlargement of the liver.

Tissues of choice for postmortem confirmation of exposure include adipose tissue, brain, and liver. Tissues should be wrapped in aluminum foil for submission, and shipped in glass containers if the laboratory will accept specimens submitted in glass containers.

CYROMAZINE

Cyromazine is an insect growth regulator. It is of very low toxicity in mammals. Toxicity as a result of exposure to cyromazine is highly unlikely.

TOXICOKINETICS

Cyromazine is poorly absorbed through skin. If ingested, it is well absorbed from the gastrointestinal tract. It undergoes limited hepatic metabolism, with most of an ingested dose being excreted as the parent compound in the urine. Most of an ingested dose is excreted within 24 hours.

Mode(s) of Action

The mode of action of mammalian toxicity is unknown.

Clinical Signs

Clinical signs in massive overdose in laboratory mammals were ataxia, hypersalivation, depression, dyspnea, and exophthalmos. Animals recovered in 9–12 days.

Diagnostic Aids

None.

Treatment

Treatment is symptomatic and supportive.

Necropsy

No information.

DIETHYLTOLUAMIDE

The correct name for this insect repellent is diethyltoluamide, but it is most commonly referred to as DEET.

Toxicokinetics

DEET is readily absorbed through intact skin and widely distributed systemically. T_{max} in the dog is $1-2$ hours. The half-life of DEET is a matter of hours. DEET is metabolized in the liver. Excretion is primarily by the renal route. Metabolites include glucuronides, but it is not clear whether this means that cats are more susceptible to DEET toxicosis.

Mode(s) of Action

The mechanism of action of DEET is unknown.

DEET increases the dermal absorption of some chemicals.

Clinical Signs

Most cases of DEET toxicosis in the medical and veterinary literature are confined to dermal or ocular irritation. However, neurotoxicity has been observed in some human beings and in laboratory studies in Beagle dogs. Examples of study findings in laboratory Beagles are as follows:

- Two-week daily oral gavage study. At ≥ 250 mg/kg bw/day, occasional emesis, hypersalivation, abnormal head movements and, at 500 mg/kg bw/day, ptosis, ataxia, and convulsions. Clinical signs occurred shortly after dosing and then resolved spontaneously.
- Eight-week daily oral capsule study. Abnormal head movements and hypersalivation within 1 hour of dosing at 400 mg/kg bw/day, and occasionally at 200 mg/kg bw/day. Other adverse effects included decreased bodyweight gain, decreased food consumption in females, and slight

increase in plasma cholesterol in males. No adverse effects at 50 or 100 mg/kg bw/day.

- Eight-week daily oral gavage study. Terminated after 5 days for humane reasons due to adverse effects. At dose levels ≥ 125 mg/kg/day, adverse effects were observed, including emesis, hypersalivation, abnormal biting and scratching, abnormal head movements, ataxia, ptosis, and convulsions. Clinical signs occurred shortly after dosing and then resolved spontaneously.
- Eight-week dietary study. The diet was unpalatable at > 3000 ppm (approximately 75 mg DEET/kg bw/day). There were no adverse clinical signs below this dose, and at this dose the only adverse clinical sign was thin body condition.

Clinical signs of suspected DEET exposure in dogs and cats have included emesis, tremors, excitement, ataxia, and seizures. Bradycardia and hypotension have also been reported.

Rarely, individual humans have developed toxic encephalopathy following ingestion or dermal application of DEET. Symptoms and clinical signs have headache, restlessness, irritability, ataxia, loss of consciousness, hypotension, and seizures. Flaccid paralysis and areflexia have also occurred in some cases. Cerebral edema, sometimes fatal, has occurred in some human cases of DEET toxicosis.

DEET is very irritating to the eyes, but not corrosive. Dermal reactions in human beings have in some cases been severe.

Diagnostic Aids

A 20 ppm DEET in blood serum is considered to be diagnostic.

The medical literature indicates that CSF may contain increased protein, glucose, and cell count, but premortem CSF collection is unlikely to be justifiable in a suspected case of DEET toxicosis in a domestic animal.

Treatment

Treatment is symptomatic and supportive. In the rare event of seizures, diazepam or barbiturates should be used to control them.

If emesis has been controlled, it is plausible that DEET may be adsorbed by activated charcoal, given that DEET has a molecular weight of 191.3. Bathing with a mild shampoo or hand dishwashing detergent may be beneficial in the case of dermal exposure.

Prognosis

Prognosis is usually good. Most animals recover within 72 hours or less.

Necropsy

There are no specific lesions. CSF may be collected and is most easily accessed postmortem by the ventral route after the tongue, larynx, trachea, and esophagus have been reflected. CSF can then be aspirated from the cisterna magna by directing the syringe needle dorso-rostrally through the foramen magnum.

Tissues that may contain DEET or metabolites include urine, skin (dermal exposure), gastrointestinal content (oral exposure), and vitreous humor.

FIPRONIL

Fipronil is used for flea and tick control of domestic pets, for home insect control, and for pest control on plants. It is often applied as a spot-on to domestic pets.

Toxicokinetics

Although it is lipid-soluble, fipronil has low systemic absorption when applied dermally. It principally remains in the skin, including stratum corneum, viable epidermis, and pilo-sebaceous units, where it has a long half-life.

If ingested, fipronil has slow absorption but appears to be widely distributed. It has been detected in the liver, kidney, muscle, and adrenal glands, with the highest concentrations and longest half-life occurring in fat. Fipronil is present in milk of lactating animals. Fipronil is largely or wholly metabolized prior to excretion. Excretion is largely by the renal route, with some fecal excretion.

Mode(s) of Action

Fipronil is a GABA agonist. The conformation of the GABA receptor in insects is quite different to that in mammals, with the result that insects are much more susceptible to the action of fipronil.

Clinical Signs

Dermal application of fipronil may cause a hypersensitivity reaction in some individual animals. Clinical signs include erythema, irritation, and alopecia. It is not clear to what extent these signs are caused or potentiated by other chemicals in the dermal formulations.

Oral exposure to fipronil, for example through grooming, appears to cause an unpleasant taste and may result in salivation and/or vomiting. Very large doses may cause some neurological effects such as ataxia, tremors, or seizures, particularly in rabbits. However, as a rule fipronil has a wide margin of safety when ingested by domestic animals.

Daily oral dosing with fipronil in a 13-week study in laboratory Beagles was not associated with any adverse signs at ≤ 0.5 mg/kg bw/day. However, at 2.0 mg/kg bw/day, dogs exhibited inappetence and decreased bodyweight gain. At 10 mg/kg bw/day, clinical signs including bodyweight loss, tremor, nodding, hyperreflexia, impaired vision, and arrhythmia, and four animals required humane euthanasia due to development of seizures.

In a 52-week chronic toxicity/carcinogenicity study in laboratory Beagles, in which fipronil was administered daily by oral capsule, intermittent adverse neurological effects at ≥ 2.0 mg/kg bw/day included twitching, tremors, nervousness, postural abnormalities, ataxia, and hyperreflexia, while three dogs were euthanased because they developed seizures. Similar neurological signs were observed in a chronic dietary study in Beagles, at doses ≥ 1.0 mg/kg bw/day. Hyperplasia of the red pulp of the spleen was found on necropsy of male dogs consuming ≥ 2.0 mg/kg bw/day.

Diagnostic Aids

If testing for fipronil is available, the tissue of choice is plasma or serum.

Treatment

For dermal exposure, fipronil may be removed by bathing with hand dishwashing detergent or a mild shampoo. Dermatitis should be treated symptomatically.

Fipronil is adsorbed by activated charcoal, which may be administered subject to the usual caveats. Treatment of oral exposure is otherwise symptomatic and supportive.

Prognosis

Prognosis is generally good, but is guarded for rabbits that develop seizures.

Necropsy

There are no specific lesions. If testing for fipronil is available, fresh tissues of choice are fat, liver, or kidney.

HYDRAMETHYLNON

Hydramethylnon is most commonly used as an ant bait in Australia and New Zealand.

Toxicokinetics

Absorption of hydramethylnon from the gastrointestinal tract is low in mammals. Trials of repeat-dosing of hydramethylnon to lactating goats and cows did not result in detectable residues in meat or milk. Small amounts of polar metabolites have been found in rat urine after oral dosing with hydramethylnon, but most of the chemical was excreted unchanged in the feces within 24 hours. Dermal absorption is very low.

Mode(s) of Action

Hydramethylnon inhibits the electron transport system in mitochondria, preventing the production of ATP.

Clinical Signs

The acute oral LD_{50} of hydramethylnon in laboratory rats is in the range of 1100−1300 mg/kg bw, making it in the "Slightly Toxic" according to the Hodge and Sterner scale.

In a laboratory study using Beagle dogs, dosed daily with hydramethylnon in oral capsules for up to 91 days, anorexia was observed at $\geq$ 6 mg/kg bw/day. There were no clinical signs at 3 mg/kg bw/day.

In veterinary practice, consumption of ant baits containing hydramethylnon may be associated with gagging and vomiting.

A number of chronic studies have found adverse effects on testicular tissue in laboratory animals.

Chronic consumption of high doses of hydramethylnon by grazing animals appears to be generally well tolerated but may have mild to moderate adverse effects on humoral immunity.

Hydramethylnon is effectively nontoxic to honeybees and birds under normal conditions of use, but is toxic to fish.

Diagnostic Aids

Samples of choice for analysis for hydramethylnon would be feed, blood, or milk.

Treatment

Treatment is supportive. Most cases of hydramethylnon may be expected to be mild and self-limiting.

Prognosis

Prognosis is excellent.

Necropsy

No specific lesions. Mortality would not be expected in an acute case. Chronic consumption would be associated with weight loss and possibly testicular atrophy.

IMIDACLOPRID

Toxicokinetics

Systemic absorption of dermally applied imidacloprid is negligible.

Imidacloprid is rapidly and extensively ($\sim 92\%$) absorbed from the gastrointestinal tract. T_{max} in the rat is around 2.5 hours. Imidacloprid absorbed from the gastrointestinal tract is widely distributed in the rat, with the exception of adipose tissue and the central nervous system. Metabolism primarily occurs in the liver. Imidacloprid may be broken by oxidative cleavage to 6-chloronicotinic acid and imidazolidine. Of these metabolites, imidazolidine is excreted in the urine, and 6-chloronicotinic acid undergoes further metabolism via glutathione conjugation to form mercaptonicotinic acid and hippuric acid. An alternative metabolic pathway of imidacloprid is hydroxylation of the imidazolidine ring, with metabolic products including 5-hydroxy and olefin derivatives. Metabolites are found in both the urine and the feces. Rats excreted 96% of radio-labeled imidacloprid within 48 hours following an unspecified oral dosing, with 90% excreted in the first 24 hours. There is no evidence of bioaccumulation.

Mode(s) of Action

Imidacloprid acts on postsynaptic nicotinic acetylcholine receptors, which are located only in the CNS in insects. Binding of imidacloprid to the nicotinic receptor causes spontaneous discharge, after which the neuron is unable to propagate any further impulses. The binding of imidacloprid to the receptor is irreversible.

Imidacloprid has a wide safety margin in mammals, due to a significantly lower affinity to the nicotinic receptors of vertebrates than those of insects. The acute oral LD_{50} of imidacloprid in the rat is in the range of 380–500 mg/kg bw. A chronic (52 weeks) dietary study in dogs established a No Observed Effect Level of 41 mg/kg bw/day, based on increased serum cholesterol and elevated hepatic cytochrome P450 levels at higher doses.

Clinical Signs

Some animals may exhibit signs of dermal hypersensitivity, such as erythema, pruritis, and alopecia, following dermal application.

Adverse effects of ingestion are likely to be limited to salivation and emesis.

Experimental administration of very high doses of imidacloprid to laboratory animals has been associated with lethargy, diarrhea, muscle weakness, ataxia, and tremor; clinical signs expected with overstimulation of nicotinic receptors. Onset was rapid, within 15 min of administration, and generally resolved within 24 hours. Fatally poisoned animals died within 24 hours of administration.

There are no reports of delayed neurotoxic effects, or persistent neurotoxic effects, of imidacloprid toxicosis.

Treatment

In the event of a dermal hypersensitivity reaction, the animal may be bathed, with use of a mild shampoo or hand dishwashing liquid to remove imidacloprid. Treatment is otherwise symptomatic.

Treatment of ingestion of imidacloprid is symptomatic and supportive.

Prognosis

Prognosis is usually excellent.

METHOPRENE

Methoprene is an insect growth regulator, used in spot-on products with insecticides that kill adult fleas. There are also some applications for methoprene for use against parasites of plants.

The acute oral LD_{50} of methoprene in the rat >34,600 mg/kg bw, meaning that methoprene is well into the least toxic ("Relatively Harmless") classification of the Hodge and Sterner scale, while in the dog the acute oral LD_{50} of methoprene is >5000 mg/kg bw.

Toxicokinetics

There is very little systemic absorption of dermally applied methoprene.

When ingested, methoprene is rapidly absorbed. The extent of metabolism varies with species. Methoprene and/or metabolites are excreted in the urine and feces. In the rat, plasma T_{max} is at about 6 hours and $T_{1/2}$ is about 48 hours.

Mode(s) of Action

Methoprene inhibits normal maturation of pupae to adult insects.

Clinical Signs

Methoprene is not irritant, toxic, or teratogenic in mammals. Dermal hypersensitivity is possible with any dermal product, but has not been observed in laboratory animals treated dermally with methoprene. Taste aversion reactions might occur.

PYRETHRINS AND PYRETHROIDS

Pyrethrins are compounds found in pyrethrum, an extract from flowers of plants in the genus *Chrysanthemum*. Pyrethroids are synthetic analogs of pyrethrins. Pyrethroids are more stable in the environment and more potent as insecticides than pyrethrins, but also tend to be more toxic to mammals.

Pyrethroids are subdivided into Type I and Type II pyrethroids on the basis that Type II pyrethroids have an α-cyano moiety and Type I pyrethroids do not. Type II pyrethroids are generally more toxic to mammals than Type I pyrethroids.

Examples of Type I pyrethroids and Type II pyrethroids are:

Type I Pyrethroids	Type II Pyrethroids
Allethrin	Cyfluthrin
Bifenthrin	Cyhalothrin
Permethrin	Cypermethrin
Phenothrin	Deltamethrin
Resmethrin	Genvalerate
Sumithrin	Flumethrin
Tefluthrin	Fluvalinate
Tetramethrin	Tralomethrin

Pyrethrins and pyrethroids are often formulated with potentiating substances, of which piperonyl butoxide is perhaps the best known. Piperonyl butoxide has negligible toxicity in its own right at the doses used, inhibits metabolizing enzymes in insects and mammals, increasing the toxicity of pyrethrins and pyrethroids to target and nontarget species.

There are a large number of insecticides of this class on the market. Of particular veterinary concern are spot-on products for dogs, that concentrations of insecticide that are toxic to cats.

Toxicokinetics

Absorption is generally around 2% from dermal exposure and in the range of 40%−60% following ingestion. Some hydrolysis to nontoxic metabolites occurs in the gastrointestinal tract, which helps to contribute to the low toxicity of these insecticides to mammals. Pyrethroids are widely distributed in the body. They are metabolized in a variety of tissues by mixed-function oxidases and by esterases. Metabolism involves hydrolysis of the central ester bond, which reduces toxicity, oxidation of some groups, and conjugation with glycine, sulfate, or glucuronide. Pyrethroids are excreted by first-order kinetics. Both the parent compound and metabolites are excreted. Pyrethroids are excreted in urine, feces, and milk.

The acute oral mammalian toxicity of pyrethrins/pyrethroids is variable, but generally in the range of 100−2000 mg/kg bw.

Mode(s) of Action

Pyrethrins/pyrethroids act on the sodium channels of axonal membranes, decreasing sodium influx and potassium efflux. They also appear to inhibit ATPases. The overall result is decrease in the amplitude of action potentials, and generation of repetitive nerve impulses.

Type 2 pyrethroids interfere with binding of GABA and glutamic acid to their receptors.

Clinical Signs

Clinical signs include salivation, emesis, excitability, severe prolonged shivering, dyspnea, cyanosis, exhaustion, and death. Seizures are rare in most species, but are common in cats treated with spot-on products intended for dogs, or that are in close contact with dogs treated with such products. Seizures are not inducible, but are severe and may be difficult to control.

Toxicosis is most often seen in cats, and signs may include paw shaking, ear twitching, tail flicking, and twitching of the skin of the dorsum. Some cats exhibit oddities of limb movement when walking.

Cattle treated with pyrethroid pour-on products may exhibit restlessness and apparent discomfort of the skin of the dorsum.

Clinical signs may develop within minutes or 2−3 hours of exposure, depending on the route. The animal usually recovers or dies within 72 hours, although longer clinical course may occur in cats.

Poisoning is always acute. Subchronic or chronic toxicosis has not been described.

Topical allergic reactions to pyrethroids are common, but anaphylactic reactions appear to be rare.

Idiosyncratic reactions to pyrethroids are recognized in veterinary medicine. These are toxic reactions in certain individuals at doses well below the usual threshold of toxicity in the population. These reactions tend to persist, so pyrethroids should not be used again on an animal that has an idiosyncratic reaction.

Diagnostic Aids

Clinical pathology findings are nonspecific and indicative of stress, e.g., neutrophilia. Blood glucose may be elevated in response to stress, but may become depressed if shivering has been present for a protracted period.

Detection of pyrethrins/pyrethroids in biological samples is not often available, and if available, can confirm exposure but not toxicosis.

Treatment

Excitability and, if present, seizures should be controlled with diazepam or barbiturates. Phenothiazine tranquillizers are contraindicated.

Methocarbamol may be required in cats. The dose is 55–220 mg/kg IV. One-third of the dose is administered as a bolus (up to 2 mL/min). This is usually sufficient to cause some relaxation, and the rest of the dose can then be titrated to effect. Methocarbamol can be administered at up to 330 mg/kg/day. Methocarbamol can be used in association with diazepam. Cats may show a disappointing response to barbiturates, reaching profound CNS depression without control of peripheral tremor and shivering. Propofol IV infusion or gas anesthesia have also been used in some cases.

Treatment is generally symptomatic and supportive. Body temperature and blood glucose should be monitored.

A low dose of atropine may assist in controlling hypersalivation.

In the case of dermal exposure, the animal should be bathed when stabilized. If a cat has been in contact with a pyrethroid such as a spot-on intended for dogs, and is not yet showing clinical signs, it should be bathed.

Activated charcoal may be administered in the event of oral exposure, subject to the usual caveats, but animals are often presented too late for activated charcoal to make much difference to the clinical course. Given the somewhat limited absorption from the gastrointestinal tract, a single dose of a cathartic may be considered 30 min after administration of activated charcoal, subject to recognition that there is no proven benefit of administering one.

Prognosis

Prognosis is usually good to excellent in most species, but may be poorer in cats.

Necropsy

There are no specific gross or microscopic lesions.

Postmortem samples for analysis are brain and liver.

ROTENONE

Rotenone is prepared from the root of plants of the genus *Derris*. Rotenone is used in a variety of products including flea control products and in domestic gardens to kill insect pests. Toxicosis in domestic mammals is rare, but may result from excessive use of topical products. Toxicosis is most commonly seen in cats.

Toxicokinetics

Oral absorption is limited. Rotenone is metabolized in the liver, and primarily excreted in the feces.

Mode(s) of Action

Rotenone forms a complex with NADH dehydrogenase, inhibiting the oxidation of NADH to NAD, and therefore blocking the oxidation by NAD of a number of substrates including glutamate, alpha-ketoglutarate, and pyruvate. Rotenone inhibits mitochondrial electron transport and also inhibits mitosis.

Clinical Signs

Clinical signs include emesis, lethargy, stupor, dyspnea, and respiratory depression. Rarely, there may be tremors or seizures.

In laboratory Beagles, consumption of rotenone for 30 days at 5 mg/kg bw/day for a month resulted incellular degeneration in the liver and kidneys, although there were no clinical signs. A dose of 10 mg/kg/day killed 3/5 dogs, although the time to death is not clear.

Diagnostic Aids

There may be hypoglycemia.

Although rotenone may be detectable in vomitus, blood, urine, or feces, there is a lack of information on how detected levels correlate with clinical effects.

Treatment

Treatment is symptomatic and supportive. Phenothiazine tranquillizers are contraindicated.

Prognosis

Prognosis is generally excellent.

Necropsy

Gross lesions may include moderate gastroenteritis, pulmonary congestion, and hepatic congestion. Chronic exposure may lead to midzonal degeneration and necrosis in the liver.

SPINOSAD

Spinosad has very low toxicity to mammals. The major components of spinosad are spinosyn A and spinosyn D.

Toxicokinetics

Spinosad is rapidly absorbed from the gastrointestinal tract, with T_{max} 2–4 hours after administration. Bioavailability is >70% and increases if spinosad is administered with food.

Spinosad undergoes extensive metabolism and is largely excreted in the feces.

Mode(s) of Action

The mechanism of action of spinosad and other spinosynson insect is not entirely clear, but they are known to act on both GABA and nicotinic acetylcholine receptors of the membranes of nerve cells of insects through pathways distinct from those of other insecticides.

The mechanism or mechanisms of mammalian toxicity are not known.

Clinical Signs

The most common clinical sign of spinosad toxicity in the dog is vomiting. Other clinical signs are inappetence, lethargy, diarrhea, coughing, and polydipsia. Rare clinical signs include erythema, salivation, pruritis, and trembling.

Spinosad may lower the seizure threshold in epileptic dogs.

Spinosad can enhance the toxicity of ivermectin when used at a high dose (e.g., 0.6 mg/kg, against demodicosis) so it should not be administered in conjunction with ivermectin.

Spinosad is a macrocyclic lactone and therefore should in theory be contraindicated for use on dogs with the MDR-1 mutation (see Chapter 5: Vulnerable Patients). However, tolerance studies have shown that dogs with the MDR-1 mutation did not suffer from adverse effects when treated with spinosad at 300 mg/kg (~4.5 times the therapeutic dose) or with spinosad and milbemycinoxime at five times the therapeutic dose.

Diagnostic Aids

No information.

Treatment

Treatment is symptomatic and supportive.

Necropsy

No information.

Chapter 9

Molluscicides

Rhian Cope

In this section, molluscicides known to be legally present in Australia and New Zealand, and those suspected of being illegally available are listed in alphabetical order. The following molluscicides are described in this section:

Bromoacetamide
Metaldehyde
Trifenmorph
  For the following molluscicides, readers are referred to other relevant sections of this book:
Allicin: see Chapter 24, Poisonous Plants.
Arsenicals (calcium arsenate, copper acetoarsenite): see Chapter 14, Metals, and Chapter 15, Metalloids.
Copper sulfate and other copper derivatives: see Chapter 14, Metals, and Chapter 15, Metalloids.
Organotins (fentin, triphenyl tin, tributyltin oxide): see Chapter 14, Metals, and Chapter 15, Metalloids.
Niclosamide: see the Parasiticides chapter.
Ferric phosphate: see Chapter 14, Metals, and Chapter 15, Metalloids.
Anticholinesterase carbamates (trimethacarb, cloethocarb, thiodicarb, tazimcarb, methiocarb, and many others): see Chapter 8, Insecticides and Acaricides.
Neonicotinoids (thiacloprid): see Chapter 8, Insecticides and Acaricides.

Most veterinary poisons involve snail and slug treatment preparations containing either metaldehyde or carbamate anticholinesterases. However, molluscicides are extensively used in marine antifouling paints and for removing molluscs from irrigation systems and dams.

BROMOACETAMIDE

Alternative Names

N-Bromoacetamide.

Veterinary Toxicology for Australia and New Zealand
DOI: http://dx.doi.org/10.1016/B978-0-12-420227-6.00009-8

Target Species

Molluscs primarily in antifouling paints but it has been used to control terrestrial snails, particularly in China.

Mode of Action in Target Species

Mitochondrial poison, particularly in the hepatopancreas.
  Developmental toxin in snail eggs.
  Voltage-gated sodium channel blocker.

Circumstances of Poisoning

Misuse of antifouling paints.

Toxicokinetics

Unknown.

Toxic Mode(s) of Action

Inhibits sodium currents in cardiac myocytes.
  Blocks voltage-gated sodium channels (used experimentally for this purpose).
  Known to be embryotoxic in rats.

Clinical Signs

Little information is available; neural and cardiac effects relating to blocking of sodium channels (i.e., Class 1 antiarrhythmic effects, flaccid paralysis resembling that induced by saxitoxin, neosaxitoxin, and tetrodotoxin) could be reasonably expected.

Diagnostic Aids

None available.

Treatment

Symptomatic and supportive; respiratory support and correction of cardiac arrhythmias may be required.

Prognosis

Unknown.

Necropsy

Likely to be nonspecific.

Public Health Considerations

Unknown.

Prevention

Outside of China the product appears to be mostly used in antifouling paints. Antifouling paints should not be used in animal facilities.

METALDEHYDE

Alternative Names

Numerous trade names and formulations.
     Was originally developed as a fuel for cooking stoves.
     Continues to be used in fire starters and solid fuel stoves.

Target Species

Garden snails and slugs.

Mode of Action in Target Species

Destruction of mucous production that decreases mobility and digestion.

Circumstances of Poisoning

A very common toxicosis in dogs: dogs readily consume metaldehyde slug and snail baits. Such baits typically contain high levels of protein that are attractant to snails (and unfortunately, dogs).
     Poisoning is more rare in other species.
     Household slug and snail baits typically contain about 3.5%−4% metaldehyde.
     Fire starters and solid fuel stove pellets are an occasional cause of poisoning (more problematic for human children).
     Metaldehyde is also extensively used in some forms of agriculture (particularly for artichokes, broccoli, cauliflower, lettuce, cabbage, and tomatoes).

Toxicokinetics

Rapidly absorbed from the gut and readily passes through the blood−brain barrier.

Toxic Mode(s) of Action

Current theory is that metaldehyde decreases brain GABA, noradrenalin, and 5HT (serotonin) resulting in a loss of neuronal inhibition in CNS.

Older theory was that the metaldehyde breaks down to acetaldehyde in the low pH of the stomach. Acetaldehyde then inhibits serotonin degradation resulting in serotonin excess. However, while metaldehyde has been detected in brain tissues following poisoning, acetaldehyde has not.

Clinical Signs

Dogs

- Early: anxiety, restlessness.
- Intermediate: salivation, mydriasis, tremors, ataxia.
- Late: opisthotonus, continuous convulsions, cyanosis, nystagmus, hyperthermia, death from respiratory failure.
- Dogs are not as hyperesthetic as with strychnine (an important differential diagnosis).
- Liver failure may develop 2–3 days following exposure in survivors.

Cats

- Similar to dogs; nystagmus is usually prominent

Ruminants

- Ataxia and tremors predominate
- Cattle my display salivation, diarrhea, and sometimes appear to be blind

Horses

- Colic, diarrhea, sweating, tremors, and hyperesthesia are the most common signs.

Metabolic acidosis is often present due to the formation of acetaldehyde

Diagnostic Aids

Blood cholinesterase levels are normal.

Acetaldehyde can be detected in stomach contents (difficult to detect in tissues).

Treatment

Induction of emesis is risky because of the potential to induce seizures.

Single-dose activated charcoal treatment is reputedly beneficial but definitive data are lacking.

Airway security is paramount, particularly in animals with reduced gag reflexes.

Benzodiazepines or methocarbamol is recommended for control of tremors and other signs of neurological hyperexcitability. Barbiturates may delay the metabolic detoxification of metaldehyde.

IV crystalloids (lactated Ringer's solution) are recommended for the control of metabolic acidosis.

Prognosis

Dependent on the dose and how soon treatment was instituted.

Necropsy

Necropsy findings are generally nonspecific:

- Hepatic, renal, and pulmonary congestion
- Nonspecific hemorrhages, GI petechiae, and eccymosis
- Gastric contents smell like acetaldehyde
- Histopathology is nonspecific: hepatocyte swelling and degeneration, CNS neuronal degeneration

Public Health Considerations

Metaldehyde poisoning is an occasional, but serious, cause of poisoning in children.

Prevention

Snail and slug baits containing metaldehyde need to be used with great caution in dog accessible areas. Fire starters and solid fuel stove pellets should be stored securely.

TRIFENMORPH

Alternative Names

Frescon
N-Tritylmorpholine
WL 8008R
Triphenmorph

Target Species

Highly selective for aquatic and semiaquatic snails.

Not toxic to terrestrial molluscs.
Used in irrigation ditches and streams.
Has been used to control *Fascioloa hepatica.*

Mode of Action in Target Species

Neurotoxic in aquatic snails.
Affects the neuronal bicarbonate-chloride exchange mechanism, resulting in increased intraneuronal chloride. This decreased neuronal excitability.

Circumstances of Poisoning

Poisoning is very rare. Preparations that use chlorinated solvents increase the risk of toxicity.

Toxicokinetics

It is slowly absorbed from the gut and through intact skin. There is substantial presystemic elimination/first pass metabolism in the gut in mammals. Chlorinated solvents greatly increase the level of absorption.
It is rapidly metabolized by gastrointestinal enzymes to triphenylcarbinol, and morpholine.
Triphenylcarbinol is oxidized by hepatic systems to primarily to parahydroxyphenyl diphenyl carbinol that is then glucuronidated and excreted mostly in urine.
Morpholine is rapidly absorbed from the gut and excreted in the urine as a glucuronic acid conjugate.

Toxic Mode(s) of Action

Poorly described in mammals.
Assumed to be similar to the target species.

Clinical Signs

Poorly described in mammals. Flaccid paralysis would be expected.

Diagnostic Aids

None readily available.

Treatment

Poorly described.
Symptomatic and supportive.

Prognosis

Unknown.

Necropsy

Unknown.

Public Health Considerations

Human poisoning is unlikely.

Prevention

Should not be used in streams or water sources that animals can access.

Chapter 10

Vertebrate Pesticides

INTRODUCTION

Vertebrate pesticides covered in this chapter are covered in alphabetical order of those targeting mammalian pests, followed by those targeting birds (avicides), as follows:

Toxicants for control of mammalian pests

- Anticoagulants
- Chloropicrin
- Cholecalciferol
- Combined cholecalciferol and an anticoagulant
- Cyanide
- Norbormide
- Para-aminopropiophenone (PAPP)
- Phosphides (Zn, Mg, or Al)
- Phosphorus
- Sodium fluoroacetate (1080)
- Sodium nitrite
- Strychnine

Avicides

- Alphachloralose
- DRC-1339 ("Starlicide")

Public Health Considerations and *Prevention* are generally not included for each toxicant, unless there are special aspects to public health considerations and/or prevention.

Omissions from this chapter, because they are covered elsewhere, are as follows:

- *Arsenic*, historically used as a rodenticide, is covered in Chapter 14, Metals.
- *Carbon monoxide*, used for fumigating rabbit burrows, is covered in Chapter 20, Smoke and Other Inhaled Toxicants.
- *Rotenone*, used as a piscicide, is covered in Chapter 8, Insecticides and Acaricides.

Veterinary Toxicology for Australia and New Zealand
DOI: http://dx.doi.org/10.1016/B978-0-12-420227-6.00010-4

TOXICANTS FOR CONTROL OF MAMMALIAN PESTS

Anticoagulants

General Remarks

Anticoagulant rodenticides are classified as first-generation or second-generation. First-generation anticoagulants are relatively rapidly excreted and may only be effective against vertebrate pests if they consume the rodenticide several times. Second-generation anticoagulant rodenticides have a substantially longer half-life in the body and are more likely to be effective after only one feeding.

First-generation anticoagulants include: warfarin, dicoumarol, pindone, and coumatetralyl.

Second-generation anticoagulants include: brodifacoum, bromadiolone, flocoumafen, and difethialone.

Diphacinone and chlorphacinone are sometimes classified as first-generation, and sometimes considered to be intermediate between first-generation and second-generation.

Circumstances of Poisoning

Domestic animals may be poisoned by consuming the rodenticide directly, or by relay toxicosis if the domestic animal consumes poisoned rodents.

Anticoagulant rodenticides are excreted in milk, so if a nursing bitch or queen consumes an anticoagulant rodenticide, the puppies or kittens will need to be treated as well.

Toxicokinetics

Bioavailability is high, >90%, and C_{max} may occur within 12 hours of ingestion. Anticoagulant rodenticides bind strongly to plasma proteins, and this helps to prolong half-life. They are metabolized by hydroxylation in the liver and excreted in the urine.

Pharmaceuticals that bind to the same plasma proteins as anticoagulant rodenticides may potentiate toxicosis by making more anticoagulant rodenticide available in the free form. Drugs known to do this include phenylbutazone, corticosteroids, diphenylhydantoin, and most sulfonamides.

Sulfa drugs and antibiotics may potentiate toxicosis by reducing the synthesis of vitamin K in the intestines. For this reason, sulfaquinoxaline is sometimes included in baits.

Ruminants are relatively resistant to anticoagulant rodenticide poisoning, compared to monogastric animals.

Mode(s) of Action

Anticoagulant rodenticides competitively inhibit vitamin K epoxide reductase, the enzyme that converts vitamin K epoxide to the reduced form.

The reduced form of vitamin K is essential for the activation of clotting factors II, VII, IX, and X. Decline of coagulating ability of the blood is delayed until natural decay of the circulating clotting factors takes place, usually 24−36 hours after ingestion of the anticoagulant.

A wide range of oral LD_{50} doses (single ingestion) have been reported for anticoagulant rodenticides in domestic species:

Species	Warfarin (mg/kg)	Diphacinone (mg/kg)	Pindone (mg/kg)	Brodifacoum[a] (mg/kg)
Cat	50−100	15		0.25−25
Dog	50	3−7.5	50	0.25−3.6
Pig	3	150		0.1−2.0
Ruminant			100	5−25

[a]Flocoumafen, bromadiolone, and difethialone are of similar toxicity to brodifacoum.

Clinical Signs

Depression and anorexia are often observed before evidence of hemorrhage. Clinical signs depend on the site(s) of hemorrhage but may include epistaxis, melena, hematemesis, gingival hemorrhages, subcutaneous hemorrhages, and/or lameness due to hemarthrosis or intramuscular hemorrhage. Hemorrhages may be slow, or sudden and massive. There may be hematuria. Hemorrhage may occur in the central nervous system, causing neurological signs, or in the placenta, leading to abortion.

The patient becomes weak and ataxic, with pale mucous membranes, anemia, irregular heart rate, dyspnea, and weak pulse.

Diagnostic Aids

Analysis of clotting factors shows marked increases. The activated prothrombin time is the first to increase, followed by the activated partial thromboplastin time. These times are at least doubled and usually increased by substantially more than that.

Hematology is that of blood loss anemia. Platelet count is not normally substantially decreased.

Samples for analysis for anticoagulants or their metabolites in the live animal are blood or urine. Stomach contents or feces are not useful for analysis because of the delayed onset of toxicosis, but the inert blue or green marker often included in anticoagulant baits may be observed in the feces.

Treatment

Note: It may seem tempting, when an animal has a history of having just consumed an anticoagulant bait, to induce emesis to prevent toxicosis. However, anticoagulant rodenticides are typically formulated in waxes to make them weatherproof. At body temperature the wax melts to oil, and oil is a specific contraindication for inducing emesis. There is no evidence that emesis + activated charcoal is more effective than activated charcoal alone, and inducing emesis delays the administration of activated charcoal. Note also that the green or blue color of any vomitus produced is not the anticoagulant rodenticide, but only an inert marker which, unlike the anticoagulant, is not absorbed from the gastrointestinal tract. Therefore the production of green or blue vomitus is *not* an indication that absorption of a toxic dose of anticoagulant has been prevented or even ameliorated.

The specific antidote for anticoagulant rodenticides is phytonadione, vitamin K_1. This is most safely administered orally to domestic pets, because parenteral administration may cause hemorrhage. Phytonadione should be administered at 3−5 mg/kg/day, split into two doses/day, and followed by a fatty meal (e.g., cheese or dog sausage) to promote absorption. Phytonadione should also be administered to any suckling puppies or kittens.

Stabilize the animal and treat for blood loss. Blood transfusion, plasma, or plasma expander may be required. Hemorrhages in specific locations, e.g., the thoracic cavity, may need to be drained.

Once the animal has stabilized and coagulation is normal or near-normal, the animal may be sent home on a daily dose of phytonadione. This treatment should continue for 14 days for warfarin, 21 days for bromadialone, and at least 30 days or for other second-generation anticoagulants. Whatever the anticoagulant, the clotting times should be checked 3 days after the last phytonadione dose, and again 3 days after that.

The total daily dose of phytonadione to horses should not exceed 2 mg/kg/day, and menadione (vitamin K_3) should never be administered to horses as it may cause renal failure.

Ruminants should be administered 0.5−1.5 mg/kg phytonadione, SC, or IM, not more than 10 mL/site. Pigs may be administered 2−5 mg/kg phytonadione, SC, or IM.

Convalescing animals should be kept quiet and not exercised.

Prognosis

Prognosis varies depending on location(s) and severity of hemorrhage(s), but is generally good with adequate and timely treatment.

Necropsy

Necropsy findings depend on the site(s) of hemorrhage but include ecchymoses, bloodstained gastrointestinal contents, pulmonary edema, and/or hemorrhage. Tissues are otherwise pale. There may be centrilobular hepatic necrosis and hemosiderin accumulation in liver and spleen. In sudden death there may be hemothorax, hemomediastinum, hemopericardium, or cerebral hemorrhage.

The tissue of choice for postmortem analysis is liver, although kidney can also be submitted.

Chloropicrin

Chloropicrin is used as a fumigant for rabbit burrows and as such is unlikely to cause toxicosis in domestic animals. However, it is discussed here in the interests of completeness.

Chloropicrin causes severe irritant to the skin, eyes, respiratory tract, and gastrointestinal tract. Exposure causes lacrimation, vomiting, sore throat, dyspnea, and lethargy. There is irritation of exposed mucous membranes, and dermal exposure can cause blisters. Inhalation or ingestion can lead to methemoglobinemia, and inhalation can lead to fatal pulmonary edema.

Chloropicrin is highly toxic to nontarget vertebrate species. It should be used only with appropriate personal protective equipment, including respirator, goggles and impervious gloves, overalls and footwear, with no skin exposed. There should be no domestic animals in the area.

Rabbits trapped in warrens that are fumigated with chloropicrin usually die within 30 minutes, but if they escape from warrens they may survive for several days before succumbing to the toxic effects of chloropicrin on the respiratory tract or other systems. However, chloropicrin is not expected to persist in their tissues.

Chloropicrin is short-lived in the environment. It is degraded by soil microbes, with degradation more rapid in warm weather. It also degrades rapidly in water provided it is exposed to light, and is degraded in the atmosphere by photolysis. It is not taken up by plants and has no detrimental effects on plants.

Cholecalciferol

General Remarks

Cholecalciferol is vitamin D_3.

Circumstances of Poisoning

Cholecalciferol is used against rats and mice in Australia, and against possums in New Zealand.

Poisoning of domestic animals is most likely if the animals consume baits. Mild, nonfatal relay toxicosis (renal damage) in dogs, but not cats, from consumption of vertebrate pests poisoned by cholecalciferol has been demonstrated experimentally.

Toxicokinetics

Cholecalciferol is rapidly absorbed from the gastrointestinal tract and is transported by a specific protein to the liver, where it is metabolized to $25(OH)D_3$ (calcifediol). Cholecalciferol in excess of that which can be metabolized in the liver is stored in adipose tissue, so although the plasma half-life is 19−24 hours, cholecalciferol actually persists in the body for weeks or months. Calcifediol is the principal metabolite in circulation, and has a functional half-life of 29 days in the circulation because of continued mobilization of cholecalciferol from adipose tissue and metabolism in the liver. Calcifediol is further metabolized in the kidneys to $1,25(OH_2)D_3$ (calcitriol) and $24,25(OH_2)D_3$. Metabolites are principally excreted by the biliary route.

Clinical signs of cholecalciferol poisoning may develop as soon as 14 hours after ingestion, but more commonly are delayed for 18−48 hours.

Mode(s) of Action

Vitamin D enhances absorption of calcium and phosphorus from the gastrointestinal tract, promotes the reabsorption of calcium in the kidneys, and induces mobilization of calcium from bone by the action of osteoclasts. In cholecalciferol toxicosis the resulting hypercalcemia leads to metastatic calcification affecting many soft tissues, including lungs, stomach, heart, skeletal muscle, kidneys, and major arteries. In addition, hypercalcemia reduces the effects of vasopressin, leading to hyposthenuric polyuria.

Death in dogs is most commonly due to renal failure, although it can ensue from gastric or pulmonary hemorrhage, or from cardiac failure.

A single dose of 2 mg/kg cholecalciferol can cause significant toxicosis in the dog, and the acute oral LD_{50} in the dog is estimated to be around 13 mg/kg. There is a lack of comparable information for other domestic species.

Clinical Signs

Early clinical signs are depression, anorexia, emesis, polyuria with compensatory polydipsia, and consequent dehydration leading to constipation. Intestinal bleeding may lead to melena, and gastric bleeding may lead to hematemesis, which can progress to fatal shock within hours. Dyspnea may be indicative of pulmonary hemorrhage. Cardiac signs of hypercalcemia include bradycardia and ventricular arrhythmia.

Diagnostic Aids

Clinical pathology findings include hypercalcemia (total and ionized Ca), hyperphosphatemia, decreased urinary specific gravity, and calciuria. Calcifediol, if the assay is available, is markedly elevated, whereas calcitriol level is normal or depressed. Intact parathyroid hormone is suppressed.

ECG may reveal shortened QY interval and prolonged PR interval.

Treatment

Activated charcoal is recommended in the event of recent consumption of bait, but in most clinical cases, any gastrointestinal decontamination is futile because of the delayed onset of clinical signs. Repeated doses of activated charcoal may promote excretion of cholecalciferol metabolites, but should only be administered if vomiting has been controlled. It has also been suggested that cholestyramine may be useful to prevent enterohepatic cycling of cholecalciferol and metabolites, but this has not been demonstrated experimentally or clinically in dogs.

Pamidronate sodium (or other bisphosphonate as available) provides long-lasting inhibition of bone resorption. Pamidronate sodium should be administered by slow (2−4 hours) intravenous infusion in saline, at 1.3−2 mg pamidronate sodium/kg bodyweight. The infusion may be repeated 3−4 days later. Serum calcium and BUN should be measured 48 and 96 hours after each infusion, and creatinine should also be monitored periodically.

Fluid therapy should be administered to treat dehydration, maintain renal throughput, and promote calcium excretion. When dehydration has been corrected, furosemide should be administered, either orally (2−4 mg/kg at 8 hour intervals) or by a 5 mg/kg IV bolus followed by IV infusion at 5 mg/kg/hour. This is because furosemide decreases renal sodium and chloride reabsorption, resulting in decreased positive potential across the renal tubule, which in turn promotes calcium excretion.

Prednisone (2 6 mg/kg IM or PO b.i.d.) or other corticosteroid should be administered to suppress osteoclast activity, reduce calcium absorption from the intestines, and promote urinary excretion of calcium. Animals should be administered a low-calcium, low-phosphate diet, and kept out of sunlight to prevent endogenous vitamin D synthesis.

Hyperphosphatemia is treated with oral phosphate binders, aluminum hydroxide or magnesium hydroxide, given orally.

Emesis should be controlled with metoclopramide, and protection of the gastrointestinal mucosa provided in the form of antacid and sucralfate.

Salmon calcitonin may be used as an alternative to bisphosphonate therapy but the two should not be used together, because the outcome appears to be worsened if both are used. The suggested dose of salmon calcitonin in dogs is 4−6 IU, IM, or SC, every 6 hours until serum calcium stabilizes. However, there is a lack of evidence of the effectiveness of salmon calcitonin in dogs, and there can be undesirable side effects such as anorexia, emesis, and risk of anaphylaxis.

Prognosis

Prognosis varies depending on how soon the animal is presented for treatment, and is poorer for puppies than for mature dogs. If severe hypercalcemia is present, prognosis is guarded to poor. If hematemesis is present, prognosis is grave.

Necropsy

The animal is usually dehydrated. The gastric mucosa is often hyperemic, sometimes gastric mucosa. The kidneys may be mottled, and the lungs may be edematous or hemorrhagic.

Histological findings are mineralization of kidneys, stomach, lungs, major arteries and heart (particularly atria), and myocardial degeneration.

Combination of Cholecalciferol and Anticoagulant

A relatively novel strategy to control vertebrate pests has been the inclusion of an anticoagulant, such as coumatetralyl or diphacinone, with cholecalciferol. One possible advantage is that the earlier onset of toxic effects of cholecalciferol, relative to anticoagulants, may tend to induce pests to withdraw to their burrows or nests, thus reducing the risk that they will be caught and consumed by nontarget species. Furthermore, cholecalciferol is less persistent in the environment than the anticoagulants.

There is a lack of information on how toxicosis from such a combination would be manifested in domestic animals. In possums, rats, and mice, the effects of cholecalciferol predominate, with the pests dying of the effects of hypercalcemia. Coumatetralyl increases the toxicity of the cholecalciferol by blocking vitamin K_2-dependent proteins involved in calcium regulation. On the other hand the combination of a low dose of cholecalciferol with a first-generation anticoagulant increases the potency of the anticoagulant to that of a second-generation anticoagulant.

Cyanide

General Remarks

Cyanide is used for the control of possums and wallabies in New Zealand. Cyanide can be used under special permit in Australia, such as for projects sampling fox or wild pig populations.

Cyanide is also used in the extraction of gold and silver ores, and many plants synthesize cyanogenic glycosides.

Circumstances of Poisoning

Cyanide baits are usually either KCN or NaCN. Cyanide is nonselective. Cyanide salts are not generally attractive to domestic animals but may be attractive if presented with foods attractive to possums, e.g., peanut butter or jam.

Relay toxicosis by the consumption of poisoned target species is considered unlikely because cyanide is readily broken down.

Toxicokinetics

Cyanide is rapidly absorbed through inhalation or ingestion. Toxicity by the dermal route is disputed because in cases in which it has been described, inhalation was also a likely route of exposure.

Onset of clinical effects is rapid, within 15 seconds if exposure is by inhalation, and usually within 10 minutes if baits are consumed. Death usually occurs within an hour, but may take as long as 3 hours if smaller amounts of bait are consumed.

In sublethal poisoning, cyanide is metabolized in the liver to thiocyanate, which is excreted in the urine. Small amounts of cyanide can be exhaled as HCN (hydrogen cyanide). The half-life of cyanide in the dog is 19 hours.

The minimum lethal oral dose of HCN or KCN in most species is approximately 2 mg HCN-equivalent/kg. The LD_{50} is 5.3 mg/kg in the dog, and 6 mg/kg in the cat.

Mode(s) of Action

Cyanide combines with iron in the mitochondrial cytochrome oxidase system, blocking the ability of cells to use oxygen in cellular respiration. Oxyhemoglobin is unable to release oxygen for electron transport, while tissues become anoxic. The brain, as the organ most dependent on oxidative phosphorylation, is the first tissue to show signs of anoxia, and the heart, also a tissue with a high dependence on oxidative phosphorylation, also shows signs of toxicity. Cyanide also has a direct toxic action on cell membranes.

Clinical Signs

Clinical signs are tachypnea, rapid loss of consciousness, mydriasis, convulsions, coma, and cardiac arrest. Prior to cardiac arrest, heart rate may be fast or slow, and there may be ventricular arrhythmias, supraventricular arrhythmias, and/or atrioventricular blocks.

In slower onset of toxicosis, there may be vomiting and evidence of nausea (i.e., hypersalivation).

Cyanosis is generally only seen terminally, because oxygenation of blood is normal until the final stages of central respiratory depression. Venous as well as arterial blood is oxygenated.

Pulmonary congestion may develop in slower progression of toxicosis or in nonfatal poisoning.

Diagnostic Aids

Some people can smell the "bitter almond" smell of exhaled HCN, but since many people cannot detect the smell, its absence does not preclude cyanide poisoning.

Medical laboratories may offer a whole blood cyanide assay, but this is more of value for retrospective confirmation of diagnosis than for emergency treatment, because of the extremely acute nature of cyanide poisoning.

There is severe lactic acidosis (serum lactate >2 mequiv./L) and an elevated anion gap.

Auscultation or ECG will reveal cardiac abnormalities.

Treatment

Warning: Treating an animal with cyanide poisoning poses a risk to veterinary personnel, who should avoid breathing exhaled cyanide. Any traces of bait on or in the mouth should be washed away with copious water.

If the animal is apprehensive and hyperventilating, but conscious, pure oxygen should be provided by mask. Establish an IV line for treating lactic acidosis.

Although a variety of antidotes are used around the world for cyanide poisoning, there is debate about which antidote is the best, and for veterinarians there are issues of availability. Furthermore, a number of antidotes have toxic effects in their own right.

In mild to moderate cyanide poisoning, *sodium thiosulfate* may be used alone, at 660 mg/kg, in a 25% solution, intravenously. Thiosulfate acts as a substrate for rhodanase, which converts cyanide to thiocyanate.

In severe cyanide poisoning, *sodium nitrite*, 16–22 mg/kg, may be administered IV and then followed by sodium thiosulfate as described above. Sodium nitrite causes methemoglobinemia, and methemoglobinemia reacts with cyanide to form cyanmethemoglobin. Sodium nitrite is a potent vasodilator and hypotensive agent. Sodium nitrite should never be used unless the diagnosis of cyanide poisoning is certain.

An alternative antidote is rapid infusion of *methylene blue*, IV, at 9–22 mg/kg. Although methylene blue is usually thought of as an antidote to methemoglobinemia, it can act as both a donor and acceptor of electrons, so while it can reduce methemoglobin in the presence of excess methemoglobin, it can induce formation of methemoglobin when only hemoglobin is present. It induces methemoglobin rather more slowly than sodium nitrite, but on the other hand it is less likely to have severe adverse effects, so it is the preferred antidote if the diagnosis is not certain. *Do not use both sodium nitrite and methylene blue.*

Methylene blue is a cost-effective treatment of cyanogenic glycoside poisoning in large herbivores.

Hydroxocobalamin, a vitamin B12 (cyanocobalamin) precursor, is considered to be preferred antidote for cyanide poisoning in human beings. It is an effective chelator of cyanide, and has few adverse side effects, so it is less harmful in the case of mistaken diagnosis. The recommended dose rate in acute cyanide poisoning in dogs is 79 mg/kg. As an antidote for use in human patients, it is presented in 2.5 g ampoules. Each ampoule should be reconstituted with 100 mL of physiological saline and administered slowly over 15 minutes, except in the case of cardiac arrest, in which case a bolus of two ampoules should be administered directly, either IV or into the heart. Each ampoule is sufficient to bind 100 mg of cyanide.

Dicobalt edetate was developed as a cyanide antidote because cobalt is able to form stable complexes with cyanide. However, experience of use in humans shows that it can cause seizures, upper airway edema, angina, hypotension, and vomiting, especially when the patient does not in fact have cyanide poisoning. It is suitable for use only in confirmed severe cyanide poisoning. Hydroxocobalamin is a preferable antidote.

Prognosis

Prognosis is grave; cyanide poisoning is usually rapidly fatal.

Animals that recover from sublethal cyanide poisoning may exhibit neurological damage. Human beings who have recovered from cyanide poisoning may also exhibit neurological damage, and/or thyroid enlargement.

Necropsy

Although the classic lesion of cyanide poisoning is cherry-red blood on necropsy, this color disappears rapidly after death so a lack of this finding does not preclude cyanide poisoning. Stomach contents may smell of bitter almonds but many people cannot detect this smell. If cyanide poisoning is suspected, the necropsy should take place in a well-ventilated area.

There may be petechial hemorrhages under the epicardium and/or endocardium, but these findings are not specific for cyanide poisoning.

Samples of choice for postmortem analysis are stomach contents, skeletal muscle, and spleen.

Norbormide

Norbormide has been registered for use against rats in New Zealand. Norbormide is specifically toxic against members of the genus *Rattus* and highly unlikely to cause toxicosis in nontarget species. A dose of 1000 mg/kg causes no toxicosis in domestic dogs or cats. Norbormide acts as a calcium channel blocker and vasoconstrictor in rats. A disadvantage of norbormide is that sublethal toxicosis in rats leads to bait shyness.

Para-aminopropiophenone

General Remarks

Originally developed in the USA, PAPP has been introduced in New Zealand for the control of mustelids and feral cats, and in Australia for the control of foxes and feral or wild dogs. It has the advantage that carnivores are more susceptible to its effects than birds are.

Circumstances of Poisoning

Domestic dogs or cats could take baits laid for target animals. Baits are designed to be attractive to carnivores. It is reasonable to suppose that baits would also be attractive to pigs, although a pig might have to consume many baits designed for stoats or cats.

Relay toxicosis is considered to be unlikely.

Toxicokinetics

PAPP is rapidly absorbed. Experimentally, dogs fed 11−43 mg/kg PAPP in baits developed clinical signs within 2 hours and 10 of the 14 dogs died within 3.5 hours, although there was no clear relationship between dose and onset of clinical signs or time to death. Most cats fed 20−112 mg/kg developed clinical signs within an hour, although some were slower to develop clinical signs. Eighteen of the 20 cats died, most within 2 hours.

In dogs, PAPP is hydroxylated in the liver. There is a lack of information on how PAPP is metabolized by cats.

PAPP is rapidly excreted, principally in the urine, and is cleared from the circulation in approximately 12 hours.

Mode(s) of Action

PAPP causes methemoglobinemia.

Clinical Signs

Clinical signs are those of weakness, "muddy" mucous membranes, loss of consciousness, and death.

Diagnostic Aids

Blood is dark or brown. Laboratory analysis confirms methemoglobinemia.

Treatment

The antidote for PAPP is methylene blue. Recommended administration to dogs is 4−22 mg/kg as a 1% solution, by slow IV infusion (i.e., via a drip). Recovery is usually complete in an hour.

Note: The use of methylene blue in cats has been controversial due to the reported risk of Heinz body hemolytic anemia. However, this risk appears to be associated only with chronic use of antiseptics containing methylene blue to treat urologic syndrome in cats. For this reason, appropriate administration regimes of methylene blue for cats are not well established. However, experimentally, methylene blue can be safely administered to cats over an acute (<12 h) timeframe with some increase in Heinz bodies but without inducing hemolytic anemia. In PAPP poisoning the use of methylene blue is indicated for cats, although it may be prudent to start at the lower end of the dose range used for dogs.

Prognosis

Because PAPP is a relatively novel vertebrate pesticide, there is a lack of clinical experience concerning prognosis. Methylene blue acts rapidly to reverse methemoglobinemia, and provided it is given in a timely manner, prognosis should be good.

Necropsy

The brown color of methemoglobin is readily apparent when the carcass is first opened, but disappears over a short time once the blood is exposed to air. Diagnostic laboratories have not yet specified the tissues of choice for analysis, but in light of the metabolism and excretion, it is likely that liver and/or kidney would be useful.

Phosphides (Zn, Mg, or Al)

General Remarks

Zinc phosphide is used in Australia against mice in crops, and has been introduced in New Zealand, principally for possum control. Aluminum phosphide canisters have washed ashore in Australia. Aluminum phosphide and magnesium phosphide are permitted as fumigants in New Zealand.

Circumstances of Poisoning

Nontarget species may be poisoned by direct consumption of zinc phosphide baits. Risk of relay poisoning by consumption of dead or dying vermin is considered to be low, but is possible.

Toxicokinetics

Zinc phosphide decomposes rapidly in the acid environment of the stomach, releasing phosphine gas that is rapidly absorbed. Phosphine is exhaled or oxidized to less toxic metabolites and excreted in the urine. Zinc phosphide can also be absorbed intact from the gastrointestinal tract, and it is thought that this may be responsible for, or contribute to, hepatic and renal toxicity.

WARNING: Veterinary personnel have developed sublethal toxicosis as a result of phosphine gas exhaled or eructated by the poisoned animal, or from phosphine gas released from vomitus.

Mode(s) of Action

Phosphine gas has a direct irritant effect on the gastrointestinal tract. Systemically absorbed phosphine causes central nervous system depression and respiratory irritation. It is not clear whether phosphide or phosphine, or both, is responsible for myocardial toxicity and degenerative changes in liver and kidneys. Phosphine is known to be a strong reducing agent that causes oxidative stress, and the high-oxygen requirements of brain, heart, liver, and kidney may be why these organs are among the target organs of phosphide poisoning.

Phosphides inhibit cytochrome C oxidase, but the toxicological significance of this is not clear. Phosphine has been shown experimentally to cause methemoglobinemia, and may inhibit acetylcholinesterase. However, these effects do not appear to be significant clinically.

The LD_{50} for domestic species is generally in the range of 20—40 mg/kg, although ruminants appear able to tolerate slightly higher doses than monogastric animals, probably because the rumen acts to slow the passage of the phosphide to the abomasum, resulting in more gradual conversion of phosphide to phosphine gas.

Clinical Signs

Clinical signs are generally observed within 15 minutes to 4 hours of ingestion, but may be delayed for up to 18 hours if a small quantity of bait is consumed. Onset of toxicosis is delayed by food in the stomach.

Vomiting, sometimes containing blood clots, is an early sign of toxicosis. The animal is often in significant pain and may bite. There is a rapid clinical course with development of apprehension, severe abdominal pain, muscular weakness, tremors, increasing dyspnea, disorientation, and eventually coma. Signs may include hyperesthesia, "running fits," tonic/clonic convulsions, or tetanus-like extensor convulsions. There may be arrhythmias.

Horses develop colic, and bloat may develop in ruminants.

Diagnostic Aids

Blood phosphate levels are not consistently elevated and may be depressed. They are not informative.

Acidosis is a consistent finding. There may be hypoglycemia and/or hypocalcemia.

Arrhythmia may be present.

Clotting times are often increased. In severe cases, disseminated intravascular coagulation may develop. Methemoglobinemia may be present.

Phosphine may be detectable by Dräger tube, if available.

Treatment

DO NOT induce vomiting. Not only are phosphides highly irritant to the gastrointestinal tract of the animal, but release of phosphine gas from vomitus is hazardous to veterinary personnel.

Examine and treat the animal *only* under conditions of excellent ventilation. The human threshold of detection of phosphine is higher than the Short-Term Exposure Limit for human exposure.

Administration of an antacid, to raise stomach pH and decrease the liberation of phosphine from the phosphide in the stomach, may be beneficial but this has not been proven. The efficacy of gastric lavage or of activated charcoal has not been proven either.

Establish an IV line and administer fluids to correct acidosis. Monitor serum calcium level and correct if necessary.

Support respiratory function as required. Steroids to treat shock and assist maintenance of pulmonary integrity, and a β2-agonist to counteract bronchospasm, may be beneficial.

The response to diazepam is generally poor, so nervous signs should be controlled with propofol, gas anesthesia, or a barbiturate. Phosphide toxicosis causes significant pain and analgesia should be provided.

Monitor cardiac function, serum calcium, and serum magnesium; correct electrolyte derangements as necessary.

Gastrointestinal protectants are recommended.

It has been suggested that *n*-acetylcysteine may be beneficial to scavenge reactive oxygen species and to combat methemoglobinemia.

Monitor liver and kidney functions and provide supportive treatment as required.

Prognosis

Because some effects may be delayed, prognosis can be difficult to predict. Prognosis is guarded if cardiac and circulatory effects are apparent within 4−6 hours of exposure. Prognosis generally improves after 24 hours, although pulmonary and hepatic effects may be delayed up to 72 hours.

Necropsy

The stomach contents may have an odor similar to acetylene, "dead fish," or garlic.

Other findings are nonspecific. Pulmonary edema and congestion are likely, but are often mild. The gastrointestinal mucosa is congested or hemorrhagic. There may be myocardial degeneration, an enlarged, pale liver, and renal congestion.

Tissues to collect for histopathology include lung, heart, gastric mucosa, liver, and kidney.

Phosphine analysis from postmortem tissues is not usually available, and results of analysis for zinc, magnesium, or aluminum have not proved to be reliable in phosphide poisoning.

Phosphorus

General Remarks

Phosphorus (also known as white phosphorus or yellow phosphorus) has been used in the past for control of feral pigs in Australia, but its use is not currently supported by state governments. Phosphorus has also been used for control of rabbits and possums in New Zealand.

Circumstances of Poisoning

Because of its reactivity, phosphorus is presented in butter or other oil-based bait.

Relay toxicosis is rare but may occur if, for example, dogs eat rabbits that have recently died of phosphorus poisoning.

Toxicokinetics

Phosphorus is rapidly absorbed from the gastrointestinal tract and can also be absorbed by inhalation or through damaged epithelium. It is excreted by the respiratory and renal routes.

Mode(s) of Action

Phosphorus has strong irritant and necrotizing properties. It coagulates protein, causing chemical burns.

Absorbed systemically, it causes fatty degeneration in multiple organs including brain, liver, and kidneys. The usual cause of death is massive hepatic failure, but cardiac failure may occur as a result of direct cardiotoxicity or as a consequence of hypocalcemia.

The acute LD_{50} of phosphorus in dogs is 2 mg/kg.

Clinical Signs

Initial clinical signs are those of violent vomiting and diarrhea, due to the direct effects on the gastrointestinal tract. Breath and vomitus have a characteristic garlic-like odor.

If the dose is high, the animal may die of shock within hours, and there may be perforation of the esophagus or stomach.

Often, the animal appears to recover for 24 or 48 hours. The animal then goes into shock due to toxic effects on liver, kidneys, heart, gastrointestinal tract, and other organs, and is likely to exhibit icterus.

In some cases animals have survived for up to 3 weeks before succumbing to convulsions and coma. It is not clear whether these effects are due to primary neurotoxicity, secondary effects on the brain from liver damage (hepatic encephalopathy), or hyperbilirubinemia (kernicterus).

Diagnostic Aids

Findings of severe hepatic damage, i.e., elevated liver enzymes and bilirubin, are nonspecific.

There may be hypoglycemia.

If the patient vomits, collect vomitus for analysis to confirm diagnosis. Freeze the vomitus if analysis is likely to be delayed.

Treatment

Do not induce emesis. Administer a nonabsorbed oil (e.g., mineral oil) to dilute and dissolve the phosphorus, and prevent its systemic absorption. Emesis should be controlled by an antiemetic, e.g., metoclopramide, before the oil is administered, and oil should be administered before using any pain relief that may cause sedation.

Other oral treatments that have been proposed to convert phosphorus to harmless phosphate include 0.1% potassium permanganate, 1% copper sulfate, or 2% hydrogen peroxide. Suggested quantity is in the region of 50 mL for an average-sized (20−430 kg) dog. There is a lack of information of which of these, if any, are effective, and all have potential adverse effects including the potential to induce emesis, with resulting irritation of the esophagus. Mineral oil is preferable because, with appropriate precaution against aspiration, it carries less risk of adverse side effects.

Otherwise, treatment is symptomatic for shock, pain, compromise of liver and kidney function, hyperbilirubinemia, and severe gastrointestinal irritation.

Prognosis

Prognosis is guarded to poor. Animals that recover are likely to have permanent damage to vital organs.

Necropsy

Lesions are those of severe fatty degeneration and necrosis of liver and kidneys. Fatty degeneration may also be present in the heart, brain, and other organs.

The intestinal tract is severely inflamed, and contents are likely to be hemorrhagic.

Postmortem findings are nonspecific, and diagnosis can only be definitively confirmed by analysis of vomitus or, in acute death, gastrointestinal contents. When death is the result of delayed hepatoxicity, gastrointestinal content analysis may not be diagnostic.

Sodium Fluoroacetate (1080)

General Remarks

Sodium fluoroacetate is registered in Australia for control of rabbits, wild or feral dogs, foxes, feral cats, and feral pigs. In New Zealand, target species include rabbits, feral cats, rats, and brushtail possums.

Circumstances of Poisoning

Poisoning occurs from direct consumption of baits or, in the case of carnivores, by relay toxicosis from the consumption of recently poisoned vermin. Sodium fluoroacetate baits are stable in cool, dry conditions, including partially mummified carcasses of target species, but are biodegraded when moisture and ambient temperature are sufficient.

Toxicokinetics

Sodium fluoroacetate is readily absorbed following ingestion or inhalation. It is not readily absorbed through intact skin. Ingested fluoroacetate is rapidly absorbed from the stomach. Plasma C_{max} is reached after approximately 30 minutes in possums and rabbits, but may be delayed in ruminants; a T_{max} of 2.5 hours has been measured in sheep.

Fluoroacetate combines with coenzyme A to form fluoroacetyl CoA. Fluoroacetyl CoA replaces acetyl CoA in the tricarboxylic acid (TCA or Krebs) cycle, and is converted by citrate synthase to fluorocitrate. Fluorocitrate binds with aconitase, halting the tricarboxylic acid cycle.

Fluoroacetate and metabolites are defluorinated in the liver and rapidly excreted by the renal route within a few days in sublethal exposure.

Mode(s) of Action

The features of fluoroacetate poisoning are primarily the consequences of severe impairment of oxidative metabolism by impairment of the tricarboxylic acid cycle, as well as inhibition of mitochondrial citrate transport leading to accumulation of citrate.

Inhibition of the tricarboxylic acid cycle means that energy production is greatly reduced, and there is depletion of the intermediates of the tricarboxylic acid cycle subsequent to citrate. One such intermediate is oxoglutarate, which is a precursor of glutamate. Glutamate is a neurotransmitter and is also required for metabolism of ammonia via the urea cycle. Lactic acidosis occurs as a result of the depression of cellular oxidative metabolism, and acidosis is exacerbated by the impairment of oxidation of fatty acids via the tricarboxylic acid cycle, which also leads to formation of ketone bodies. ATP, which is essential for gluconeogenesis, is depleted. There is rapid hydrolysis of glycogen in the liver, skeletal muscles, and cardiac muscle. Organs with high metabolic rates including brain and heart are the most severely affected by fluoroacetate toxicosis.

High levels of citrate bind to serum calcium, leading to hypocalcemia that may result in heart failure, and also inhibit phosphofructokinase that is an important glycolytic enzyme. Citrate also inhibits the production of acetylcholine.

Death may be due to neurotoxicity and/or cardiotoxicity. Acute oral $LD_{50}s$, in mg/kg bodyweight of various domestic species are as follows:

	mg/kg		mg/kg
Dog	0.06−0.35	Cat	0.07−0.49
Pig	1−1.04	Sheep	0.25−0.52
Cow	0.22−0.39	Horse	0.35−1.00
Human being	2.00−5.00		

Birds appear to be more tolerant of sodium fluoroacetate. The acute oral LD_{50} for the domestic duck is in the region of 9 mg/kg, while that of the hen is 14 mg/kg.

Clinical Signs

Clinical signs usually become evident 30 minutes to 3 hours after ingestion of sodium fluoroacetate. Clinical signs tend to be those of neurotoxicity in carnivores but those of cardiotoxicity in herbivores.

Dogs

Dogs develop agitation, followed by vomiting, vocalization, hypersalivation, defecation, urination, tenesmus, and sudden muscle contractions. Dogs typically have mydriasis and photophobia, and tend to appear oblivious to their surroundings and their owners. They also exhibit dyspnea. The neurological signs progress to wild running fits and tonic-clonic seizures, which increase in severity and frequency until death. Death usually occurs within 2−12 hours of ingestion, but some dogs survive up to 48 hours. Death generally appears to be a result of respiratory failure.

Cats

Clinical signs in the cat are less severe than in the dog, and usually begin with vomiting at 1−2 hours after ingestion. Other clinical signs may include disorientation, either excitement or depression, vocalization, hypersalivation, diarrhea, mydriasis and photophobia, hyperesthesia, hypothermia, bradycardia with arrhythmias, and convulsions. Cats usually succumb to either respiratory failure or cardiac failure between 4 and 24 hours after ingestion.

Pigs

Clinical signs reported for pigs include vomiting, tremors, either agitation or lethargy, violent convulsions, and death due to either respiratory failure or cardiac failure.

Ruminants and Horses

Toxicosis in herbivores is generally less dramatic than in carnivores. Sudden death from cardiac failure is common, but recumbency with grunting may occur. Disorientation, agitation, bruxism, apparent blindness, weakness, ataxia, and coma have been reported in sheep. Nonfatal poisoning cattle has been associated with listlessness, anorexia, visual impairment, incoordination, tachycardia, polypnea, and exercise intolerance. Ventricular arrhythmias, myocardial depression, and ventricular fibrillation have been reported in horses.

Other Species

Birds have survived up to 10 days after dosing with sodium fluoroacetate, and reptiles have survived up to 22 days.

Diagnostic Aids

Clinical pathology findings typically include increased serum citrate, hyperglycemia, hypocalcemia, azotemia, and lactic acidosis.

Vomitus may contain green marker.

Treatment

Because of the rapid absorption of fluoroacetate, decontamination efforts are likely to be futile by the time an animal is presented for treatment. Gastric lavage followed by activated charcoal may be beneficial if there are no clinical signs.

Some antidotes have been suggested but their effectiveness is debated. They are unlikely to be effective unless given before any neurological signs develop. They are:

- glycerol monoacetate (monoacetin), 0.55 g/kg hourly IM to a total dose of 2−4 g/kg
- 50% ethanol and 5% acetic acid, 8 mL of each orally.

Prognosis is generally considered to be hopeless if neurological signs are evident, and owners should be warned of that fact before costs of intensive treatment are incurred.

Convulsions should be controlled with diazepam and/or pentobarbitone. Muscle relaxants such as methocarbamol may be helpful. Monitor for respiratory depression. Oxygen should be administered.

Establish an IV line and supply bicarbonate and electrolytes. Use the IV fluid line to supply calcium gluconate at 0.2−0.5 mL/kg IV (5% solution, slowly, in fluids) to correct hypocalcemia.

Correct any arrhythmias with lidocaine or procainamide.

Maintain core body temperature.

Prognosis

Prognosis is guarded to poor if there are any clinical signs, and grave to hopeless if there are any neurological signs.

Necropsy

Necropsy findings are nonspecific. The stomach, colon, and urinary bladder of carnivores will be empty. The heart is often flaccid and pale.

Severe necrosis if skeletal muscles has been reported in birds.

Samples of choice include blood, skeletal and/or muscle tissue, rumen contents, and vomit.

Public Health Considerations

There has been a great deal of unfortunate scaremongering about risk to human beings, when in fact the risk is remote.

Accidental consumption of poisoned livestock or wildlife is unlikely to pose any risks to human beings. Sodium fluoroacetate baits are rapidly broken down in water. Only traces of sodium fluoroacetate have been found in honey from bees intentionally fed large amounts of sodium fluoroacetate. The average person would have to consume 2.2 tonnes of watercress to be poisoned by sodium fluoroacetate taken up by watercress.

There is no evidence that acute exposure to sodium fluoroacetate by human beings (e.g., being in the vicinity of an aerial bait drop), without any clinical signs of acute toxicosis, is likely to lead to any chronic effects or carcinogenicity.

There is *no* valid evidence that sodium fluoroacetate is a teratogen at doses that do not cause maternal toxicity. One New Zealand study concluded that sodium fluoroacetate is a teratogen on the basis of findings in fetal rats of "slightly curved forelimbs, and bent or 'wavy' ribs." As a result of this conclusion, some women in New Zealand have been scared into leaving their homes during aerial spreading of sodium fluoroacetate baits. However, curved forelimb bones and wavy ribs are both well-recognized and well-documented, by researchers experienced in developmental toxicity studies in rats, to be normal variants that do *not* indicate teratogenic potential.

Sodium Nitrite

General Remarks

The target species for sodium nitrite are feral pigs and, in New Zealand, brushtail possums.

Circumstances of Poisoning

Nontarget species could be poisoned by consumption of baits. The likelihood of relay toxicosis from consumption of a poisoned animal appears to be very low.

Toxicokinetics

Sodium nitrite acts quickly. Clinical signs may be evident in pigs in 20–40 minutes. If a sublethal dose is consumed, the nitrite is reduced to ammonia in the rumen of ruminants, or the large intestine of monogastric animals.

The LD_{50} in pigs is in the region of 250 mg/kg.

Mode(s) of Action

Sodium nitrite converts hemoglobin to methemoglobin. Death results from hypoxia.

Clinical Signs

Clinical signs include restlessness, vomiting, urination, lethargy, incoordination, and dyspnea with rapid, shallow breathing. The conjunctival vessels may appear brown and the mucous membranes are "muddy" due to both methemoglobinemia and cyanosis. Terminally there may be paddling and seizures.

Pigs are particularly sensitive to sodium nitrite. Time to death in pigs is 1–3 hours. However if pigs consume a sublethal dose, they are likely to show signs of recovery after 4–6 hours and recover fully within 12–14 hours.

Diagnostic Aids

Blood is dark or brown. Laboratory analysis confirms methemoglobinemia.

Treatment

Methylene blue, as for PAPP (q.v.)

Prognosis

Prognosis is variable depending on the severity of methemoglobinemia, but is good with prompt treatment.

Necropsy

The brown color of methemoglobin is readily apparent when the carcass is first opened, but disappears over a short time once the blood is exposed to air.

Strychnine

General Remarks

Strychnine has been withdrawn from general use in both Australia and New Zealand. It is covered here because of the possibility that some old baits may still exist.

Circumstances of Poisoning

Consumption of baits or of recently poisoned vermin.

Toxicokinetics

Strychnine is rapidly absorbed from ingestion or inhalation, and can be absorbed through mucous membranes, but not through intact skin. It is rapidly detoxified by the liver, with a half-life of 10−16 hours. It is also rapidly excreted unchanged in the urine, and can be detected in urine within minutes of ingestion. Urinary excretion is practically complete in 72 hours. Because strychnine is an alkaloid, urinary excretion is enhanced by acidification of urine.

Mode(s) of Action

Strychnine is a competitive antagonist of the inhibitory neurotransmitter glycine. This is the same neurotransmitter as that inhibited by tetanus toxin. Toxicosis reflects the effects of strychnine on the recurrent inhibitory interneurons (Renshaw cells) of the reflex arc of the medulla oblongata and spinal cord. The inhibitory effects of the reflex arc are lost. The consequences are extensor rigidity and tonic seizures, with death from rigid paralysis of the respiratory muscles. Consciousness is retained until just before death, and as with tetanus, the toxicosis is extremely painful.

The LD_{50} in most domestic species is approximately 0.5 mg/kg, but cats are slightly more tolerant at 2.0 mg/kg, and poultry at 5.0 mg/kg.

Clinical Signs

Clinical signs usually begin 10−30 minutes after ingestion, but can commence sooner. Food in the stomach may moderately delay onset of clinical signs.

Initial signs are those of apprehension, muscle tremors, erect ears, and muscle tics, which are inducible. These signs suddenly progress to tonic to tetanic seizures with opisthotonus and, in quadrupeds, extensor rigidity of all limbs (in humans, the flexors of the arms are stronger than the extensors, so the arms are flexed). Seizures are characteristically highly inducible by light or sound. Intervals between seizures become progressively shorter, and seizures may be practically continuous by the time death ensues. Consequent to the seizures are hyperthermia, myoglobinemia and myoglobinuria, acidosis, cyanosis, and mydriasis.

In practical terms, strychnine poisoning resembles a peracute case of tetanus, because the toxins share the same mechanism. However, the *risus sardonicus* observed in dogs with early tetanus is not so characteristic of strychnine poisoning.

Diagnostic Aids

Clinical pathology findings are nonspecific consequences of seizures: myoglobinuria, acidosis, and elevated creatine phosphokinase.

Strychnine is likely to be present in urine.

Treatment

Do not induce emesis. The very rapid absorption means that emesis is highly unlikely to alter the extent of absorption, and emetics may trigger seizures. Gastric lavage with infusion of activated charcoal may be considered only under general anesthesia with a cuffed endotracheal tube in place, but is unlikely to make a significant difference to clinical course, because of the rapid absorption and metabolism.

Barbiturate anesthesia should be supplemented with an appropriate muscle relaxant such as methocarbamol (150 mg/kg initially, with 90 mg/kg top-ups as required) or glyceryl guiacolate (110 mg/kg).

Respiratory support may be required.

Ketamine and morphine are *contraindicated*.

Establish an IV fluid line to promote urinary excretion of strychnine (strychnine-*N*-oxide) and myoglobin, and treat for acidosis if present. If acidosis is not present, acidify the urine with ammonium chloride. Catheterize the patient and monitor urinary output.

The animal should be kept in a warm, very quiet environment, with ambient light as low as compatible with monitoring and treatment. Sudden changes in light intensity should be avoided.

Prognosis

Prognosis is good if the animal survives for 24–48 hours, because of the rapid excretion of strychnine.

Necropsy

Findings are nonspecific consequences of seizures and hypoxia.

Dogs commonly have baits in the stomach. Samples for postmortem analysis include stomach contents, liver, and urine.

AVICIDES

Alphachloralose

General Remarks

Alphachloralose is formed by condensing chloral hydrate, a basal narcotic, with glucose.

Circumstances of Poisoning

Poisoning may result from the consumption of baits, or by relay toxicosis due to the consumption of poisoned birds.

Toxicokinetics

Alphachloralose is rapidly absorbed, and rapidly metabolized to chloral and then to trichloroethanol, to which the clinical signs are attributed. Trichloroethanol is glucuronidated to urochloralic acid, which is excreted in the urine.

Mode(s) of Action

The active metabolite, trichloroethanol, acts as an anesthetic. However, dogs and cats may manifest clinical signs of involuntary excitement, such as that observed when a barbiturate anesthetic is administered too slowly. Depending on the dose, this excitement may be followed by a phase of profound sedation and anesthesia. If death occurs, it is likely to be due to hypothermia or respiratory depression.

The acute oral LD_{50} in the cat is 100 mg/kg, whereas in the dog it is 600−1000 mg/kg.

Clinical Signs

Clinical onset is generally rapid, within 1−2 hours.

Signs of excitation include agitation, hyperesthesia, hypersalivation, miosis, muscle tremors, and convulsions.

Clinical signs of the anesthetized phase are central nervous depression, hypotension, hypothermia, and coma.

Diagnostic Aids

The sample of choice for analysis is urine.

Treatment

Treatment is symptomatic and supportive.

The use of sedatives during the excitation phase should be avoided if possible because the animal may progress to a state of profound sedation or anesthesia. If the animal is so excited that it is hyperthermic or convulsing, consider the use of rapidly reversible anesthesia, e.g., inhaled anesthetic such as isoflurane.

Generally, management and monitoring of the sedated/comatose phase is as for an anesthetized animal. Body temperature should be monitored.

Prognosis

Prognosis is generally good, although recovery from the anesthetized phase can be 24–48 hours.

Necropsy

There are no specific lesions.

DRC-1339 ("Starlicide")

General Remarks

Chemical names for DRC-1339 include 2-chloro-4-aminotoluene, 3-chloro-p-toluidine, 3-chloro-4-methylaniline, and 3-chloro-4-ethylbenzenamine. However, these are all the same toxicant.

Circumstances of Poisoning

The risk of a cat developing toxicosis as a result of consuming poisoned birds is considered to be low.

Toxicokinetics

There is very little information on the toxicokinetics of DRC-1339 in domestic mammals. Absorption in cats appears to be rapid, because the first clinical sign, methemoglobinemia, reaches its maximum level in the first hour. Metabolism and excretion of DRC-1339 appears to be rapid in mammals.

Mode(s) of Action

The mode of action of DRC-1339 in mammals is not clear. It is only moderately to mildly toxic to mammals, with LD_{50}s in the range of 100–1000 mg/kg.

Clinical Signs

The first clinical sign in cats is methemoglobinemia, which is usually moderate (up to 55%) and not life-threatening. This is followed by central nervous system depression, flaccid paralysis, hypothermia, and respiratory depression.

Diagnostic Aids

Clinical pathology findings include methemoglobinemia, hyperkalemia, and hemoconcentration.

Treatment

Keep the animal warm and monitor vital functions. Establish an IV fluid line and correct hyperkalemia. Methemoglobinemia generally does not require correction, but may be treated with 30 mg/kg ascorbic acid, four times daily, in the conscious animal.

Prognosis

There are insufficient case reports in the literature to estimate prognosis. It is reported that once hypothermia has developed, it can be difficult to reverse.

Necropsy

There are no specific lesions.

The tissue of choice for postmortem analysis is kidney.

Chapter 11

Herbicides and Fungicides

INTRODUCTION

In both Australia and New Zealand, there are a large number of herbicides and fungicides that are approved for use. For many of these chemicals, toxicological information is limited to LD_{50} values in rodents, and toxic effects in human beings involved in the manufacture or handling of the concentrates. Furthermore, only a few chemicals are significantly associated with veterinary poisonings. For these reasons, this chapter is largely limited to those herbicides and fungicides that have been frequently associated with veterinary and/or human poisoning.

HERBICIDES: GENERAL COMMENTS

Most herbicides are unlikely to be toxic to domestic animals when diluted for application, or after application to plants. Inadvertent consumption of concentrated herbicide is rare in veterinary medicine. Domestic livestock should not be allowed to graze plants to which herbicides have been applied until the recommended withholding period has been observed. Poisonous plants may become more palatable to livestock when dying or dead as a result of herbicide application.

DIPYRIDYL HERBICIDES: PARAQUAT AND DIQUAT

General Remarks

Paraquat is the most significant herbicide in veterinary toxicology, in terms of number of reports of serious clinical toxicoses.

Circumstances of Poisoning

These herbicides are readily available for residential and farming use. Livestock are most commonly poisoned by access to the concentrate or to diluted herbicide in the spraying tank. Once applied, dipyridyl herbicides bind strongly to soil and are degraded by sunlight and, because the application rate is low, toxicosis as a result of grazing is unlikely.

Veterinary Toxicology for Australia and New Zealand.
DOI: http://dx.doi.org/10.1016/B978-0-12-420227-6.00011-6

Dipyridyl herbicides are often incriminated in malicious poisoning of domestic dogs.

Toxicokinetics

Gastrointestinal absorption of ingested dipyridyl herbicide is <30%, and dermal absorption is minimal. Systemic toxicosis as a result of inhaling spray drift is unlikely because formulations generally form droplets that do not reach the lower respiratory tract.

Gastrointestinal absorption is rapid, with C_{max} at approximately 75 minutes in dogs.

Paraquat, but not diquat, concentrates in lung tissue, specifically in the Types I and II alveolar cells and in Clara cells.

The herbicides are primarily excreted unmetabolized in the urine.

Mode(s) of Action

Paraquat undergoes cyclic oxidation—reduction reactions. Electron transfer occurs from paraquat to oxygen, forming the superoxide radical which reacts with lipids in cell membranes to form lipid hydroperoxides. A lipid free radical chain reaction follows, leading to cellular degeneration and necrosis.

Clinical Signs

Early signs may be mild and unnoticed, although if a high dose is consumed, there may be vomiting, evidence of gastrointestinal pain, and oral lesions. However, the most severe and eventually fatal respiratory signs of paraquat poisoning are generally delayed for at least 2—7 days. The animal develops dyspnea, moist rales, and cyanosis, as well as evidence of renal insufficiency. In the final phase of paraquat poisoning, progressive pulmonary fibrosis eventually leads to death.

Exposure to spray drift may lead to sore throat and epistaxis, but is unlikely to lead to systemic toxicosis.

Dermal exposure may lead to irritation and vesication of skin and mucous membranes. Paraquat is extremely irritant to the eyes.

Diagnostic Aids

The pulmonary fibrosis evident on radiograph often appears milder than the clinical signs would suggest. Pneumomediastinum may be present.

Serology concurrent with the development of respiratory and renal clinical signs may reveal elevated liver enzymes, indicative of centrilobular hepatocellular necrosis.

Herbicide is generally only detectable in the urine for 2—3 days following ingestion, so it may be absent by the time clinical signs develop.

Treatment

Given the serious nature of paraquat poisoning, gastric lavage is justified if the animal is presented within an hour of ingestion. However, the rapid absorption of ingested paraquat means that this measure may be futile.

Activated charcoal, bentonite, or Fuller's earth should be administered as soon as possible. Of these three, activated charcoal appears to be the most effective adsorbent.

Paraquat is frequently used in suicide attempts in Asia, and published reports do not support the efficacy of gastrointestinal decontamination in these human cases.

Charcoal hemoperfusion has been successfully used to prevent toxicosis in dogs experimentally dosed with paraquat, but is not available to most veterinary practices.

Forced diuresis is recommended to maintain urine flow and promote herbicide excretion.

Assisted ventilation may prolong life. Pure oxygen should not be administered, even if cyanosis is present, because it will promote oxidative damage. Renal function should be monitored and fluids may be used to maintain renal function.

Prognosis

The prognosis in paraquat poisoning is guarded to hopeless.

The prognosis in diquat poisoning is more favorable than that in paraquat poisoning.

Necropsy

Gross findings include erosive lesions in the mouth and esophagus. In paraquat poisoning, pulmonary congestion and/or hemorrhage, atelectasis, and bullous emphysema may be grossly evident.

Histological lesions in paraquat poisoning include necrosis of alveolar Type I epithelium, alveolar emphysema, and both alveolar and interstitial fibrosis. Degeneration may also be present in proximal convoluted tubules of the kidney and in centrilobular hepatocytes.

In diquat poisoning, typical lesions are those of ulcerative lesions in the mouth and gastrointestinal tract, cerebral hemorrhages and infarcts, and renal tubular degeneration and necrosis.

In acute poisoning, specimens to collect for analysis are urine, lung, and kidney. Lung, liver, and kidney should be fixed for histopathology. Paraquat may no longer be present at detectable concentrations if the animal succumbs slowly to pulmonary fibrosis.

Public Health Considerations

The dipyridyl herbicides do not reach high concentrations in edible tissues of livestock, and have a short half-life.

Prevention

Because of the poor prognosis of paraquat poisoning, exposure to concentrated or mixed herbicide must be prevented.

PHENOXY HERBICIDES

The best known of these are:

- 2,4-Dichlorophenoxyacetic acid (2,4-D)
- 2-Methyl-4-chlorophenoxyacetic acid
- Methylchlorophenoxypropionic acid

Circumstances of Poisoning

Animals may consume concentrates or diluted herbicide in spraying tanks. Toxicosis from exposure to sprayed pasture or lawn is highly unlikely.

The acute toxic dose is 200 mg/kg in cattle and 100 mg/kg in pigs. An acute oral LD_{50} of 100 mg/kg has been claimed for dogs, but more recent research indicates that the LD_{50} in dogs is likely to be higher than 200 mg/kg.

A daily oral dose of 25 mg/kg was fatal to dogs after 6 days. However, dogs can tolerate a dietary dose of 500 ppm for 2 years with no adverse effects.

A daily dose of 100 mg/kg is toxic to cattle after 10–30 days, but cattle can tolerate a long-term dietary intake of 2000 ppm.

Toxicokinetics

Phenoxy herbicides are rapidly absorbed from the gastrointestinal tract, with high bioavailability. They are protein-bound in the circulation. Most of a dose of phenoxy herbicide is excreted unchanged in the urine. The half-life of 2,4-D in the circulation is approximately 18 hours.

Mode(s) of Action

The toxic mechanism(s) of the phenoxy herbicides in mammals are not well understood.

Clinical Signs

Reported clinical signs in dogs have included vomiting, diarrhea, anorexia, depression, myotonia, ataxia, and posterior weakness. Opisthotonus may occur. Dogs may have ulcerations in the oral cavity. In severe cases, dogs may progress through periodic clonic spasms to coma.

Clinical signs in cattle are those of anorexia, ruminal atony, oral ulcerations, bloat, diarrhea, depression, and weakness.

Pigs also exhibit tremors, ataxia, and weakness, in addition to vomiting and diarrhea.

An association between 2,4-D and malignant lymphoma in dogs has been claimed, but is not considered to be convincing. A link between phenoxy herbicide use on lawns, and transitional cell carcinoma of the bladder in Scottish Terriers, has also been claimed but awaits replication.

An association between phenoxy herbicide use, with or without use of picolinic acid herbicide, and small intestinal adenocarcinoma in sheep has also been asserted.

Diagnostic Aids

Serological findings are likely to include elevations in alkaline phosphatase, lactic dehydrogenase, and creatine phosphokinase.

Phenoxy herbicide may be present in the urine.

Treatment

Decontamination with activated charcoal is helpful if exposure is recent. Gastrointestinal clinical signs should be treated as appropriate. Renal function should be monitored, and fluid therapy instituted to promote diuresis. Animals should be provided with a bland high-quality diet because of hepatic injury.

Prognosis

Prognosis is generally good with supportive care.

Necropsy

Oral ulcerations may be present. The liver and kidneys are typically swollen and the liver may be friable. Mesenteric lymph nodes may be enlarged and congested. Hydropericardium and/or epicardial hemorrhages may be present.

Fresh or frozen specimens for analysis are kidney and urine. Liver, kidney, and lesions may be fixed for histopathology.

Public Health Considerations

The tissue half-life of phenoxy herbicides in livestock is short.

Prevention

Livestock and domestic pets should not be allowed access to phenoxy herbicide concentrates or solutions prepared for use.

OTHER HERBICIDES: SHORT NOTES

Short notes on some other herbicides are presented in Table 11.1.

TABLE 11.1 Short Notes on Miscellaneous Herbicides

Name	Comments
Atrazine	Atrazine is classified as slightly toxic in mammals. Activated charcoal has been found to be beneficial in experimental atrazine toxicosis in cattle
Dicamba	Has been reported to cause mild icterus in dogs
Dichlobenil	Clinical signs in ruminants include anorexia, hypersalivation, and depression. On necropsy, findings include hemorrhages in skeletal muscle and epicardium, and congestion of liver, kidney, and intestinal tract
Fluometuron	Experimental fluometuron poisoning in sheep was characterized by grinding of the teeth, ruminal tympany, mydriasis, dyspnea, staggering, paresis, and recumbency. Lesions included hepatic lipdosis, enteritis renal tubular degeneration
Glyphosate	Glyphosate is of low mammalian toxicity. Poisoning has not been reported in domestic animals. Dermal absorption is negligible. Surfactants in commercial preparations of glyphosate may cause mild gastrointestinal irritation. There is considerable misinformation about glyphosate on social media, disseminated by opponents of genetically modified crops that are glyphosate-resistant
Metolachlor	Clinical signs in experimental metolachlor poisoning of goats included convulsions, ataxia, tremors, muscle spasms, hypersalivation, dyspnea, and recumbency. Liver enzymes were elevated
Nitrofen	Clinical signs in ruminants are those of anorexia, depression, ataxia, diarrhea, and hematuria. Necropsy findings include pulmonary edemia, hydropericardium, and epicardial hemorrhages
Propachlor	Clinical signs in ruminants include anorexia, depression, hypersalivation, muscle tremors, and recumbency. Lesions include enlarged pale liver, enlarged adrenals, congested kidneys, and petechiae in the urinary bladder
Simazine	Simazine toxicosis in sheep featured generalized muscle tremors and mild tetany followed by collapse of the hind legs. Other signs included a short prancing gait with head tucked. Death occurred within 2–3 days of the appearance of clinical signs. Lesions included myocardial degeneration and hepatic lipidosis
Sodium chlorate	Sodium chlorate causes methemoglobinemia, with clinical signs and necropsy findings as for nitrate/nitrite poisoning, and should be treated with methylene blue according to the same protocol as in nitrate/nitrite poisoning
Thiocarbamate herbicides	Some, but not all, members of this group have anticholinesterase activity that may respond to atropine
Triclopyr	May cause mild nephrosis in dogs

TABLE 11.2 Short Notes on Miscellaneous Fungicides

Name	Comments
Benomyl	Of low toxicity, with a dietary No Observed Effect Level (NOEL) of 500 ppm in the dog. Toxic effects are on the liver
Captan	A 250 mg/kg oral dose is acutely lethal to sheep. Clinical signs in mammals include hypothermia, depression, diarrhea, anorexia, and polydipsia
Chlorothalonil	Dietary NOEL 120 ppm in the dog
Dicloran	Chronic dietary No Observed Adverse Effect Level in the dog is 100 ppm, equal to 1.7 mg/kg/day. Up to 3000 ppm was tolerated by dogs for 2 years, but dogs at the high dose developed hepatocyte hypertrophy and pleomorphism
Metiram	May affect thyroid function
Thiophanate-methyl	Acute oral LD_{50} in the dog is 4000 mg/kg. Clinical signs in the dog include decreased respiratory rate, mydriasis, and prostration
Thiram (tetramethylthiuram disulfide)	Moderately toxic, with effects on the liver
Zineb	Low oral toxicity. Toxicosis in sheep features yellow, watery diarrhea

FUNGICIDES

Fungicide poisoning is a rare problem in veterinary toxicology. Notes on some fungicides currently or formerly approved in Australia and/or New Zealand are presented in Table 11.2.

For fungicides not listed in Table 11.2, further data on toxicity may be found online, for example through the New Zealand Environmental Protection Authority. However, mammalian toxicity information may be limited to rodents. It cannot be assumed that an LD_{50} or NOEL established in the mouse or the rat will be the same in other mammalian species.

Chapter 12

Human Pharmaceuticals

PRESCRIPTION DRUGS FOR HUMAN BEINGS

Toxicity from consumption of prescription drugs, when not iatrogenic, is most common in young dogs and cats.

The toxicology of prescription drugs for human use is a very large body of information that can, and does, fill reference books in its own right. However, information on treating overdose is generally readily available to the practitioner via helplines and in packet inserts. Furthermore, helplines for human poisoning cases generally have considerable information on the effects of overdoses of prescription drugs. For these reasons, only brief notes are provided here (Table 12.1). Treatment is in most cases purely symptomatic, and *only specific antidotes or contraindications are mentioned below*. As always the use of a specific antidote does not replace the need for nonspecific supportive therapy.

The toxic effects summarized below are for acute overdose and do not include toxic effects from repeat-dose or chronic use as part of veterinary treatment.

Volatile anesthetics and neuromuscular blocking agents used in a surgical setting are not discussed, because it is assumed that the veterinary practitioner is familiar with the risks and safe uses of these agents.

Similarly, the toxicology of antibiotics and parasiticides commonly used in veterinary practice is not covered here.

OVER THE COUNTER PHARMACEUTICALS

Introduction

Over the counter (OTC) pharmaceuticals for human use pose a threat to animals, particularly domestic pets, if they are administered in error to animals, or if animals gain access to them and consume them.

OTC pharmaceuticals covered in this section include the following:

Antacids
Antifungals
Antihistamines
Aspirin

TABLE 12.1

Drug or Class	Toxic Effects, Clinical Signs	Treatment Comments
Nervous System		
Anticholinergics: atropine, hyoscamine, scopolamine, and analogs	Anticholinergic toxidrome: delirium, tachycardia, hyperthermia, mydriasis, dry mouth, convulsions	Physostigmine IV is the antidote
	mnemonic: mad as a hatter, hot as hell, red as a beet, dry as a bone, and blind as a bat	
Antihistamines	Convulsions, coma	*Do not use stimulants*
Antinausea drugs: ondansetron and metoclopramide	Both of these drugs can cause serotonin syndrome in human beings. For clinical signs and antidote, see Selective serotonin reuptake inhibitors (SSRIs), below	
Lithium	Depression, tremor, emesis, diarrhea, hyperreflexia, seizures, coma	Saline diuresis may enhance excretion
	NOTE: Lithium can cause serotonin syndrome in human beings. For clinical signs and antidote, see SSRIs, below	
Local anesthetics, e.g., lidocaine, benzocaine	Methemoglobinemia, hypotension, convulsions	
Monoamine oxidase inhibitors, e.g., tranylcypromine, phenelzine, iproniazid, isocarboxazid, pargyline, pheniprazine, nialimide	Signs of catecholamine excess followed by catecholamine depletion, i.e., initial stimulation and hyperthermia, progressing to hypotension, coma, and death	
	Also hepatotoxic	

(Continued)

TABLE 12.1 (Continued)

Drug or Class	Toxic Effects, Clinical Signs	Treatment Comments
Narcotic analgesics	CNS depression, coma, respiratory failure. Some can be convulsant, e.g., codeine, apomorphine, oxymorphone	Naloxone HCl is the antidote
	NOTE: fentanyl, tramadol, and methadone can cause serotonin syndrome in human beings. For clinical signs and antidote, see SSRIs, below	
Parasympathomimetics, e.g., physostigmine, pilocarpine	Clinical signs as for organophosphate/carbamate poisoning (q.v.)	Atropine is the antidote. Pralidoxime is only useful for echothiophate
Phenothiazine derivatives, e.g., promazine, chlorpromazine	Initial hyperactivity followed by sedation, hypotension, hypothermia, ventricular arrhythmia	
Polycyclic antidepressants (e.g., clomipramine, imipramine, amitriptyline, protriptyline, nortriptyline doxypin) and related drugs, e.g., cyclobenzaprine, amoxaprine, loxapine, bupropion, trazodone, nefazodone, mirtazapine	CNS stimulation, arrhythmia, mydriasis, hypotension, respiratory depression	*Physostigmine, quinidine, procainamide, disopyramide, corticosteroids, propranolol and atropine are all contraindicated*
	NOTE: clomipramine, trazodone, buspirone can all cause serotonin syndrome in human beings. For clinical signs and antidote, see SSRIs, below	
Sedatives, hypnotics, and anticonvulsants	Clinical signs general to these drugs are drowsiness, ataxia, hypotension, hyporeflexia, coma, respiratory depression, and cyanosis. Most cause hypothermia; some cause hyperthermia. There are possible additional clinical signs for specific drugs; seek advice from a poison advisory service	*Do not use stimulants*

(Continued)

TABLE 12.1 (Continued)

Drug or Class	Toxic Effects, Clinical Signs	Treatment Comments
SSRIs e.g., citalopram, fluoxetinem, sertraline, escitalopram paroxetine	Overdose causes "serotonin syndrome" characterized by cognitive changes (agitation, hallucinations, coma), autonomic dysfunction (arrhythmia, hypertension, hyperthermia, mydriasis, emesis), and neuromuscular abnormalities (ataxia, convulsions, hyperreflexia, nystagmus, tremor, possible rhabdomyolysis)	Treat with cyproheptadine, orally or per rectum, divided into three or four doses/24 hours, 1.1 mg/kg for dogs, or a total dose of 2−4 mg to a cat
Serotonin−norepinephrine reuptake inhibitors, e.g., venlafaxine, duloxetine	As for SSRIs, above	As for SSRIs, above
Sympathomimetics: epinephrine, ephedrine, albuterol, etc.	Principal toxic effect is convulsions	Chlorpromazine is *contraindicated* except for amphetamine poisoning
Cardiovascular Agents		
Angiotensin-converting enzyme inhibitors, e.g., captopril, enalapril, and other drugs ending in -pril	Hypotension, renal failure, hemolytic anemia	This class of drug appears to be of low toxicity in dogs
Angiotensin II receptor blockers, e.g., cilexetil, valsartan, and other drugs ending in −sartan	Hypotension, renal failure	
Anticoagulants, e.g., warfarin, heparin	As for anticoagulant rodenticides	Warfarin and other coumarin-related: phytonadione as for anticoagulant rodenticides
		The antidote for heparin is 1% protamine sulfate by slow IV push. This drug will antagonize heparin at a 1:1 ratio by mass

TABLE 12.1 (Continued)

Drug or Class	Toxic Effects, Clinical Signs	Treatment Comments
B-sympathetic blocking agents, e.g., propranolol, metaprolol, atenolol, etc. Note -olol suffix	Hypotension, bradycardia, arrhythmia, respiratory depression, coma	Insulin IV or amrinone (4 mg/kg bolus) has been suggested as alternative antidotes in the dog rather than the recommended human antidote, glucagon
Calcium channel blocking agents, e.g., amlodipine and other -dipines, mibbefradil, pepridil, diltiazem, and verapamil	Bradycardia and hypotension	IV calcium gluconate or calcium chloride, 10% solution in saline
		AV block and bradycardia may respond to atropine or isoproterenol. Treat hypotension with fluids by preference, use dopamine with caution. Digoxin improves BP in verapamil-poisoned dogs
		Insulin if hyperglycemic
		Intravenous fat emulsion improves survival in verapamil toxicosis in dogs
Cholestyramine and colestipol (resins)	Constipation, electrolyte derangement, may bind Vitamin K leading to hemorrhagic diathesis	
Diazoxide	Hyperglycemia. Has caused arrhythmia and shock in human beings	
Digitalis and analogs	Increase the irritability of the ventricular myocardium, leading to extrasystoles, ventricular tachycardia, and ventricular fibrillation. Also stimulate the CNS	Digibind, digoxin-specific antibody, is the antidote
		Monitor ECG, serum K and Mg
		Cholestyramine resin, orally, will reduce half-life of digitoxin. IV

(Continued)

TABLE 12.1 (Continued)

Drug or Class	Toxic Effects, Clinical Signs	Treatment Comments
Disopyramide	Hypotension, anticholinergic effects. Has caused cardiac block in human beings	
Doftilide	Increased QT(c) interval, premature ventricular contractions, and right bundle branch block	Dogs are more sensitive to the cardiovascular effects than humans
Ergot alkaloid derivatives, e.g., ergotamine, methysergide, pergolide, bromocriptine	Convulsions and gangrene	Antidote is a vasodilator such as IV nitroprusside or phentolamine to effect; monitor heart rate and blood pressure. Maintain blood clotting time at approximately twice normal with heparin. Vasopressors are *contraindicated*
Ethacrynic acid	Nephrotoxic and ototoxic in dogs. Toxic effects in humans include acute pancreatitis, ventricular fibrillation due to potassium loss, agranulocytosis, thrombocytopenia	
Fenoldopam	Arterial lesions in dogs. Reflex tachycardia and increased intraocular pressure reported in humans	
Flecainide	Exaggerated arrhythmias. Liver damage reported in humans	
Furosemide and related drugs	Hypotension, dehydration, hypokalemia, and ototoxicity. Acute pancreatitis has been reported in humans	

(Continued)

TABLE 12.1 (Continued)

Drug or Class	Toxic Effects, Clinical Signs	Treatment Comments
Hydralazine	Vasculitis of coronary arteries, epicardial hemorrhage, and papillary muscle necrosis in dogs. Dogs do not appear to develop all the characteristics of "hydralazine syndrome" seen in humans	Vasopressors are *contraindicated* in acute poisoning although dopamine may be used with caution if hypotension is severe
Ibutilide	Hypotension	
Mecamylamine	Hypotension, renal failure	
Metolazone	Hypoglycemia, hyperkalemia	
Mexilitene	Tremor, hypotension, decreased cardiac contraction, may be arrhythmia	
Milrinone	Hypotension, may be arrhythmia	
Minoxidil	Myocardial necrosis, epicardial and endocardial hemorrhage, and coronary arteritis in the dog	
Moricizine	Arrhythmia, hypotension. Toxic effects on liver and bone marrow in humans	
Nitrites and nitrates, e.g., nitroglycerin, amyl nitrite, sodium nitrite	Vasodilation through direct action on smooth muscle. Some also cause methemoglobinemia	Antidote for methemoglobinemia is methylene blue
Nitroprusside	Hypotension, tachycardia, hyperventilation. See also cyanide	
Potassium chloride (in coated tablets)	Ulceration and possible perforation of small intestine, hyperkalaemic cardiac arrest	

(Continued)

TABLE 12.1 (Continued)

Drug or Class	Toxic Effects, Clinical Signs	Treatment Comments
Procainamide HCl	Hypotension and irregular heartbeat	Treat cardiac arrhythmia with bolus dose of sodium bicarbonate, 1–2 mequiv./kg
Quinazoline α1-adrenoreceptor antagonists (prazosin, doxazosin, terazosin)	Hypotension, may be gastrointestinal, sedation, tachycardia, dyspnea	
Quinidine	Hypotension, decreased cardiac conduction and bradycardia, respiratory failure	Antidote is IV sodium bicarbonate to increase serum binding of quinidine and reverse its effects on sodium-dependent membrane channels. Monitor serum potassium
Reserpine, deserpine, rescinnamine (derivatives of *Rauwolfia*)	Diarrhea, miosis, sedation, hypotension	
Sotalol	Hypotension, bradycardia, QT prolongation, can lead to torsades de pointes ventricular tachycardia in the dog	
Tocainide	Anorexia and gastrointestinal disturbance	
Antiinfectives		
Acyclovir	GI toxicity. Has caused encephalopathy in humans	
Adefovir	GI toxicity, nephrotoxicity	
Albendazole	Hepatotoxicity	
Amantidine	CNS toxicity	
Amprenavir	GI toxicity	
Cidofovir	Hepatotoxicity	

(*Continued*)

TABLE 12.1 (Continued)

Drug or Class	Toxic Effects, Clinical Signs	Treatment Comments
Clofazamine	GI and renal toxicity	
Clotrimazole	Irritant	
Delavirdine	Hypotension	
Didanosine	Pancreatic toxicity, hepatotoxicity, optic neuritis	
Efavirenz	Hepatotoxicity	
Emetine	Emesis, hypotension, myocardial damage	
Ethionamide	Hepatotoxicity, neurotoxicity	
Famciclovir	CNS toxicity in humans, testicular toxicity in experimental animals	
Fluconazole	Hepatotoxicity	
Flucytosine	CNS disturbances in humans	
Foscarnet	Nephrotoxicity, neurotoxicity	
Isoniazid	Seizures	
Ketoconazole	Hepatotoxicity, CNS effects	
Lamivudine	Pancreatic toxicity in humans	
Linezolid	Can cause serotonin syndrome in human beings. For clinical signs and antidote, see SSRIs, above	
Mefloquine	GI, cardiac, and CNS toxicity	
Methenamine	Renal irritation and hematuria	
Nelfinavir	Seizures	
Nevirapine	Hepatotoxicity	

(*Continued*)

TABLE 12.1 (Continued)

Drug or Class	Toxic Effects, Clinical Signs	Treatment Comments
Oseltamivir	Hepatotoxicity and nephrotoxicity	
Pentamidine	Hypotension, bronchospasm, CNS toxicity, hepatotoxicity, nephrotoxicity	
Phenazopyridine	Methemoglobinemia	
Pyrazinamide	Hepatotoxicity	
Quinine, chloroquine quinacrine, hydroxychloroquine	Emesis, hypotension, hepatitis. May also have toxic effects in liver, kidneys, nervous system, and retina	
Ribavirin	Pulmonary toxicity, cardiac arrest	
Rifapentine	Hepatotoxicity	
Rimantidine	CNS depression	
Ritonavir	GI and CNS effects	
Saquinavir	GI and CNS effects	
Stavudine	GI and respiratory effects	
Trifluridine	Increased intraocular pressure	
Trimetrexate	GI, liver, kidney, and bone marrow effects	
Valacyclovir	Thrombocytopenia	
Vidarabine	GI effects, CNS effects, hepatotoxicity, may be hematopoietic effects	
Zalcitabine	Pancreatic and hepatic toxicity	
Zanamavir	Hypoglycemia, nephrotoxicity, may be hematopoietic toxicity	
Zidovudine	Hepatotoxicity, myopathy, hematopoietic effects	

Decongestants
Enemas (hypertonic phosphate)
H_2-receptor antagonists
Insect repellents (principally concerns diethyl toluamide (DEET))
Loperamide
Mineral supplements
Paracetamol
NSAIDs (other than aspirin and paracetamol)
Opioid cough suppressants
Vitamins
Zinc oxide

Antacids

Antacids may be pills or suspensions of calcium carbonate, aluminum hydroxide, or magnesium hydroxide (milk of magnesia).

Absorption, Distribution, Metabolism, and Excretion

Systemic absorption of antacids is low.

Mode(s) of Action

Antacids decrease the acidity of the stomach and are used to reduce gastric pain (heartburn) or esophagitis resulting from reflux or hiatus hernia.

Clinical Signs

Toxicity of antacids to domestic pets is low. Calcium carbonate and aluminum hydroxide may cause constipation, while magnesium hydroxide may cause diarrhea. Calcium carbonate may cause transient hypercalcemia. Magnesium hydroxide may be hazardous in pets with kidney failure that have decreased ability to excrete magnesium.

Diagnostic Aids

Generally not required. The radiodensity of antacids may be useful to confirm consumption.

Treatment

Generally not required.

Prognosis

Prognosis is excellent.

Antifungals

There are a number of antifungals available OTC for the treatment of dermal mycoses such as Athlete's Foot, Jock Itch, and oral candidiasis in infants. Common OTC antifungals in Australia and New Zealand include the imidazole antifungals miconazole, ketaconazole, clotrimazole, and the allylamine antifungal terbinafine HCl.

Absorption, Distribution, Metabolism, and Excretion

Imidazole antifungals are rapidly absorbed by the oral route, and widely distributed in the body. Most imidazoles do not readily cross the blood—brain barrier. They are generally highly protein-bound in circulation. They are metabolized in the liver and most are principally excreted by the biliary route.

Terbinafine HCl is also readily bioavailable by the oral route. T_{max} is <2 hours in man. It is widely distributed in the body and is mostly protein-bound in circulation. It is extensively metabolized in the liver to a number of metabolites that are excreted in the urine.

Mode(s) of Action

Imidazoles and terbinafine block the synthesis of ergosterol, the primary cell sterol of fungi, leading to cell membrane disruption and cell death.

Clinical Signs

Clinical signs associated with overdose of imidazole antifungals in domestic pets include anorexia, nausea, vomiting, and, particularly in cats, hepatic dysfunction. Endocrine effects have been reported with ketaconazole, including alterations in metabolism of testosterone and cortisol, and decreased adrenal response to ACTH. Ketaconazole inhibits sperm motility in dogs.

Reported adverse effects of terbinafine administration to dogs include anorexia, nausea, vomiting, and incoordination. Vomiting and blood-stained feces have been reported in cats. Terbinafine HCl levels in the pancreas are relatively high, and the drug has been associated with rare cases of severe pancreatitis in human beings.

Diagnostic Aids

Clinical pathology may reveal elevated liver enzymes in hapatopathy due to imidazole antifungals. Because the common OTC antifungals are highly protein-bound in circulation, they will be present in serum, but toxic levels are not defined.

Treatment

There is no specific antidote. Treatment is symptomatic and supportive.

Prognosis

Mild hepatotoxicosis is generally reversible.

Necropsy

Hepatotoxicity is centrilobular with cholestasis. Fresh tissue samples for confirmation of diagnosis should include liver, kidney, and urine.

Antihistamines

Introduction

Antihistamines are H_1-receptor antagonists usually used in allergic rhinitis or allergic pruritis, although they may be taken as antiemetics or as mild sedatives.

Commonly used OTC antihistamines include chlorpheniramine, diphenhydramine, loratidine, cetirizine, and promethazine.

Absorption, Distribution, Metabolism, and Excretion

Antihistamines are generally rapidly absorbed with a T_{max} of 3 hours or less. First-generation antihistamines such as chlorpheniramine, diphenhydramine, and promethazine cross the blood−brain barrier whereas second-generation antihistamines such as loratidine and cetirizine do not. Antihistamines are metabolized in the liver and the metabolites excreted in the urine, with the exception of cetirizine that is excreted unchanged in the urine.

Mode(s) of Action

Antihistamines are competitive H_1-receptor antagonists. They therefore inhibit the increased capillary permeability, bronchoconstriction, pain, and itch of allergic responses. First-generation antihistamines tend to have sedative effects and also have anticholinergic effects. Promethazine, being a phenothiazine antihistamine, has also α-adrenergic blocking proterties.

Clinical Signs

Clinical signs of antihistamine overdose typically develop within 30 minutes of ingestion. They may include central nervous system (CNS) depression, vomiting, diarrhea, xerostomia, and urinary retention. Signs of toxicity are more likely following ingestion of first-generation antihistamines than second-generation antihistamines. In severe overdose, respiratory depression may develop.

CNS excitation has been reported in children and in young animals, and may include hyperactivity, anxiety, aggression, or seizures.

Anticholinergic effects are similar to those seen in atropine poisoning and include disorientation, hyperthermia, tachycardia, arrhythmia, xerostomia, hypertension, and mydriasis.

Diagnostic Aids

There are no specific clinical pathology findings. Antihistamines or their metabolites can be measured in serum or urine, but toxic levels are not defined.

Treatment

Activated charcoal, subject to the caveats and contraindications described in Chapter 3, Emergency Care and Stabilization of the Poisoned Patient, may be administered to adsorb antihistamines. Otherwise, treatment is supportive, with particular attention to control of seizures, maintenance of respiratory function, and treatment of arrhythmias. Mild to moderate arrhythmia may respond to fluid therapy alone. Monitor acid—base and electrolyte status, blood pressure, and body temperature. Intravenous fluid therapy should be instituted to promote urine production and elimination of antihistamines or their metabolites.

Prognosis

Prognosis depends on the dose and the aggressiveness of supportive therapy. Clinical signs may persist for up to 72 hours, although most animals show clinical improvement within 24 hours. Seizures or coma signify a guarded prognosis.

Necropsy

There are no specific lesions. Fresh tissue samples for confirmation of diagnosis should include liver, kidney, and urine.

Aspirin

The information in this section also applies to other salicylates such as methyl salicylate (oil of wintergreen).

Absorption, Distribution, Metabolism, and Excretion

Aspirin is readily absorbed from both the stomach and the small intestine, with a T_{max} between 0.5 and 3 hours. It is 50%—70% protein-bound in serum, principally to albumin, and distributed widely in the body. Aspirin is conjugated with either glycine or glucuronic acid and excreted in the urine.

Because of their limited capacity for glucuronidation, cats excrete salicylates very slowly when compared with other species, and are at particular risk of toxicity. Cats have been shown to be able to tolerate 25 mg/kg of aspirin every 48 hours for up to 4 weeks, but 325 mg bid may be lethal in to cats.

Mode(s) of Action

Aspirin is a cyclooxygenase (COX) inhibitor, reducing prostaglandin and thromboxane synthesis. Acetylation of platelet COX inhibits platelet aggregation. Aspirin also uncouples mitochondrial oxidative phosphorylation, leading to hyperthermia.

Aspirin may cause gastric mucosal damage, leading to gastric ulcers. COX inhibition may also lead to renal medullary ischemia.

At high doses, aspirin inhibits glycolysis, leading to metabolic acidosis. Hepatic toxicity from aspirin is observed at excessive doses, particularly in cats.

Clinical Signs

Clinical signs are those of vomiting, anorexia, depression, pyrexia, metabolic acidosis with compensatory respiratory alkalosis, and hepatotoxicity. Seizures have been reported in dogs with salicylate toxicosis.

Diagnostic Aids

Clinical pathology may reveal metabolic acidosis, elevated serum sodium, decreased serum potassium, thrombocytopaenia, Heinz body anemia, and elevated liver enzymes. Oliguria may be present.

Endoscopy may confirm gastric irritation with or without ulceration.

Salicylates are readily measured in serum or urine, but toxic levels are not defined for domestic animals.

Treatment

Salicylates are absorbed by activated charcoal, which should be administered if exposure is recent (see Chapter 3: Emergency Care and Stabilization of the Poisoned Patient). Intraveous fluid therapy with sodium bicarbonate, 1−3 mequiv./L, should be instituted to correct metabolic acidosis, to maintain renal throughput, and to promote alkaline urine in order to enhance salicylate excretion. The animal on fluid therapy should be subject to monitoring for pulmonary edema. Furosemide may be administered to promote diuresis if there is evidence of pulmonary edema. Measures to cool the hyperthermic patient are addressed in Chapter 3, Emergency Care and Stabilization of the Poisoned Patient. Histamine-receptor antagonists such as cimetidine may be administered to reduce acid secretion by the stomach, and sucralfate may be administered if gastric irritation or ulceration is present. Blood transfusion may be indicated in severe anemia.

Prognosis

Prognosis is poor if gastric perforation occurs, if hepatitis is severe or if renal papillary necrosis develops. Nonperforating gastric lesions usually resolve.

Necropsy

Lesions may include gastric irritation with or without ulceration, toxic hepatitis, and renal medullary necrosis.

Decongestants

Decongestants sold OTC generally fall into one of two classes; the imidazoline derivative class and the ephedrine class.

Of the imidazoline derivatives, oxymetazoline and xylometazoline are used in OTC topical nasal decongestants in Australia and New Zealand, while tetrahydrozoline and naphazoline are present in some ocular preparations.

The ephedrine class include ephedrine and pseudoephedrine. Quantities of these active ingredients are subject to controls because they can be used in the manufacture of metamphetamine.

Absorption, Distribution, Metabolism, and Excretion

Imidazoline compounds are weakly basic and lipophillic. They are rapidly absorbed, with high bioavailability, from the gastrointestinal tract, and are widely distributed throughout the body. They cross the blood—brain barrier. They undergo some hepatic metabolism but large proportions of the ingested dose may be excreted unchanged in the urine. In humans the elimination half-life is 2—4 hours for tetrahydrozoline, 5—8 hours for oxymetazoline, and 10—12 hours for xylometazoline.

Ephedrine and pseudoephedrine are also rapidly and extensively absorbed, and widely distributed including into milk. They undergo limited hepatic metabolism but are largely excreted unchanged in the urine. Urinary excretion is enhanced by urinary acidification.

Mode of Action

Imidazoline derivatives are sympathomimetic agents which act almost exclusively on α-adrenergic receptors. Their therapeutic action is to cause vasoconstriction in nasal mucosa. Ephedrine and pseudoephedrine, in contrast, have both α-adrenergic and β-adrenergic effects.

Clinical Signs

Clinical signs of imidazoline derivative toxicity in dogs develop in 0.5—4 hours of ingestion and include vomiting, depression, weakness, anxiety/hyperactivity, panting, and bradycardia with or without cardiac arrhythmia. Capillary refill time is often impaired and there may be increased respiratory sounds.

Clinical signs of toxicosis due to ephedrine or pseudoephedrine include mydriasis, vomiting, tachycardia, agitation/hyperactivity, hypertension, sinus arrhythmia, tremor, and hyperthermia. Doses of $10-12$ mg/kg may be lethal in dogs.

Diagnostic Aids

Analysis of serum or urine may confirm exposure, but toxic levels are not defined for domestic animals.

Treatment

Imidazoline Derivatives

Decontamination is unlikely to be useful because of the rapid absorption and onset of clinical signs. An intravenous fluid line should be placed, and used to administer 0.02 mg/kg atropine if bradycardia develops. Diazepam at up to 0.5 mg/kg IV may be used to treat CNS signs. Serum electrolytes should be monitored and corrected as necessary. Yohimbine, which is a specific α_2-adrenergic antagonist, may be administered at 0.1 mg/kg IV, and can be repeated in $2-3$ hours as necessary.

Ephedrine and Pseudoephedrine

Administration of activated charcoal may be helpful if ingestion was very recent and the patient is asymptomatic. An intravenous fluid line should be established. CNS signs may be treated with barbiturates, but diazepam is contraindicated and phemothiazine derivatives such as acepromazine and chlorpromazine should be used with caution because they can lower the sei- zure threshold and are also hypotensive. Cardiac function and blood pressure should be monitored. Tachycardia can be controlled with propranolol. Urinary acidification with ammonium chloride or ascorbic acid, subject to monitoring of acid–base balance, may enhance urinary excretion of pseudo- ephedrine. Tremors should be controlled to avoid myoglobinuria, and hyper- thermia treated to avoid disseminated intravascular coagulation.

Prognosis

Prognosis is variable depending on dose ingested and aggressiveness of ther- apy. Imidazoline toxicity in dogs should be considered to be a veterinary emergency. Clinical course of ephedrine or pseudoephedrine toxicosis may be protracted, lasting up to 4 days.

Necropsy

There are no characteristic lesions on necropsy.

H₂-Receptor Antagonists

These drugs are used to treat erosive lesions of the esophagus and stomach. H_2-receptor antagonists approved for use in Australia and/or New Zealand include cimetidine, ranitidine, nizatidine, and famotidine.

Absorption, Distribution, Metabolism, and Excretion

These drugs are typically rapidly absorbed, with a T_{max} within 3 hours. They are widely distributed in the body and metabolized in the liver. With the exception of cimetidine, they are excreted in the urine. Cimetidine is excreted in feces. They have a short elimination half-life.

Mode(s) of Action

Drugs in this class act on the H_2 receptors of the parietal cells of the gastric mucosa, reducing gastric acid secretions.

Clinical Signs

These drugs have a wide margin of safety when ingested. Clinical signs are generally limited to vomiting, diarrhea, anorexia, and xerostomia. The oral lethal dose of famotidine in dogs is greater than 2 g/kg, and that of nizatidine, greater than 800 mg/kg.

Diagnostic Aids

There are no specific diagnostic aids.

Treatment

Treatment is symptomatic and supportive.

Prognosis

Prognosis is generally excellent.

Necropsy

No specific lesions would be expected.

Insect Repellents

The most significant insect repellent toxicity problem in small animals arises from DEET but it should be recognized that a wide range of plant oils used as insect repellents, including citronella oil, are hepatotoxic to cats. Plant-derived oils should never be applied to the fur of a cat.

Absorption, Distribution, Metabolism, and Excretion of Diethyl Toluamide

DEET is readily absorbed through the skin and widely distributed systemically. It may be persistent in the skin. It appears to be primarily excreted by the renal route.

Mode(s) of Action

The toxic mechanism is not well understood.

Clinical Signs

Dermal applications of DEET to domestic pets have been associated with dermal and ocular reactions. Repeated dermal applications of DEET to horses have been associated with sweating, irritation, and exfoliation.

Oral administration of DEET to dogs and cats has led to vomiting, anorexia, excitement, ataxia, tremors, seizures, hypotension, and bradycardia.

DEET may also increase the dermal absorption of some chemicals with which it is delivered.

Diagnostic Aids

DEET may be present in urine or blood, but toxic levels are not well established for domestic animals.

Treatment

Activated charcoal may be useful following recent DEET ingestion. Bathing with a mild detergent may be helpful in dermal exposure. Seizures should be controlled with diazepam or barbiturates. Monitor cardiac function and blood pressure, and treat as necessary.

Prognosis

Prognosis is generally favorable.

Necropsy

Lesions of DEET toxicity in domestic animals are not defined.

Loperamide

Loperamide is a weak opioid used as an antidiarrheal agent in human beings and dogs, and is sometimes used in cats although it may cause excitement in cats.

Toxicity may occur in dogs, usually as a result of consuming large quantities of loperamide formulated for human use. Collies appear to have a particular susceptibility.

Absorption, Distribution, Metabolism, and Excretion

Systemic absorption of loperamide is low in human beings but appears to be higher in domestic animals. Although loperamide is not considered to penetrate the blood−brain barrier to any significant extent in human beings, clinical signs of toxicity in cats and dogs are those of an effect on the central nervous system. Loperamide is metabolized in the liver and excreted in the feces.

Mode(s) of Action

Loperamide binds to the opiate receptor in the intestinal wall and inhibits the release of acetylcholine and prostaglandins, resulting in reduced peristalsis and increased intestinal transit time. Loperamide also increases the tone of the anal sphincter.

Clinical Signs

Cats may become agitated at therapeutic doses.

Clinical signs of poisoning in dogs, particularly Collie breeds, are those of sedation, stupor, and coma, as well as miosis, bradycardia, respiratory depression, and hypothermia. Prolonged use of loperamide in dogs has been associated with hemorrhagic diarrhea.

Diagnostic Aids

There are no specific diagnostic aids.

Treatment

Activated charcoal should not administered because it may exacerbate constipation.

If miosis and/or nervous signs are present, opioid reversal with naloxone, 0.04−1.0 mg/kg IV, IM, or SC, generally results in prompt response. It may be necessary to administer repeat doses of naloxone.

Prognosis

Prognosis is generally good.

Necropsy

There are no specific lesions on necropsy.

Mineral Supplements

The reader is referred to Chapter 14, Metals. The most common problem is iron toxicosis from ingestion of iron tablets.

Paracetamol

Paracetamol is known as acetaminophen in the USA.

Absorption, Distribution, Metabolism, and Excretion

Paracetamol is rapidly absorbed after ingestion, and metabolized in the liver by a variety of pathways. At low doses, metabolism is primarily by conjugation with glucuronic acid or sulfates. However, the capacity of these pathways is limited, particularly in cats which have significantly lower glucuronidation capacity than other domestic species. When these conjugation pathways are saturated, metabolism through N-hydroxylation leads to the formation of toxic metabolites, including the hepatotoxic metabolite N-acetyl-p-benzoquinoneimine. This metabolite may be detoxified by conjugation with glutathione, glutathione stores are limited and readily depleted when large amounts of N-acetyl-p-benzoquinoneimine are generated.

Mode(s) of Action

N-Acetyl benzoquinoneimine covalently binds to cellular proteins and damages cellular membranes. Furthermore, glutathione depletion increases the susceptibility of cells to oxidative injury. In dogs the primary target organ is the liver, whereas in cats, the primary target cells are erythrocytes. Feline erythrocytes are particularly susceptible to oxidative injury, leading to methemoglobinemia, than those of other species because feline hemoglobin molecules have eight sulfhydryl groups rather than four as in other species.

The lethal dosage in cats is in the rage of 50–100 mg/kg while that for dogs is around 600 mg/kg.

Clinical Signs

In dogs the clinical signs are usually those of hepatic injury and necrosis, although at high doses methemoglobinemia may also develop. Clinical signs include vomiting, anorexia, tachycardia, tachypnea, and abdominal pain. Mucous membranes may be cyanotic, or later, icteric. Edema of the face and paws are commonly observed.

Clinical signs in cats include depression, vomiting, hypothermia, cyanotic mucous membranes, edema of face and paws, and dyspnea. Edematous face and paws may be accompanied by pruritis and lacrimation. Icterus may be present but is more commonly a result of hemolysis than of hepatotoxicity. Hepatotoxicosis appears to be more common in male cats than in females.

Cyanosis is generally an early sign. Hemaglobinuria or hematuria is evidence that the blood methemoglobin is 20% or greater.

Diagnostic Aids

Clinical pathology findings include methemoglobinemia, hemolytic anemia, hemoglobinuria, decreased PCV, elevations in serum ALT, AST and bilirubin, and decreases in serum cholesterol, albumin, and BUN. Cats in particular may have Heinz body anemia. In severe hepatoxicity, increases in prothrombin time and activated partial thromboplastin time may develop.

If measurement of reduced glutathione in erythrocytes is available, this will be decreased.

Exposure to paracetamol can be confirmed through analysis of plasma, serum, or urine, but toxic levels are not well defined for domestic animals.

Treatment

Administration of activated charcoal may reduce absorption of paracetamol if ingestion is very recent.

Antidotal therapy with *N*-acetylcysteine is directed toward repletion of glutathione stores in the liver. *N*-Acetyl cysteine is administered orally or intravenously at a dose of 140 mg/kg, followed by doses of 70 mg/kg every 6 hours for five to seven treatments. *N*-Acetylcysteine should be administered regardless of time since ingestion of paracetamol.

An alternative treatment, if *N*-acetyl cysteine is not available, is *S*-adenosylmethionine. The suggested treatment regime for dogs is 40 mg/kg orally, followed by 20 mg/kg every 24 hours for 9 days, while a tentative regime for cats is 180 mg orally, every 12 hours for 3 days, followed by 90 mg orally every 12 hours for 14 days.

Another treatment regime that has been shown to have beneficial effects is sodium sulfate at 50 mg/kg IV, every 4 hours for six treatments, in a 1.6% solution.

Reduction of methemoglobin to hemoglobin may be promoted by oral administration of ascorbic acid at 30 mg/kg every 6 hours for six treatments, or methylene blue at 1 mg/kg IV, using a 1% solution, every 2 or 3 hours for up to three treatments. Methylene blue acts more rapidly than ascorbic acid.

Corticosteroids and antihistamines are contraindicated.

Prognosis

Paracetamol poisoning, particularly of cats, is a serious toxicosis and prognosis is guarded, although prompt and aggressive treatment improves the prognosis.

Necropsy

Lesions include methemoglobinemia and pulmonary edema. Dogs in particular may have congested and/or mottled livers and, on histopathology, centrilobular necrosis. Icterus may be present. Renal tubular degeneration has also been observed in dogs. Focal lymphoid necrosis has been reported.

NSAIDs (Other Than Aspirin and Paracetamol)

NSAIDs other aspirin and paracetamol include ibuprofen, naproxen, ketoprofen, phenylbutazone, piroxicam, meloxicam, and a number of other NSAIDs for human and/or veterinary use. Some NSAIDs are available OTC while others are prescription-only. For the sake of simplicity, they are covered together in this section.

Absorption, Distribution, Metabolism, and Excretion

NSAIDs are generally weak acids. Absorption after ingestion is generally rapid and complete. Most NSAIDs are highly protein-bound in circulation, and may be potentiated by agents that displace them from protein binding sites, such as sulfonamides. NSAIDs are generally metabolized in the liver, with excretion of metabolites in the urine.

Mode(s) of Action

NSAIDs are COX inhibitors that decrease prostaglandin levels. This can lead to reduced blood flow to susceptible tissues including the renal medullae and papillae, and the gastric mucosa. Other target organs include liver, hematopoietic system, hemostatic system, and central nervous system.

Clinical Signs

Clinical signs are usually those of gastrointestinal injury, although renal injury may also develop at higher doses. Early clinical signs are those of anorexia, depression, vomiting, abdominal pain, ataxia, and stupor or coma. Gastric ulcers may develop, resulting in melena. Oliguria and azotemia indicate renal degeneration and necrosis. Hypotension may develop.

Liver toxicity may be manifested as icterus and elevated liver enzymes. Hematopoietic effects may include aplastic anemia, thrombocytopenia, and/ or neutropenia. Blood clotting may be impaired.

Administration of 100 mg/kg ibuprofen to the dog, or 50 mg/kg to the cat, is likely to cause moderate to severe toxicosis affecting the gastrointestinal tract. Dosages of 300 mg/kg to the dog, or 150 mg/kg to the cat, are likely to cause severe toxicosis with significant renal necrosis.

The lethal dose of naproxen in the dog is around 15 mg/kg.

Subchronic exposure to 44 mg/kg/day phenylbutazone has been lethal in cats.

Diagnostic Aids

Clinical pathology changes include hyperkalemia, azotemia, blood loss anemia, and metabolic acidosis. Increased clotting time may be evident.

Analysis of plasma or urine may confirm exposure, but toxic levels are not well defined for domestic animals.

Treatment

Misoprostol inhibits the gastrointestinal toxicity of NSAIDs. A suggested treatment regime for dogs is 2.5 µg/kg orally, every 8 hours. An intravenous fluid line should be established to maintain urinary output, to prevent or treat hypotension, and to enable administration of bicarbonate to treat metabolic acidosis. Administration of bicarbonate may also enhance urinary elimination of NSAIDs.

Monitor for hyperkalemia and treat as necessary using 20% dextrose solution at 1 mL/kg IV, with or without insulin. If there is evidence of impending hyperkalaemic heart failure, slow IV administration of calcium gluconate, 0.5−1.0 mL/kg in 10% solution, is indicated.

Dopamine may be administered IV if fluids alone do not correct hypotension and/or oliguria.

Treatment of gastric ulcers may include cimetidine, sucralfate, or a combination of the two. An alternative approach for dogs, but not cats, is omeprazole. The dosage of cimetidine for the dog or cat is 10 mg/kg every 6−8 hours, either IV, IM or orally, unless renal failure is evident, in which case the dose should be 2.5 mg/kg every 12 hours. Sucralfate is administered orally every 8−12 hours, 0.5−1.0 g for the dog and 0.25 g for the cat.

It may be necessary to assist ventilation in the severely poisoned animal. Anemia, whether aplastic or due to blood loss, may require correction by blood transfusion.

Prognosis

Prognosis is guarded, but may be improved by aggressive therapy.

Necropsy

Gross findings on necropsy include gastric ulcers and intestinal inflammation. At high doses there may be visible renal papillary necrosis.

Opioid Cough Suppressants

Examples of opioid cough suppressants are dextromethorphan and pholcodine.

Absorption, Distribution, Metabolism, and Excretion

These cough suppressants are rapidly absorbed by the oral route, and cross the blood−brain barrier to raise the cough threshold centrally. Both are metabolized in the liver with metabolites excreted in the urine.

Mode(s) of Action

Pholcodine and dextromethorphan act centrally to raise the cough threshold.

Clinical Signs

Overdoses can affect the gastrointestinal tract and/or the central nervous system.

Gastrointestinal signs include nausea, vomiting, and either constipation or diarrhea.

Animals may be drowsy and ataxic with respiratory depression, but on the other hand they may exhibit agitation and disorientation. These clinical signs may be related to the dissociative euphoriac and mildly hallucinogenic effects reported in people who deliberately overdose on dextromethorphan for recreational reasons.

Diagnostic Aids

A positive response to opioid assay of the plasma or urine confirms exposure.

Treatment

Treatment is supportive. Naloxone may be used to reverse severe clinical signs.

Prognosis

Prognosis is generally favorable.

Vitamins

The risk of vitamin overdose by accidental ingestion of vitamin supplements is low. Although the toxicity of Vitamin A, particularly to cats, is well known by veterinarians, it is unlikely to result from a single acute dose. The greater risk is from Vitamin D. The reader is referred to the section on cholecalciferol in Chapter 10, Vertebrate Pesticides.

Zinc Oxide

Zinc oxide is often included in nappy rash creams, creams for treatment of mild skin abrasions, or sunscreens.

Clinical Signs

Ingestion of zinc oxide causes gastrointestinal irritation, manifested as vomiting and diarrhea, but does not usually lead to the effects on liver, kidney and blood that result from ingestion of elemental zinc.

Facial edema, consistent with hypersensitivity, has been reported in some dogs.

Treatment
Treatment is supportive. Hypersensitivity reactions respond to antihistamines.

Prognosis
Prognosis is favorable.

ALTERNATIVE MEDICINES

Introduction

Alternative medicines are popular with consumers who erroneously suppose that "natural" substances are sure to be less toxic than chemicals synthesized by mankind. These remedies may be administered to animals by misguided owners, or may be voluntarily eaten by animals that gain access to them.

General concerns about alternative medicines, which apply equally to human use and veterinary use, include the following:

- Lack of evidence of the claimed therapeutic effect.
- Botanical misindentification or mislabeling, resulting in consumption of toxic plants rather than the intended species.
- The absence of Good Manufacturing Practice in processing, particularly the lack of quality control to prevent the contamination of natural remedies with microorganisms, bacterial or fungal toxins, or toxic metals.
- Lack of standardization of the quantity of active constituent present.
- Lack of preclinical and clinical toxicity testing, including lack of testing for genotoxicity or for developmental and reproductive toxicity.
- Interaction of herbal remedies with prescribed or OTC pharmaceuticals.

These concerns are not merely theoretical, but based on numerous real-life examples.

As a generalization, homeopathic and Bach flower remedies may be assumed to be nontoxic, although also lacking in any therapeutic effect. Also as a generalization the topical use of any oil, including essential oils, should be avoided in the cat, because of the risk of ingestion following self-grooming.

Alternative medicines covered in this section include the following:

5-Hydroxytryptophan (*Griffonia* extract)
Artemisia absinthium (absinthe; wormwood)
Aconite
Aloe

Aristolochia
Black cohosh
Bladderwrack, and other kelp and seaweed products
Camphor
Chromium piconolate
Citrus oils
Comfrey
Dong quai
Echinacea
Ephedra (Ma Huang)
Essential oils, general
Garlic
Gingko
Golden seal (*Hydrastis*)
Guarana
Kava kava
Melaleuca oil (tea tree oil)
Oil of wintergreen
Pennyroyal oil
St. John's Wort (*Hypericum*)
Saw palmetto (*Serenoa repens*)
Uva ursi (*Arctostaphylos*)
Valerian

This is not intended to be an exhaustive list. The reader is also referred to Chapter 24, Poisonous Plants, because some herbs used in herbal remedies are covered in that chapter.

5-Hydroxytryptophan (*Griffonia* Extract)

A number of cases of intoxication with this alternative medicine have been reported in dogs. Clinical signs included vomiting, diarrhea, depression, ataxia, hyperesthesia, hyperthermia, tremors, and seizures. This remedy is believed to increase serotonin levels in the brain. The ASPCA Animal Poison Control Centre estimated that the oral toxic threshold is 23.6 mg/kg, and the minimum lethal dose is 128 mg/kg, but these figures are based on a small number of cases.

Artemisia absinthium (Absinthe; Wormwood)

The name wormwood is derived from historical use of *A. absinthium* as a treatment for intestinal worms, and some people still attempt to use it for this purpose in dogs. Wormwood oil may also be applied as a dermal insecticide or for treatment of skin disorders. The active principles are α-thujone and β-thujone, which cause seizures in animals. Consumption of the liqueur absinthe has been associated with delirium and hallucinations in human beings.

Aconite

Aconite, derived from *Aconitum* root, was traditionally used for topical analgesia, as well as for neuralgia, asthma, and cardiac disease. Toxic principles include aconine, aconitine, picraconitine, and napelline, which increase the passage of sodium through sodium channels. However, acute toxicosis can be induced in human beings by approximately 1 g of plant material. Principal clinical signs are hypotension and slow respiration.

Aloe

The leaf gel of various species of *Aloe* is popular as a topical treatment for minor skin disorders such as dry skin, grazes, or sunburn. However, the latex from cells immediately below the skin of the leaves contains chemicals that are extremely irritating to the gastrointestinal tract. Inadvertent consumption of aloe preparations intended for topical use may result in severe gastrointestinal discomfort and diarrhea.

Aristolochia

The genus *Aristolochia* gained notoriety among toxicologists when a member of the species was inadvertently included in a weight loss medication made from Chinese herbs, in the place of a nontoxic species. A number of consumers of the medication developed renal failure and there were some mortalities. Besides being nephrotoxic, aristolochic acid is also carcinogenic and mutagenic, and some of the people who escaped fatal nephrotoxicity have subsequently developed urothelial malignancies. The use of herbal remedies containing *Aristolochia* species is widespread in Taiwan, and Taiwan also has the highest incidence of urothelial cancer in the world. All herbal remedies containing members of this genus should be considered toxic and carcinogenic.

Black Cohosh

This may be derived from the genera *Cimicifuga* or *Actaea*. Toxic effects reported in human beings include bradycardia and convulsions.

Bladderwrack, and Other Kelp and Seaweed Products

Seaweeds generally are high in iodine, and may cause congenital hypothyroidism in the offspring of pregnant female animals. This because the thyroid gland responds to high I exposure by halting the organification of I, a response called the Wolff−Chaikoff effect. In adult animals, the Wolff−Chaikoff effect only lasts a few days, but in fetuses and neonates, the normal escape from the Wolff−Chaikoff effect is lacking, and so they remain unable to use iodine to form thyroid hormones, and become hypothyroid.

Bladderwrack and other seaweeds are also high in sodium.

Camphor Oil

Camphor oil may be used in aromatherapy, or as a topical agent. Camphor oil is readily absorbed following ingestion or dermal exposure. Human toddlers have been fatally poisoned by as little as 1 mL of camphor oil, and chronic exposure in children has been associated with neurotoxicity and hepatotoxicity. Clinical signs reported in human beings include emesis, abdominal pain, excitement, tremors, and seizures, followed by coma and apnea.

Chromium Picolinate

Excessive intake is associated with thrombocytopaenia, renal failure, and hepatitis in human beings.

Citrus Oils

Citrus oils or their extracts, D-limonene or linalool, have insecticidal properties. Toxicity and fatalities have been reported in cats following the use of citrus oil, D-limonene or linalool, most commonly when cats were treated at the dosages recommended for dogs. Piperonyl butoxide potentiates toxicity due to those chemicals. The toxic dose for cats is only about five times the recommended dose for therapeutic effect. Clinical signs include hypersalivation, tremors, ataxia, weakness, hypotension, hypothermia, general paralysis, and coma.

Comfrey

Comfrey has traditionally been used topically on wounds or hemorrhoids, and occasionally internally as a "blood purifier." However, comfrey contains pyrrolizidine alkaloids that are hepatoxic and carcinogenic. Systemic exposure to pyrrolizidine alkaloids following dermal application of comfrey been demonstrated in rats. Comfrey is not safe for consumption or topical application.

Echinacea

Effects of overconsumption of Echinacea may include fever, dizziness, and weakness.

Ephedra

Extracts of plants of this genus have been used in weight loss formulations. The plants contain ephedrine and pseudoephedrine, which are sympathomimetics. Toxic effects in dogs include vomiting, agitation, tachycardia, cardiac arrhythmia, hyperthermia, tremors, and seizures.

Essential Oils, General

Aspiration of vomitus containing essential oils may lead to pneumonia. Other general clinical signs include circulatory collapse, emesis, diarrhea, coma, convulsions, and evidence of renal toxicity including hematuria and dysuria. The use of essential oils on domestic pets should be strongly discouraged because of the risk that the animal will groom itself. Milk may be useful to allay gastric irritation. Fluid diuresis may be indicated to maintain renal throughput but may be hazardous in the first 24 hours because of risk of pulmonary edema.

See also specific notes on citrus oils, *Melaleuca* oil, oil of wintergreen, and pennyroyal oil.

Garlic (*Allium sativum*)

Garlic has been promoted for "natural" flea control in cats, and has been used to inhibit platelet aggregation in human beings. The toxic principles are disulfides, such as allicin, that denature hemoglobin, leading to hemolysis and Heinz body anemia. Chronic use of garlic in dogs has been shown to cause anemia. Because of the susceptibility of cat hemoglobin to oxidative damage, cats are particularly susceptible to toxic effects of garlic. Clinical signs include weakness, polypnea, icterus, cyanosis, and hemoglobinuria.

Topical application of garlic oil may cause moderate to severe irritation. Garlic inhibits spermatogenesis in the rat.

Gingko

Toxic effects of Gingko reported in human beings have included nausea, vomiting, diarrhea, seizures and retrobulbar or vitreous hemorrhage.

Golden Seal (*Hydrastis*)

Toxic effects in human beings have included cardiac toxicity and convulsions.

Guarana

Guarana contains methylxanthine alkaloids (q.v.) including caffeine, theobromine, and theophylline.

Kava Kava

Kava kava (*Piper methysticum*) is gaining popularity as a treatment for stress and anxiety, but is associated with idiosyncratic hepatotoxicity in human beings. The safety of kava kava in domestic animals is unknown.

Melaleuca Oil (Tea Tree Oil)

Toxicosis from the use of this oil has been reported in dogs and cats. Systemic toxicity has resulted from dermal exposure as well as from ingestion. Clinical signs in cats include ataxia, hypothermia, agitation, tremor, and coma. Clinical signs in dogs include depression, ataxia, and partial paralysis. *Melaleuca* oil may also cause skin rashes.

Oil of Wintergreen

Oil of wintergreen contains a glycoside that is readily hydrolyzed to methyl salicylate, resulting in toxicity similar to that caused by aspirin (q.v.)

Pennyroyal Oil

Pennyroyal oil has a history of use as a flea treatment. Dermal application of 2 g/kg pennyroyal oil to a dog resulted in vomiting, depression, diarrhea, epistaxis, seizures, and death. On necropsy the dog was found to have massive hepatocellular necrosis.

St. John's Wort (*Hypericum*)

Toxic effects reported in human beings include mania, neuropathy, sedation, primary photosensitivity, and possible serotonin syndrome.

Saw Palmetto (*Serenoa repens*)

Saw palmetto may cause toxic hepatitis.

Uva Ursi (*Arctostaphylos*)

Uva ursi has caused cyanosis, convlusions, renal damage, and liver damage in human beings.

Valerian

Valerian is associated with headache, tremor, cramps, and possible liver damage in human beings.

RECREATIONAL AND ILLICIT DRUGS

Amphetamines

Alternative Names

Numerous amphetamines have been marketed as prescription drugs at various times for the treatment of Attention Deficit Disorder or narcolepsy, as stimulants or as weight loss aids. In addition, illegal synthesis of methamphetamine, in particular, is widespread. Besides amphetamine and methamphetamine, prescription amphetamines have included benzphetamine, dextroamphetamine, diethylpropion, fenfluramine, mazindol, methylphenidate, pemoline, phendimetrazine, phenmetrazine, and phentamine. Substituted amphetamines used for illegal recreational use include "Ecstasy" (3,4-methylenedioxymethamphetamine), 3,4-methylenedioxyamphetamine, and cathinone (Khat). Cathinone is a natural metabolite of the shrub *Catha edulis*.

Circumstances of Poisoning

Poisoning is most likely to be seen in domestic pets that consume prescription amphetamines or illicitly prepared amphetamines.

Absorption, Distribution, Metabolism, and Excretion

Amphetamines as a class are rapidly absorbed by the oral route, with C_{max} within 3 hours of ingestion, except in the case of a sustained-release prescription amphetamine. Amphetamines are metabolized in the liver, although some metabolites may be pharmacologically active. Both the parent compound and metabolites are excreted in the urine. Elimination is increased in acidic urine, with the result that the half-life in dogs is approximately 3.5—6 hours, significantly shorter than that in humans.

Mode(s) of Action

Amphetamines act as stimulants on both the central and peripheral nervous system. Their central stimulatory effect includes agonist activity on dopamine excitatory receptors. Peripherally, they act as stimulants both by direct action on α- and β-adrenergic receptors, and indirectly by promoting release of noradrenalin from adrenergic axon terminals. They also inhibit metabolism of catecholamines by inhibiting monoamine oxidase.

Clinical Signs

Clinical signs include agitation, hyperactivity, tachypnea, mydriasis, hyperreflexia, hyperesthesia, hyperthermia, hypertension, tachycardia with arrhythmia, and tremors or seizures. Dehydration is commonly observed. Vomiting, diarrhea, and abdominal pain may occur. Methylphenidate (Ritalin) may cause prolonged painful penile erections in male dogs. Amphetamines increase the sphincter tone of the urinary bladder, resulting in acute urinary retention.

Occasional animals respond to amphetamines with depression and bradycardia.

Diagnostic Aids

Amphetamines or their metabolites may be present in blood, urine, or saliva, although levels are not well correlated to severity of toxicosis.

Lactic acidosis and hypoglycemia are typically present. Both hyperkalemia and hypokalemia have been reported.

Treatment

Gastric lavage is unlikely to be helpful because amphetamines are rapidly absorbed. Amphetamines are adsorbed by activated charcoal, and it may be useful subject to the limitations and precautions stated in Chapter 3, Emergency Care and Stabilization of the Poisoned Patient.

Seizures should be controlled by means of propofol or a barbiturate. Benzodiazapines, including diazepam, are not recommended because they may exacerbate the neurological effects of amphetamines. Intravenous chlorpromazine has been shown experimentally to control amphetamine-induced excitation and seizures in dogs and is known to be an antagonist of dopamine excitatory receptors. Intravenous haloperidol is an alternative means of controlling hyperactivity.

A beta blocker such as propranolol may be required to control tachyarrhythmia, while lidocaine may be used to control ventricular dysrhythmia.

Body temperature should be monitored and hyperthermia treated with chilled intravenous fluid, ice-water enema, or cold packs or fans as required.

Intravenous fluids should be administered to relieve or prevent dehydration and to maintain renal throughput, particularly if there is evidence of myoglobinuria, with a urinary catheter placed to overcome urinary retention and prevent fatal hyperkalemia.

Although in the experimental situation urinary acidification may result in more rapid elimination of amphetamines, it is probably not important in domestic pets given their naturally acidic urinary pH. It should be considered only if acid–base balance can be closely monitored and if there is no evidence of myoglobinuria.

Prognosis

The oral LD_{50} of amphetamine sulfate in the dog is in the range of 20–27 mg/kg, while that of methamphetamine hydrochloride is 9–11 mg/kg.

Necropsy

There are usually no characteristic lesions, although rhabdomyolysis is a rare complication of severe poisoning. Myocardial infarctions have been reported in human beings with amphetamine poisoning. Amphetamines tend to be widely distributed in the body postmortem, but fresh liver, kidney, urine, and cardiac blood are recommended for postmortem confirmation.

Barbiturates

Alternative Names

There are numerous prescription barbiturates. Most barbiturate names end in "barbital" (e.g., pentobarbital, secobarbital) with the exceptions of thiamylal, thiopental, and methohexital. In addition, there are a range of euthanasia solutions in which a barbiturate is the sole or major active compound.

Sources

Barbiturates are both prescription drugs in human and veterinary medicine, and drugs of abuse.

Circumstances of Poisoning

Most veterinary barbiturate toxicoses, other than iatrogenic overdoses during veterinary treatment, occur in small animals and are the result of ingestion of human or veterinary prescription drugs. Ingestion of meat or other tissues from large animals that have been euthanased using barbiturates is also a significant cause of toxicoses. Veterinarians using barbiturates to terminate large animals are responsible for ensuring that the carcass is disposed of safely.

Absorption, Distribution, Metabolism, and Excretion

Barbiturates are readily absorbed orally and are initially widely distributed in the body, including the brain, before redistributing into adipose tissue. Barbiturates are metabolized by hepatic microsomal enzymes, and chronic use induces increased activity of these enzymes. Barbiturates are eliminated primarily in the urine. About 25%–50% of the barbiturate is eliminated unchanged in the urine.

Mode(s) of Action

Barbiturates activate inhibitory GABA receptors, and inhibit excitatory glutamate receptors. They can also inhibit the release of acetylcholine and noradrenalin. High doses of barbiturates cause central respiratory depression. In overdose, direct depression of cardiac contractility may result from effects on calcium and potassium channels. Barbiturates also cause hypotension, which can result in oliguria or anuria.

Clinical Signs

Clinical signs generally include depression, ataxia, disorientation, recumbency, stupor or coma, hypothermia, respiratory failure, and death. Both bradycardia and tachycardia have been reported. Marked hypotension is common.

Diagnostic Aids

Barbiturates and/or their metabolites can be detected in urine and blood.

Treatment

Activated charcoal, subject to the caveats and contraindications described in Chapter 3, Emergency Care and Stabilization of the Poisoned Patient, may be administered to adsorb barbiturates.

The major cause of death is respiratory depression. Respiratory function must be maintained, by mechanical assistance if required. Body temperature and cardiac function must also be monitored and maintained. Blood pressure, acid−base balance, and urinary output should be monitored. Intravenous fluid therapy with urinary catheterization should be established to maintain blood pressure and urinary throughput. Forced alkaline diuresis is indicated in severe barbiturate toxicosis.

Prognosis

Prognosis depends on the dose and the aggressiveness of supportive therapy.

Necropsy

There are no specific lesions. Fresh tissue samples for confirmation of diagnosis should include liver, kidney, and urine.

Benzodiazepines

Alternative Names

There are numerous prescription benzodiazepines in human and veterinary medicine, although not all of them are licensed in Australia and/or New Zealand. Prescription benzodiazapines include alprazolam, chlordiazepoxide, clobazam, clonazepam, chlorazepate, diazepam, estazolam, flunitrazepam, flurazepam, halazepam, lorazepam, midazolam, oxazepam, quazepam, temazepam, triazolam, zolazepam.

Circumstances of Poisoning

Poisoning most often occurs when domestic pets consume human prescription medications.

Absorption, Distribution, Metabolism, and Excretion

Benzodiazepines are rapidly absorbed from the gastrointestinal tract and are protein-bound in the circulation. They are metabolized in the liver, although some are metabolized to pharmacologically active metabolites with a greater half-life than the parent compound. They are conjugated with glucuronide and excreted in the urine. Because cats have limited capacity for glucuronidation relative to other species, the half-life of benzodiazepines in cats is significantly longer for any given compound than it is in dogs.

Mode(s) of Action

Benzodiazepine receptors are widely distributed in the body although the function of the receptors outside the CNS is unknown. Within the CNS, benzodiazepine receptors modulate GABA, which is an inhibitory neurotransmitter. It appears that benzodiazepines may also affect the activity of some other neurotransmitters.

Clinical Signs

Clinical signs of overdose generally include depression, ataxia, and disorientation. Severe toxicosis may feature hypothermia, stupor, or coma.

Diagnostic Aids

Samples for comfirmation of exposure in the live animal are blood and urine.

Treatment

Benzodiazepines are adsorbed by activated charcoal, but are rapidly absorbed from the gastrointestinal tract so activated charcoal is only indicated if ingestion is very recent. In severe toxicosis, flumazenil 0.1 mg/kg IV is indicated. Flumazenil is a competitive benzodiazepine blocker, but repeated doses may be required because it has a short half-life relative to most benzodiazepines. Body temperature should be monitored and maintained.

Prognosis

Prognosis is usually good provided adequate supportive care is given.

Necropsy

There are no characteristic lesions. Fresh samples for postmortem analysis are liver, kidney, and urine.

Cocaine

Source

Cocaine (benzoylmethylecgonine) is an alkaloid derived from the leaves of *Erythroxylon coca*, which grows in Mexico, South America, the West Indies, and Indonesia.

As in illicit drug, cocaine is often adulterated with other substances which may be inert (e.g., corn-starch, lactose, or sugar) or may have pharmacological/toxicological effects in their own right (e.g., lidocaine, amphetamines, caffeine, heroin, phencyclidine). The powdered form of cocaine is a water-soluble hydrochloride salt. "Free base" is pure cocaine in crystals. "Crack" cocaine refers to the cracking sound that large crystals ("rocks") of free base cocaine make when heated. Free base forms of cocaine can be taken orally or heated and inhaled.

Circumstances of Poisoning

Domestic pets may be exposed to cocaine by inhalation or by ingestion. Powdered cocaine adulterated with substances such as sugar or lactose may be palatable to dogs.

Absorption, Distribution, Metabolism, and Excretion

Cocaine is rapidly absorbed from mucosa. T_{max} for nasal inhaled cocaine occurs 15 minutes to 2 hours in human beings. Cocaine is hydrolyzed by serum esterases and is demethylated in the liver. Small proportions of unchanged cocaine, and a number of metabolites, are excreted in urine.

Mode of Action

Cocaine blocks the reuptake of noradrenalin and serotonin at adrenergic synapses, resulting in excessive levels of these neurotransmitters. In addition cocaine increases the response to catecholamines.

Clinical Signs

Clinical signs include agitation, hyperesthesia, mydriasis, hypersalivation, vomiting, tachycardia, tachyarrhythmia, ventricular premature contractions, tachypnea, tremors, and seizures.

Diagnostic Aids

Cocaine or metabolites may be detectable in serum and/or plasma, stomach contents or urine.

Treatment

Treatment is supportive. Decontamination is unlikely to be useful, given the very rapid absorption.

The sedative of choice is diazepam, although a barbiturate may be required in severe toxicosis.

Propanolol or other beta blocker may be indicated for tachyarrhythmia. An IV fluid line should be established to maintain renal throughput and support urinary elimination.

Acid—base balance and body temperature should be monitored and treated as necessary.

Prognosis

Prognosis is generally favorable provided supportive treatment is given.

Necropsy

There are no characteristic lesions. Fresh kidney or urine is most useful for postmortem confirmation.

Ethanol

Alternative Names

Alcohol.

Circumstances of Poisoning

Ethanol poisoning is fairly common in dogs and may arise from drinking alcoholic beverages, from eating fermented material in garbage, such as bread dough or rotten apples, or from drinking substances in which ethanol is the carrier solvent. Owners may offer alcohol to a dog as a joke, or as a home-made sedative (e.g., milk laced with brandy) on Guy Fawkes night to promote sleep.

Pigs, goats, and donkeys have been reported to enjoy alcoholic drinks such as beer. Inebriation has been reported in pigs and ruminants, but equids have extremely high levels of alcohol dehydrogenase in their livers and ingested ethanol is detoxified on first pass.

Absorption, Distribution, Metabolism, and Excretion

Absorption is rapid on an empty stomach, with clinical signs developing within 30 minutes, but may be substantially delayed if the stomach is full.

Ethanol is primarily metabolized in the liver to aldehyde by the enzyme alcohol dehydrogenase. Aldehyde is further metabolized by aldehyde dehydrogenase to acetate, which is eventually metabolized to carbon dioxide and water. A small proportion of ethanol is excreted unchanged in the urine and in exhaled air.

Mode(s) of Action

Ethanol is believed to inhibit NMDA glutamate receptors and cyclic GMP production in the brain.

Clinical Signs

Clinical signs usually include central nervous depression, ataxia, disorientation and apparent confusion, vomiting, sedation, hypothermia, and metabolic acidosis, although occasionally dogs become excited. Involuntary defecation or urination may occur. Bradycardia and depressed respiratory rate are common, as is dehydration.

Diagnostic Aids

Blood is the specimen of choice for confirmation of diagnosis in the live animal.

Hypoglycemia is a common finding.

Treatment

Treatment is supportive and includes fluid therapy and correction of hypoglycemia and/or acidosis if present. The animal should be monitored for cardiac and respiratory depression and for hypothermia.

It is common to see the advice given that a person who has gone to sleep while drunk should be kept warm and "allowed to sleep it off." This is dangerously flippant advice because the range of blood alcohol levels at which a person may be "passed out drunk" and the range of blood alcohol levels at which ethanol paralyses the respiratory center show considerable overlap in human beings. The same is likely to be true in animals. Although in human cases in which a person dies of acute ethanol poisoning and there is no evidence of choking on vomitus, the death is typically attributed to hypothermia, in fact it is quite possible that many of these deaths may be due to respiratory paralysis. For this reason an inebriated person or animal that has gone to sleep should not be simply covered with a blanket and left to "sleep it off" but treated as a patient with a life-threatening toxicosis.

Prognosis

Prognosis is generally good with thorough supportive care.

Necropsy

There are no characteristic lesions on necropsy.

Ketamine

Because ketamine is a commonly used veterinary drug, veterinarians are already familiar with the action, pharmacokinetics and effects of this drug. This entry is included only to remind veterinarians that ketamine is a popular recreational drug and that ketamine is chemically related to phencyclidine (q.v.) although substantially less potent and with a shorter half-life. Treatment of ketamine overdose is supportive, as for phencyclidine.

Lysergic Acid Diethylamide

Sources

Lysergic acid diethylamide (LSD) is readily synthesized in illicit laboratories, although it is generally a mix of four stereoisomers of which only one, L-iso LSD, has hallucinogenic activity and synthesis of "pure" LSD that is predominantly this isomer, with little of the other three, is technically difficult.

Dogs in particular may eat sufficient quantities of the seeds of Morning Glory (*Ipomea* spp.) to have apparent hallucinations. The form of lysergic acid in Morning Glory seeds is lysergic acid hydroxyethylamide, which is estimated to be only one-tenth as potent as LSD.

Circumstances of Poisoning

Dogs in particular may ingest LSD on impregnated blotter paper, in tablets or in gelatin squares, or may ingest Morning Glory seeds.

Absorption, Distribution, Metabolism, and Excretion

LSD is rapidly absorbed. T_{max} may occur within 30 minutes and is not greater than 5 hours. LSD is distributed in the circulation largely in the protein-bound form. In human beings, effects are first perceived approximately 40−60 minutes after ingestion, reach their maximum after 2−4 hours, and pass off after 6−8 hours. LSD is hydroxylated and conjugated with glucuronide in the liver, and primarily excreted in the bile. Elimination half-life is 2−5 hours.

Mode(s) of Action

LSD appears to act in multiple sites in the central nervous system, particularly at the serotonin (5-HT) receptors. However, other neurotransmitters, such as glutamate and dopamine, may also be involved.

Clinical Signs

Clinical signs reported in animals include mydriasis, apparent confusion and disorientation, ataxia. Animals may be depressed or excited. Dogs appear to hallucinate, growling and barking, and turning their heads as if to watch threats that apparently only they can see. Sudden displays of aggression toward a usually loved owner have been reported.

Diagnostic Aids

LSD may be detectable in serum, urine, or feces, although it is rapidly metabolized and levels are not well correlated to clinical effects.

Treatment

Treatment is supportive. Activated charcoal may be helpful in the asymptomatic patient that is known to have recently ingested a large number of Morning Glory seeds, but is contraindicated if clinical signs are already present and unlikely to be effective if the animal has ingested LSD as pills or on blotter paper or gelatin squares. Gastric lavage is also contraindicated because it is likely to exacerbate psychosis. Diazepam may be used if the animal is dangerously agitated. The animal should be kept calm and monitored for tachycardia and hyperthermia. Restraint should be the minimum required to keep the animal safe.

Prognosis

Prognosis depends on the dose ingested and the quality of supportive treatment.

Necropsy

There are no characteristic lesions.

Marijuana (Cannabis)

Sources

Marijuana consists of plant material, or extracts of plant material, from *Cannabis sativa*. The predominant active ingredient in marijuana is tetrahydrocannabinol (THC).

Circumstances of Poisoning

Small animal poisonings usually result from the pet eating a person's "stash" of marijuana.

In areas where *C. sativa* grows wild, cattle may consume the tops of plants, and this could also conceivably happen if cattle gained access to an illegal crop of *C. sativa*.

Dried plant material generally has a THC content of approximately 5%, while that of hashish, the dried resin from flower tops, can be up to 10% and hashish oil may comprise up to 20% THC.

Absorption, Distribution, Metabolism, and Excretion

THC is readily absorbed by the oral route and by inhalation. Oral absorption is increased if the material is consumed with food that has a high lipid content. THC is widely distributed in the body and is readily soluble into lipids including those of liver, brain, and adipose tissue. THC undergoes hepatic metabolism to 11-hydroxy-delta-9-THC, which is more potent than THC and, like THC, crosses the blood barrier. THC and its metabolites are largely excreted by the biliary route and may undergo enterohepatic circulation, while approximately 10% is excreted in urine. THC has a short plasma half-life, because it rapidly diffuses into lipid "sinks," but the biological half-life is prolonged.

Mode(s) of Action

There are two cannabinoid receptors, designated CB1 and CB2. CB1 is widely distributed in the brain, whereas CB2 has only been detected in peripheral tissues.

Clinical Signs

The most frequently reported clinical signs in dogs include depression, ataxia, dry mucous membranes, mydriasis, tremor, hypothermia, and bradycardia. Nystagmus has been observed in some cases. Some dogs become excited and appear to have hallucinations, and develop tachycardia, tachypnea and hyperthermia. Dogs may cycle between excitement and sedation.

Clinical signs reported in cattle that graze on high-THC hemp include moderate neurological signs and diarrhea.

Diagnostic Aids

The sample of choice from the live animal is urine.

Treatment

Multiple-dose activated charcoal may be given to interrupt enterohepatic cycling.

Treatment is supportive. Body temperature and cardiac function should be monitored. Diazepam should be given to those dogs that become excited.

Prognosis

The minimum lethal oral dose (LD_{10}) for THC in the dog is >3 g/kg, meaning that marijuana has a wide safety margin. Mortality is unlikely, but recovery may take 72 hours.

Necropsy

There are no characteristic lesions. Urine is the diagnostic sample of choice, but in light of the excellent prognosis and the slow elimination, a positive result on THC assay of the urine should be interpreted with caution, and consideration given to the possibility that the death was due to another xenobiotic consumed at the same time, or to another cause.

Methylxanthine Alkaloids

Caffeine is one of the most popular recreational drugs in the world. However, since most cases of methylxanthine alkaloid poisoning in veterinary practice are associated with the consumption of chocolate, methylxanthine alkaloid toxicosis is covered in Chapter 13, Household Foods and Products (q.v.).

Opioids

Sources

Opium, harvested from *Papaver somniferum*, contains at least 24 opium alkaloids, and a number of synthetic analogs have been developed. Opioids are classified as agonists, partial agonists, or antagonists based on their action on opioid receptors. Opioid agonists include codeine, diphenoxylate, etorphine, fentanyl, heroin, hydrocodone, hydromorphone, levorphanol, loperamide, methadone, oxycodone, oxymorphone, pethidine (meperidine), and propoxyphene. Partial agonists include buprenorphine, butophanol, nalbuphine, and pentazoncine. Antagonists include dipreorphine, nalorphine, naloxone, and naltrexone.

Circumstances of Poisoning

Most animal poisonings are the result of household pets consuming pharmaceuticals that contain opioids.

Absorption, Distribution, Metabolism, and Excretion

Opioids are generally readily absorbed and undergo rapid hepatic metabolism. Metabolic pathways vary depending on the specific opioid involved, but glucuronidation is a common step in metabolism. Cats, having relatively low activity of glucuronyl-St-transferase, are therefore relatively sensitive to opioids. Opioids are largely excreted in urine but some biliary excretion, with enterohepatic cycling, occurs.

Mode(s) of Action

Four major types of opioid receptor, and a number of subtypes, have been identified, and are widely distributed in the body. Opioids vary in their affinity and activity at different opioid receptors.

Clinical Signs

Clinical signs reported in dogs include salivation, vomiting, defecation, miosis, ataxia, and depression. In severe cases there may be hypothermia, respiratory depression, cyanosis, coma, and seizures may develop. Cats, in contrast, often exhibit excited behaviur.

Diagnostic Aids

Samples for opioid detection in the live patient include urine or serum. Administration of naloxone may also be used as a diagnostic test. Naloxone has a shorter half-life than many opioids and therefore the patient is likely to relapse.

Treatment

The most common cause of death in opioid toxicosis is respiratory depression. Assisted ventilation may be required. Naloxone at a dose of 0.01—0.02 mg/kg should be given, and may be administered IV, IM, or SC. Naloxone is generally effective for reversing respiratory depression but the patient may remain in a stupor.

The patient should be kept warm, and blood gases monitored.

Opioids tend to cause pylorospasm, with the result that gastric emptying is delayed. Gastric lavage may be considered, and activated charcoal may be administered, both procedures subject to the caveats and contraindications specified in Chapter 3, Emergency Care and Stabilization of the Poisoned Patient.

Prognosis

Prognosis depends on the dose ingested and the quality of supportive treatment.

Necropsy

There are no characteristic lesions. Fresh samples for confirmation of diagnosis include liver, kidney, and urine.

Phencyclidine

Alternative Names

1-[1-Phenylcyclohexyl] piperidine (PCP).

Circumstances of Poisoning

Animal poisoning may occur if household pets are given PCP or ingest a person's supply.

Absorption, Distribution, Metabolism, and Excretion

Being a weak base, PCP is poorly absorbed from the stomach but readily absorbed in the small intestine. Absorbed PCP is secreted in the stomach and then reabsorbed in the duodenum, leading to extensive recirculation. In humans, PCP takes effect in 30–60 minutes and effects may last up to 48 hours. PCP is lipophilic and readily distributes into the brain and into adipose tissue.

In dogs, most PCP undergoes hepatic metabolism whereas in cats, most PCP is excreted unchanged. Excretion is primarily renal.

Mode(s) of Action

PCP, like its analog ketamine, dissociates the somatosensory cortex from higher centers, although the precise mechanism is unclear. PCP blocks NMDA receptors and may also stimulate α-adrenergic and opiate receptors.

Clinical Signs

Clinical signs reported in dogs include mydriasis, hypersalivation, jaw snapping, hyperactivity, stereotypical circling, muscle rigidity, seizures, hypertension, tachycardia, and arrhythmia. Animals appear to succumb to cardiovascular and respiratory failure.

Diagnostic Aids

The diagnostic sample of choice from the live animal is urine.

Treatment

Animals should be kept in a quiet place, and stimulation avoided. Diazepam may be used to control excitement or seizures, or general anesthesia may be required. Activated charcoal is useful, subject to the caveats specified in Chapter 3, Emergency Care and Stabilization of the Poisoned Patient.

Fluid therapy to promote diuresis can increase the clearance of PCP. Urinary acidification may be helpful but should only be performed if acid–base status can be monitored, and is contraindicated if there is myoglobinuria.

Blood glucose and body temperature should be monitored and corrected as necessary.

Prognosis

Prognosis depends on the dose ingested, the severity of self-trauma or rhabdomyolysis at time of presentation, and the quality of supportive treatment.

Marked clinical signs occur in dogs at oral doses in the range of 2.5–10 mg/kg, and in the range of 1.1–12 mg/kg in cats. An oral dose of 25 mg/kg is lethal in most dogs.

Necropsy

There are no characteristic lesions. Fresh tissues for postmortem analytical toxicology include liver, kidney, urine, and adipose tissue.

Psilocybin

Alternative Names

Magic mushrooms.

The chemical name of Psilocybin is 4-phosphoryl0xy-*N,N*-dimethyltryptamine.

Sources

Mushrooms of the genus *Psilocybe* are found worldwide.

Appearance or Identification

Most species of *Psilocybe* are small mushrooms with brown caps. Hallucinogenic species typically have a blue-staining reaction when the fruit body is bruised.

Circumstances of Poisoning

Ingestion of psilocybin is most likely to occur in household pets who consume magic mushrooms collected or purchased by a person in the household. Voluntary ingestion by grazing animals seems to occur only when they are unable to avoid the mushrooms due to heavy infiltration of the pasture.

Absorption, Distribution, Metabolism, and Excretion

Oral absorption of pure psilocybin is approximately 50%, and it is absorbed rapidly. Most psilocybin is metabolized on first pass through the liver, with four metabolites, of which psilocin is the predominant, and possibly the only, hallucinogenic metabolite. It is thought that psilocybin itself is not hallucinogenic and that all the hallucinogenic activity is attributable to psilocin. Psilocin can be detected in plasma approximately 30 minutes after ingestion of psilocybin and is distributed throughout the body. T_{max} occurs after approximately 80 minutes in human beings. A small proportion of psilocybin is not converted to psilocin, but is excreted unchanged in the kidneys. Most excretion is of glucuronidated metabolites. In human beings, approximately the mean elimination of psilocin is 50 minutes, but there are considerable interindividual differences.

Mode(s) of Action

Psilocin is structurally similar to serotonin and has a high affinity for the 5-HT2A serotonin receptors in the brain, where it mimics the effects of serotonin (5-hydroxytryptamine or 5-HT). Psilocin also binds with less avidity to other serotonergic receptors.

Clinical Signs

Reported clinical signs in dogs include ataxia, aggression, barking, aggression, nystagmus, and pyrexia. Human beings experience hallucinations, hyperesthesia, incoordination, tachycardia, hypertension, mydriasis, and tremors.

Diagnostic Aids

Theoretically urine and serum would be samples of choice from the live animal, but analysis is not widely available.

Treatment

Treatment is supportive only. The animal should be kept safe from accidents, and body temperature monitored. The rapid absorption and short time to T_{max} mean that gastrointestinal decontamination is unlikely to be of any value.

Prognosis

Prognosis is excellent provided the animal is kept safe. Psilocybin has a large therapeutic index. Very little human mortality associated with psilocybin use has been reported, although some people have died or been injured in accidents as a result of a "bad trip." Of the rare cases in which trauma was not involved, most involved use of combinations of mind-altering substances means that it is difficult to determine which xenobiotic was responsible for death.

Necropsy

Death due to psilocybin is highly unlikely, unless due to trauma. There are no characteristic lesions. Kidney or urine may be collected fresh for postmortem confirmation of diagnosis.

Chapter 13

Household Foods and Products

INTRODUCTION

The following hazardous substances are addressed in this chapter:

- Agene
- *Allium* species
- Batteries
- Bleaches
- Boric acid
- Clay pigeons
- Deodorants/antiperspirants
- Disinfectants
  - Phenol disinfectants
  - Pine oil disinfectants
- Ethylene glycol
- Fertilizer
- Food waste
- Glow-in-the dark items
- Hops, spent
- Macadamia nuts
- Melamine
- Methylxanthine alkaloids (caffeine, theobromine, and theophylline)
- Mothballs
- Paintballs
- Perfumes
- Play dough
- Propylene glycol
- Road salts
- Soaps and shampoos
- Teflon/PTFE
- Turpentine
- Xylitol
- Miscellaneous household items that may contain acids or bases (table)
- Miscellaneous household items that may contain aliphatic or aromatic hydrocarbons, including petroleum hydrocarbons (list)

Veterinary Toxicology for Australia and New Zealand
DOI: http://dx.doi.org/10.1016/B978-0-12-420227-6.00012-8
© 2017 Elsevier Inc. All rights reserved

AGENE

Toxicosis in dogs due to agene (nitrogen trichloride) is of historical interest only, but is mentioned here because clients may be misled by articles on the internet.

Agene was used in the first half of the twentieth century in the processing of flour. It acted as an "improving agent" to alter the baking characteristics. Consumption of bread or other products made with agene-treated flour resulted in a condition called "canine hysteria," "fright fits," or "running fits." Mild toxicosis caused signs of lethargy and incoordination, but more severely poisoned dogs would exhibit sudden onset of apparent panic, with howling, clawing at the air, and wild running. Such episodes would stop as suddenly as they began. In the worst cases of poisoning, dogs would develop recurrent tonic-clonic seizures which would become more and more frequent and could become continuous. Fatalities due to exhaustion and acidosis could occur. Similar toxicosis was induced experimentally in rabbits, cats, and guinea pigs, but not nonhuman primates.

ALLIUM SPECIES (GARLIC AND ONION)

Allium species, which include garlic and onion, are covered in the chapter on introduced plants. However, they are cross-referenced here because they may pose a threat to domestic pets. Onion is commonly used in cooking and may be present in food scraps offered to pets. Garlic is sometimes promoted as an alternative remedy to rid cats of fleas. It should be noted that the *N*-propyl disulfide in *Allium* bulbs can cause hemolytic anemia, and that toxicosis has been reported in dogs. If owners report that they are using garlic as an alternative remedy or flea treatment in pets, regular blood sampling for hematology should be suggested.

BATTERIES

Circumstances of Poisoning

Batteries that fall from devices, including toys, may be ingested by pets.

Mode(s) of Action

Mechanisms of toxicity resulting from battery ingestion include acid or alkaline burns and metal toxicity from the casings. Metals in the casings of batteries may include lead, mercury, zinc, cobalt, or cadmium. Other hazards of battery ingestion include gastrointestinal obstruction and tissue necrosis from electrical currents. Disk batteries may not pass from the esophagus to the stomach, and cause burns and possibly perforation in the terminal esophagus with consequent pleurisy.

Clinical Signs

Clinical signs usually become apparent within a few hours of ingestion. Signs of oral and gastrointestinal discomfort include hypersalivation, abnormal movements of the lips or tongue, depression, dysphagia, anorexia, and vomiting. There may be oral inflammation or ulceration. Hyperthermia may be present. Dyspnea and coughing may be present.

Further information on clinical signs of acid or alkaline burns, and on metal poisonings, can be found elsewhere in this book.

Diagnostic Aids

The leukocyte count may be elevated.

Batteries are visible on plain radiographs. Inflammatory and corrosive changes in the esophagus and stomach are apparent in endoscopy, but may not be fully evident until at least 12 hours after injury commences.

Treatment

In acute ingestion, multiple small boluses of water or milk should be administered to minimize injury by acids or bases. Clients reporting possible acute ingestion of batteries should be advised to commence this treatment before transporting the animal to the veterinary facility.

Radiography should be performed promptly and any batteries lodged in the esophagus should be removed by endoscopy.

The mouth should be examined for evidence of chemical burns. Grey residue on the teeth supports the conclusion that the casing of the battery has been punctured, but it should not be assumed that the absence of such residue indicates that the casing has not been punctured.

Further information on the management of acid and alkaline burns, and metal poisonings, can be found elsewhere in this book.

Treatment of gastrointestinal chemical injury from a leaking battery should include antibiotic cover, as well as pain relief as indicated. It may be necessary to provide nutritional and hydration support. Chemical injury may be minimized by sucralfate, but severe chemical injury may necessitate surgical resection if there is risk of full-thickness necrosis and perforation.

If a small battery is swallowed whole by a large dog, it may not cause any problems. However, the animal should be hospitalized until the battery is passed in the feces, and radiographs taken at intervals to ensure that it is progressing normally through the gastrointestinal tract. Any battery that has not progressed beyond the stomach within 48 hours should be removed by endoscopy if intact, or surgery if punctured.

Treatment of metal poisonings from battery casings is presented elsewhere in this book.

Prognosis

The prognosis varies with the severity of injury, but is guarded if there is severe injury to the terminal esophagus, because perforation of the esophagus may lead to life-threatening pleurisy, and because there is risk of esophageal stricture if the animal survives.

Necropsy

Lesions may include chemical burns and/or findings consistent with metal poisonings.

Public Health Considerations

Batteries present the same hazards to small children as to domestic pets. If a small battery is missing and cannot be found on radiograph of the pet, the client should consider examination and radiography of any infants or pre-schoolers in the household.

Toys from which batteries readily fall out should be discarded.

Prevention

Batteries should not be stored where pets, particularly young animals, can find them, and should be located and picked up promptly if it is noticed that they have gone missing from devices.

BLEACHES

Synonyms

A variety of chemicals are used in household bleaches, including hypochlorites, perborates, and peroxides.

Mode(s) of Action

Depending on pH, bleaches may be irritating or corrosive. Peroxides release a large amount of oxygen, and ingestion of hydrogen peroxide has been associated with life-threatening gas emboli. Perborates break down to peroxide and borate (q.v.). Sodium hypochlorite bleaches may break down to release chlorine or chloramine gas.

Clinical Signs

Clinical signs include hypersalivation, vomiting, depression, and anorexia. The oral mucosa may be ulcerated and the animal may paw at the mouth.

Dermal exposures may result in skin irritation and bleaching of the hair. Ocular exposure to vapor or to the liquid bleach itself may cause blepharospasm and lacrimation. Alkaline bleaches are the most harmful to the eyes, any may cause corneal ulceration. Inhalation of chlorine or chloramine gas is acutely irritating to the respiratory tract and may lead to pulmonary edema.

Diagnostic Aids

Ingestion of sodium hypochlorite bleach may cause hyperchloremia and/or hypernatremia. Metabolic acidosis may be present.

Treatment

Both induction of emesis and gastric lavage are *contraindicated* if bleach has been ingested, and activated charcoal will not be effective. Dilution of ingested bleach should be attempted with water or milk.

Supportive hydration and nutrition may be necessary if there is extensive irritation of the mouth, pharynx, and/or esophagus. Administration of a slurry of sucralfate may provide relief by coating mucous membranes. Butorphanol tartrate is recommended for pain. The animal should be monitored for secondary infection and given antibiotics as necessary. Corticosteroids are controversial and if they are used, only short-acted corticosteroids should be administered.

In the event of esophageal perforation, surgical correction via thoracotomy is indicated.

In the case of dermal exposure the animal should be bathed as soon as possible with copious water and a mild detergent such as hand-dishwashing liquid. Treatment of dermal irritation is symptomatic.

In the case of direct ocular exposure, irrigation for at least 30 minutes with tepid tap water is recommended, after which the eye should be carefully examined for corneal damage and treated as necessary.

In the event of inhalation of chlorine or chloramine gas, the animal should be monitored for pulmonary edema and treated with corticosteroids and respiratory support if necessary.

Prognosis

Prognosis is generally favorable if only small amounts of bleach are involved. Prognosis is guarded if there is esophageal perforation or pulmonary edema.

Necropsy

Necropsy findings may include corrosive lesions in the mouth, pharynx, esophagus and stomach, esophageal perforation, or pulmonary edema, depending on the route of exposure.

Public Health Considerations

Bleaches pose the same risk to human beings, especially preschool children, as they do to domestic pets.

Prevention

Bleaches should be stored out of reach of small children or pets, and used with caution in accordance with the manufacturer's directions.

BORIC ACID

Boric acid is covered elsewhere in this book.

Household products that may contain boric acid include cleaners, water softeners, insect killers, topical astringents, glazes, and tanning compounds.

CLAY PIGEONS

Circumstances of Poisoning

Although ingestion of clay pigeons is of greatest risk to livestock, particularly grazing pigs, they are covered here because they contaminate pastures as a consequence of hobby activity.

Mode(s) of Action

Clay pigeons are often made out of pitch, which like phenol is produced from distillation of bituminous coal. The metabolism of pitch leads to centrilobular hepatic necrosis, liver cirrhosis, and liver and/or cardiac insufficiency.

Clinical Signs

Animals that ingest fragments of clay pigeon may be found dead, or develop signs of chronic hepatopathy.

Diagnostic Aids

Liver enzymes will be elevated in the serum.

Treatment

Animals may be salvaged if provided with a diet containing high-quality proteins, and given supplements of vitamin E and B vitamins.

Prognosis

In severe acute liver failure, prognosis is hopeless. In less severe toxicosis, animals may be salvaged with supportive care.

Necropsy

In acute death, lesions are those of massive hemorrhagic liver necrosis. A centrilobular pattern may be evident. In chronic toxicosis, lesions are those of liver cirrhosis and nodular hyperplasia ("hobnail liver"), and ascites. There may be evidence of congestive heart failure.

Prevention

Pigs in particular should not be grazed on land that has fragments of clay pigeon on it. Clay pigeons should not be used as toys for dogs, particularly large dogs that could break the clay pigeons and ingest fragments.

DETERGENTS

Detergents are classified according to their chemistry when in solution: nonionic, anionic, or cationic. The nonionic and anionic detergents are of low toxicity although they may be mildly to moderately irritant. Most serious toxicoses are associated with the cationic detergents.

Circumstances of Poisoning

Anionic and nonionic detergents are found in shampoos, hand-dishwashing detergents, and laundry detergents.

Cationic detergents include benzalkonium chloride, benzethonium chloride, methylbenzethonium, and cetylpyridinium chloride. They are quaternary ammonium compounds that often contain a halide. They may be present in automatic dishwashing powders, fabric softeners, some hair products, sanitizers, and disinfectants.

Automatic dishwashing powders and tablets are also typically extremely *alkaline*. Toxicity of bases is covered elsewhere in this book.

Poisoning is most likely to occur if pets, particularly puppies, consume household products. Cats may be poisoned if the detergent is spilt on their coat and they attempt to groom themselves to remove it.

Mode(s) of Action

Nonionic detergents are of minimal to negligible toxicity, even when swallowed.

The mode of action is direct irritation. Quaternary ammonium compounds are irritating and harmful to mucous membranes at concentrations as low as 1%.

Clinical Signs

Ingestion may result in vomiting, diarrhea, hypersalivation due to nausea, anorexia, and depression. The gastrointestinal tract may become distended, resulting in abdominal distension. If the animal has ingested a quaternary ammonium compound, there may be corrosive injury to the gastrointestinal tract leading to shock.

Dermal exposure may result in erythema, exudation, pruritis, or vesiculation.

Diagnostic Aids

There are no specific diagnostic aids. Gastrointestinal distension may be evident on radiograph but is not always present. In the event of quaternary ammonium compound ingestion, careful endoscopy may reveal the extent of esophageal or gastric injury.

Treatment

Dilution of ingested detergent with water or milk should be commenced as soon as possible.

Induction of emesis, and gastric lavage, is *contraindicated*. Activated charcoal may be helpful. Sucralfate in slurry may be administered to provide mucosal protection. Analgesia may be indicated. In the case of cationic detergent ingestion, treatment of shock may be required.

Dermal exposure should be treated by washing with copious water and with soap, taking appropriate care to ensure veterinary personnel are not dermally exposed to quaternary ammonium compounds.

Prognosis

Prognosis depends on the severity of exposure and the nature of the detergent.

Necropsy

Necropsy findings are those of irritation or corrosion of the gastrointestinal tract.

Public Health Considerations

Detergents pose the same risk to human beings, especially preschool children, as they do to domestic pets.

Prevention

Detergents should be stored out of reach of small children or pets, and used in accordance with the manufacturer's directions.

DEODORANTS/ANTIPERSPIRANTS

There is little information on the toxicity of these products, but ingestion has been associated with gingival necrosis, hemorrhagic gastroenteritis, and nephrosis in domestic pets.

DISINFECTANTS

Disinfectants may include quaternary ammonium compounds, phenols, pine oils, bleaches, and alcohols. Bleaches have already been covered in this chapter. Quaternary ammonium compounds are discussed in the section above on detergents. Alcohols are discussed elsewhere in this book. The types of disinfectant discussed in this section are phenols and pine oil disinfectants.

Phenol Disinfectants

Phenol is an aromatic alcohol derived from coal tar. Phenol may be present in disinfectants as chlorophenol and/or phenyl phenol. Phenol is also present in creosote.

Toxicokinetics

Phenol is rapidly absorbed, detoxified and conjugated with glucuronide or sulfate in the liver, and excreted in the urine in the conjugated form. The oral LD_{50} in dogs is approximately 0.5 g/kg BW, but cats are more susceptible to phenol poisoning because of their relatively limited capacity for glucuronidation.

Mode of Action

Phenol is corrosive and is highly reactive on contact with tissues, denaturing and precipitating proteins to cause a chemical burn.

Clinical Signs

Initially, phenol burns cause intense pain.

Signs of ingestions are hypersalivation, vomiting, agitation, ataxia, and panting. Corrosive lesions may be found in the mouth. Toxicosis may progress to tremors, muscle fasciculations, shock, cardiac arrhythmias, methemoglobinemia, and coma. If the animal survives for 12–24 hours, it may develop clinical signs of hepatic and renal damage.

Dermal exposure may result in dermal burns with coagulative necrosis.

Ocular lesions are characteristically those of severe corneal damage, possibly penetrating.

Diagnostic Aids

Phenols or their metabolites may be present in urine. This can be confirmed by mixing 10 mL urine with 1 mL 20% ferric chloride. A positive result is indicated by development of a purple color.

Endoscopy to assess the severity of damage to the esophagus and stomach should be performed with great caution.

Phenol may cause intravascular hemolysis or methemoglobinemia.

Icterus may be present as a result of intravascular hemolysis and/or hepatic damage, and liver enzymes will be elevated in the event of hepatic damage.

Urine may contain protein, heme, and epithelial cells or casts.

Treatment

Milk or eggs should be administered orally, as soon as possible. Administration of water is controversial because it may increase systemic absorption. Induction of emesis, and gastric lavage, is *contraindicated*. Activated charcoal should not be administered unless the possibility of penetrating lesions of the esophagus or stomach has been eliminated. Shock should be treated symptomatically. Acid–base status and cardiovascular function must be monitored. Phenol initially causes hyperventilation and may cause metabolic acidosis, but if the animal goes into shock or coma, respiratory support may be required. After 12 hours, hepatic and renal function should be monitored and supported as necessary. Administration of *n*-acetylcysteine may limit hepatic and renal toxicity if administered four times daily for at least 3 days, at an initial loading dose of 140 mg/kg IV, and follow-up doses of 70 mg/kg orally.

If methemoglobinemia develops, a single dose of 1% methylene blue, at 4 mg/kg IV to dogs and 1.5 mg/kg IV in cats, should be administered. Oral ascorbic acid, 20 mg/kg, may also be helpful.

In the case of dermal exposure, the skin and hair should be washed with glycerol or polyethylene glycol, followed by a second wash with copious water and a mild hand-dishwashing detergent. Veterinary personnel should wear appropriate personal protective equipment. After the phenol or phenolic compound has been removed, dressings soaked in 5% sodium bicarbonate may be applied to dermal lesions.

In the case of ocular exposure, the eye should be flushed with physiological saline or water for at least 20 minutes.

Prognosis

Phenol ingestion is a serious toxicosis and prognosis is guarded to poor if a large amount has been ingested.

Necropsy

Gross lesions include necrosis or ulceration of the mouth; pharynx and esophagus, and/or stomach; swollen pale kidneys; and mottled liver. Histologically there is coagulative necrosis of the affected parts of the gastrointestinal tract, centrilobular necrosis in the liver, and proximal renal tubular necrosis.

Public Health Considerations

Phenol poses the same risk to human beings, especially preschool children, as it does to domestic pets.

Prevention

Phenol and phenolic compounds should be stored out of reach of small children or pets, and used in accordance with the manufacturer's directions.

PINE OIL DISINFECTANTS

Toxicokinetics

Pine oil is readily absorbed from the gastrointestinal tract and metabolized, with glucuronide conjugation, in the liver. Inhalation, or systemic distribution, of absorbed pine oil to the lungs may cause chemical pneumonitis. Conjugates are excreted in the urine, although if a large amount has been ingested, there may be a pine or turpentine odor to the breath. The LD_{50} of pine oil is in the range $1-2.5$ mL/kg BW. Cats, because of their limited capacity for glucuronidation, are particularly susceptible to toxicosis.

Mode(s) of Action

Pine oil is directly irritating to mucous membranes, and is also a central nervous system (CNS) and respiratory depressant.

Clinical Signs

Clinical signs include nausea, hypersalivation, vomiting, and evidence of abdominal pain. Vomitus may contain blood. Systemic clinical signs include CNS depression, weakness, ataxia, hypotension, respiratory depression, pneumonitis, pulmonary edema, myoglobinuria, renal failure, and hepatic failure.

Clinical signs of ocular exposure are those of blepharospasm, epiphora and injected conjunctiva, and sclera.

Treatment

Administer egg white, milk, and/or water to dilute the toxicant. Induction of emesis is *contraindicated* and gastric lavage is hazardous and unlikely to be justified. Activated charcoal may be helpful. Acid—base and electrolyte balance should be monitored, and renal perfusion maintained. Care for other clinical signs is symptomatic and supportive.

Animals that have been subject to dermal exposure should be washed with copious water and with soap. Ocular exposure should be treated with irrigation with physiological saline or water for at least 20 minutes.

Prognosis

Prognosis depends on magnitude of exposure and aggressiveness of treatment, but may be poor to hopeless if there is extensive renal and/or hepatic damage.

Necropsy

Lesions may include pulmonary edema, pneumonitis, renal cortical necrosis, and centrilobular hepatic necrosis.

Public Health Considerations

Pine oil poses the same risk to human beings, especially preschool children, as it does to domestic pets.

Prevention

Pine oil and pine oil-based compounds should be stored out of reach of small children or pets, and used in accordance with the manufacturer's directions.

ETHYLENE GLYCOL

Synonyms

Because domestic pets are most often exposed to ethylene glycol as antifreeze for motor vehicles, ethylene glycol toxicosis is often referred to as "antifreeze poisoning."

Circumstances of Poisoning

Dogs and cats find ethylene glycol, or water containing ethylene glycol that has leaked or been drained from radiators, palatable.

Toxicokinetics

Ethylene glycol is rapidly absorbed. Metabolism occurs primarily in the liver and kidneys. The parent compound is first metabolized to glycoaldehyde by alcohol dehydrogenase. Glycoadehyde is further metabolized by alcohol dehydrogenase to glycolic acid and, to a lesser extent, glyoxal. Metabolism of glycolic acid proceeds to glyoxylic acid while glyoxal may be metabolized to glycolic acid or directly to glyoxylic acid. Glyoxylic acid has a number of metabolites of which the most toxicologically significant is oxalic acid. Others are formic acid, which is expired as carbon dioxide, glycine which is further metabolized to hippuric acid, and α-hydroxy, β-keto adipate. Oxalic acid tends to precipitate as calcium oxalate in the renal tubules. Ethylene glycol and most of its metabolites are excreted in urine.

Modes of Action

Ethylene glycol toxicosis occurs in stages, although Stage I may not be observed clinically and animals are often presented in later stages. Also, there is likely to be overlap of stages in the clinical signs, or one stage may predominate so that other stages are not observed.

Stage I is caused by the parent compound, which is an alcohol, and the aldehyde metabolite. These cause central nervous effects. Because ethylene glycol is a small (62 Da) water-soluble molecule, it causes an increase in serum osmolality. Polyuria and polydipsia may occur in Stage I due to this increase in serum osmolality, an osmotic diuretic effect of ethylene glycol, or direct inhibition of vasopressin.

Stage II is characterized as the cardiopulmonary or acidotic stage. The acidic metabolites of ethylene glycol cause acidosis. In addition, as oxalic acid converts to calcium oxalate crystals, hypocalcemia develops. Acidosis is exacerbated by the accumulation of lactic acid, because the metabolism of ethylene glycol increases the NADH:NAD ratio, and metabolism of lactic acid is catalyzed by NAD-dependent enzymes.

Stage III features renal toxicity. Calcium oxalate crystals precipitate in the renal tubules, and glycolic and gloxylic acids cause an increased anion gap and an increase in the serum osmolal gap, resulting in renal edema, which in turn compromises renal blood glow.

Stage IV, a delayed neuropathy stage, has not been reported in animals but has been observed in human beings.

Serum phosphorus may be elevated as a result of uncoupling of oxidative phosphorylation, and hypoglycemia, an inconsistent sign, may be due to inhibition of glycolysis by aldehydes. Ethylene glycol is slightly hepatotoxic.

Pulmonary irritation from inhaled ethylene glycol has been observed in animals. Ethylene glycol is a reproductive toxicant in mice, and has been found to be teratogenic in several laboratory species.

An oral dose of 4.4 mL/kg is lethal in dogs if untreated. The minimum lethal dose in the cat is 0.9 mL/kg. This greater sensitivity of the cat is attributed to its higher baseline production of oxalic acid.

An oral dose of 2 mL/kg exceeds the toxic threshold in preruminant calves, but in adult cattle the corresponding dose is 5−10 mL/kg. The lethal dose is 6.7 mL/kg in chickens, but appears to be considerably lower in ducks. The LD_{50} in the guinea pig is in the range of 6.6−8.2 g/kg.

Clinical Signs

Stage I clinical signs usually become evident 1−3 hours after ingestion and include depression, polydipsia, progressive ataxia, and possible vomiting.

Stage II clinical signs usually develop 4−6 hours after Stage I and include tachypnea, vomiting, depression, hypothermia, and miosis. Coma may ensue.

Stage III clinical signs are those of oliguric renal failure, including lethargy, vomiting, oral ulcerations, and convulsions.

Anterior uveitis and vitreal hemorrhage have been observed in the dog.

Reported clinical signs in cattle are progressive paraparesis and ataxia, tachypnea, hemoglobinuria, epistaxis, and dypnea. Depression, ataxia, and weakness particularly affecting the hind legs have been observed in swine. Chickens become ataxic and adopt a characteristic posture in recumbency with drooping wings, closed eyes, and beak used to prop the head up. The comb may be cyanotic.

Diagnostic Aids

The anion gap is typically 40−50 mequiv./L. Other clinical pathology findings include decreased blood pH, increased serum phosphorus but decreased calcium, decreased bicarbonate, hyperglycemia, neutrophilia, and lymphopenia. As renal failure develops, serum BUN, creatinine, and potassium increase.

Oxalate crystalluria becomes evident 6−8 hours after ingestion of ethylene glycol. Other urinary findings include proteinuria, glycosuria, and hematuria.

Many antifreezes contain fluoroscein, which is added to help mechanics find small leaks in radiators. Fluorescence of the urine may assist in early diagnosis in the dog, but is not helpful in cats which naturally have fluorescent urine. It should be borne in mind that the presence of fluorescein does not indicate that a toxic dose of ethylene glycol has been ingested, and that the absence of fluorescein does not preclude ethylene glycol toxicosis.

Intravascular hemolysis has been observed in cattle.

Laboratory test kits for ethylene glycol are available.

Glycolic acid is considerably more persistent than ethylene glycol in serum, persisting for up to 60 hours after ingestion.

The "halo sign" on ultrasonography, a marked increase in both cortical and medullary echogenicity with hypoechoic areas in the corticomedullary region, appears to be reasonably unique to ethylene glycol toxicosis, but signifies a grave prognosis. Renal cortical echogenicity increases within 4 hours in ethylene glycol toxicosis but is not pathognomonic.

Treatment

Early detoxification markedly improves outcome. Activated charcoal should be administered as soon as possible.

Intravenous fluid should also be started as soon as possible, and urinary output monitored. If the animal is already oliguric or anuric, urinary through-put should be established with physiological saline, with no potassium-containing fluids administered until renal flow has been established and hyperkalemia relieved. Water should be available *ad libitum.*

The best antidote in dogs is 4-methylpyrazole (fomipazole), a specific inhibitor of alcohol dehydrogenase, but this is not sufficiently effective in cats. The recommended dose regime is 20 mg/kg BW initially, followed by 15 mg/kg at 12 and 24 hours, and 5 mg/kg at 36 hours.

The traditional antidote is ethanol, administered intravenously as a 20% solution, which is an alternative substrate for alcohol dehydrogenase. If metabolism of ethylene glycol can be prevented, it is excreted as the parent compound. This can be achieved if a serum ethanol of 50 mg/dL can be maintained. Domestic pets should be maintained in stupor for at least 72 hours. One suggested treatment regime for dogs is 5.5 mL/kg BW every 4 hours for five treatments then every 6 hours for four treatments. The serum ethanol concentration should be maintained at 50−100 mg/dL. For cats, 5 mL/kg BW every 6 hours for five treatments followed by four treatments at 8 hour intervals. An alternative treatment regime is 1.3 mL/kg of a 30% ethanol solution as an IV bolus, followed by 0.42 mL/kg/hour for 48 hours.

Clear alcohols such as vodka, gin, or white rum can be used as a source of ethanol. The "proof" can be converted to percent ethanol content by dividing by 2.

Deleterious side effects of ethanol include hypothermia and risk of respiratory arrest. It may exacerbate acidosis, osmotic diuresis, and serum hyperosmolality.

4-Methylpyrazole and ethanol should never be used together or ethanol poisoning is likely to result.

Acidosis should be corrected with intravenous bicarbonate. If hypocalcemia becomes clinically significant, 0.25 mL/kg calcium borogluconate can be administered daily in 10% solution.

Peritoneal dialysis may be helpful as an adjunct until renal function is restored, and has some effect in removing ethylene glycol and its toxic metabolites. While peritoneal dialysis has been shown to lower serum levels of ethylene glycol, this has not been shown to improve clinical outcome.

Administration of pyridoxine and thiamine, 100 mg each/day, has been used in human beings. The theoretical rationale for this is to promote the detoxification of glyoxylic acid to glycine and α-hydroxy, β-keto adipate.

Prognosis

Prognosis varies depending on how promptly treatment is instituted after ingestion. The prognosis becomes guarded to poor if renal failure has developed.

Necropsy

Kidneys are pale and firm, and may have pale streaks at the corticomedullary junction. There may be pulmonary edema, and hyperemia of lungs, gastric mucosa, and intestinal mucosa. Cats may have frank hemorrhage in the stomach or small intestine.

The specimen of choice is kidney. The distinctive and diagnostic findings are birefringent calcium oxalate crystals in and around the proximal and distal convoluted tubules. Other findings are degeneration and atrophy of tubules. There may be diffuse interstitial fibrosis of the renal cortex and mineralization of the basement membrane of tubules. Glomeruli may be atrophied, and there may be adhesions between capillary tufts and Bowman's capsules.

Ruminal content may be useful as a diagnostic specimen in ruminants. Glycolic acid also persists for some time in ocular fluid.

Prevention

Owners should be warned that when they drain radiators, they should dispose of the drained fluid immediately. Spilled concentrated ethylene glycol, or radiator fluid that has spilled or leaked from radiators, should be absorbed with bentonite-based kittylitter and then the site of the spill should be washed with copious water.

FERTILIZER

Circumstances of Poisoning

Fertilizers are generally of low toxicity. The principal components that may cause toxicity are the "NPK" triad of nitrogen, phosphorus, and potassium, but some fertilizers may contain iron (q.v.), insecticides (q.v.), or calcium cyanamide.

Dogs may consume excessive amounts if the fertilizer contains bone meal or blood meal. Ruminants and less commonly horses may develop toxicosis from the nitrates (q.v.) in fertilizers, and urea (q.v.) is particularly toxic to ruminants.

Mode(s) of Action and Clinical Signs

Phosphorus and potassium compounds may cause gastrointestinal irritation. Excessive intake of blood meal or bone meal may cause pancreatitis in dogs.

Nitrates cause methemoglobinemia, as covered elsewhere in this book. Ammonium salts and urea are predominantly gastrointestinal irritants in monogastric animals but may cause systemic ammonia poisoning in ruminants, as covered elsewhere in this book. Iron toxicosis may occur if the fertilizer contains a high iron content. Calcium cyanamide is a dermal irritant and, if ingested, may cause ataxia, pulmonary edema, hypotension, and shock.

Treatment

Activated charcoal may be helpful in recent ingestion. Treatment is otherwise symptomatic. Treatment of toxicosis due to nitrates, iron, ammonium salts/urea, and insecticides is covered under the relevant sections elsewhere in this book.

Prognosis

Prognosis is generally favorable.

Necropsy

Lesions are those of gastrointestinal irritation, as well as lesions due to specific contents (e.g., methemoglobinemia if nitrite toxicosis has developed).

Prevention

Access to fertilizers or recently fertilized ground should be prevented.

FOOD WASTE

It is commonly assumed that food that has spoiled and is unfit for human consumption can be safely fed to dogs, cats, swine, or poultry. However, it should be recognized that animals can be affected by the same bacterial pathogens (*Clostridum botulinum*, *Listeria monocytogenes*, *Salmonella* spp., *Staphylococcus* spp., *Bacillis cereus*, *Escherichia coli*, etc.) that cause food poisoning in human beings, although susceptibility to a given pathogen may vary between species. Furthermore molds that render food unfit for human consumption may synthesize mycotoxins such as penitrem A and roquefortine, both of which are tremorgens and both of which have caused toxicosis in dogs. The practitioner should be alert to the possibility of food poisoning in animals that are fed spoiled human foodstuffs, and owners should be warned that dogs that tear open rubbish bags or otherwise help themselves to food waste are not merely a nuisance, but may be at risk of sickness. It is possible that multiple bacterial and fungal toxins may be present in spoiled food, with the result that the clinical manifestations of "garbage poisoning," as it is commonly called in the USA, are difficult to predict.

GLOW-IN-THE-DARK ITEMS

Glow-in-the-dark novelties and jewelry contain dibutyl phthalate, which is of low systemic toxicity. There have been cases of domestic pets chewing on these items and releasing the contents, and developing hypersalivation, agitation, and sometimes aggressive behavior. The mouth may be rinsed with water to dilute the poison, and the animal should be placed in a safe place to prevent injury. Clinical signs usually resolve within a few hours.

HOPS, SPENT

Ingestion of spent hops, left over from beer-making, has been associated with life-threatening hyperthermia in dogs. There may be breed susceptibilities, including susceptibility of greyhounds and golden retrievers. Urgent steps should be taken to cool affected animals. Introducing intravenous fluid that is chilled by running a loop of the IV line through a bowl of ice and water is highly effective. If an IV line cannot be promptly established, or for home first aid, introduction of iced water into the rectum is another method for rapidly cooling an animal.

MACADAMIA NUTS

Circumstances of Poisoning

Toxicosis resulting from consumption of the nuts of *Macadamia integrifolia* and *Macadamia tetraphylla*, both of which are native to Australia, has only been reported in dogs. Dog owners should be alert to the risks of confectionery or baked goods containing these nuts as well as to the nuts themselves.

Toxicokinetics

There is a little information on the toxicokinetics of macadamia nuts in dogs. It is not known what the toxic principle is, or which fraction of the nut (lipophillic or lipophobic) it would extract into, although there is some evidence that the timing of clinical signs correlates with the pharmacokinetics of the triglyceride fraction of the nuts. Clinical signs usually develop within 3–24 hours of ingestion.

The toxic threshold in dogs is estimated to be in the range of 0.7–4.9 g nuts/kg BW, regardless of whether the nuts are raw or roasted. This translates to between 5 and 40 nuts in a 20 kg dog.

Mode(s) of Action

The mode of action is unknown.

Clinical Signs

Clinical signs include weakness with reluctance to rise, depression, vomiting, ataxia, tremors, and occasionally hyperthermia. Dogs may exhibit signs of joint or muscle pain. Slight exaggeration of patellar reflexes has been reported. Weakness usually peaks within 12 hours and resolves by 48 hours after ingestion. Depression may be evident as early as 3 hours after ingestion but resolves within 24 hours. Hyperthermia tends to peak at approximately 8 hours.

Diagnostic Aids

Dogs characteristically develop a marked increase in serum lipase. Neutrophilia and elevations in serum triglycerides and serum alkaline phosphatase have also been observed in experimental cases.

Treatment

If a dog is known to have ingested macadamia nuts, administration of activated charcoal may be beneficial, although it is not known whether the toxic principle would be adsorbed. Treatment is otherwise symptomatic.

Prognosis

Toxicosis is usually mild and dogs usually recover within 48 hours of ingestion.

Necropsy

No gross or histopathological lesions have been reported. The nature of the clinical signs suggests that lesions would not be expected.

Public Health Considerations

Toxicosis from macadamia nuts has only been observed in dogs.

Prevention

Owners should be made aware that macadamia nuts, that are popular snacks and ingredients for human food, may cause toxicosis in dogs.

MATCHES

Matches contain potassium chlorate, which may cause methemoglobinemia. Ingestion of sufficient matches to cause this toxic effect is unlikely.

MELAMINE

The adulteration with melamine and cynauric acid, by a Chinese company, of wheat gluten, corn gluten, and rice protein used in wet pet foods led to renal failure in hundreds of domestic cats and dogs in North America, Europe, and South Africa in 2007. Melamine by itself is considered to be of low toxicity, but current research indicates that the combination of melamine and cyanuric acid is hazardous. Postmortem histopathology of the kidney revealed the presence of characteristic crystals in the kidneys. Unfortunately these crystals are radiolucent in the live animal.

METHYLXANTHINE ALKALOIDS (CAFFEINE, THEOBROMINE, AND THEOPHYLLINE)

Synonyms

Chocolate poisoning.

Circumstances of Poisoning

Dogs are the domestic species most likely to be poisoned, and this occurs most frequently when they consume baking chocolate, which contains the highest levels of theobromine. Theophylline is used as a human pharmaceutical for a variety of respiratory conditions such as asthma and chronic obstructive pulmonary disease, and pets may be poisoned if they consume spilled theophylline tablets. Coffee, coffee beans, coffee powders, and caffeine tablets are not generally palatable to pets.

Chocolate typically contains approximately 80% theobromine and 20% caffeine, although the two substances are equivalent in toxicity. The typical contents of cacao beans and chocolate are as follows:

Product	Theobromine and/or Caffeine Content per 100 g of Product
Cacao beans	14−28 g
Baking chocolate	1.411 g
Dark chocolate	0.53 g
Milk chocolate	0.18 g
White chocolate	Negligible

Toxicokinetics

Methylxanthine alkaloids are readily absorbed and widely distributed. They are metabolized in the liver by *N*-demethylation, and conjugated. They are rapidly excreted by the renal route. Because they are alkaloids, urinary excretion may be enhanced by urinary acidification.

Mode(s) of Action

The methylxanthine alkaloids stimulate the CNS and cardiac muscle. They also act as diuretics and promote smooth muscle relaxation. They competitively antagonize adenosine receptors, resulting in CNS stimulation, vasoconstriction, tachycardia, and accumulation of cyclic nucleotides.

The acute oral LD_{50} of caffeine and theobromine is $100-200$ mg/kg in dogs and $80-150$ mg/kg in cats. Theophylline is less toxic, with an acute oral LD_{50} of 300 mg/kg in dogs and 700 mg/kg in cats.

Mild toxicosis, limited to polyuria and gastrointestinal signs, occurs at about 20 mg/kg. Cardiotoxic effects may occur at $40-50$ mg/kg, and seizures may develop at dosages ≥ 60 mg/kg.

Clinical Signs

Clinical signs include agitation, hyperactivity, mild hyperreflexia, diuresis with or without urinary incontinence, vomiting and diarrhea, tachycardia, polypnea, and hyperthermia. In advanced toxicosis, there may be tonic to tetanic convulsive seizures.

Diagnostic Aids

The presence of methylxanthine alkaloids can be confirmed in vomitus, serum, or urine, but the clinical course is rapid, so there is generally insufficient time to wait for laboratory results.

Treatment

Methylxanthine alkaloids are adsorbed by activated charcoal, but it should only be administered with a cuffed endotracheal tube in place, because methylxanthine alkaloids are also emetic. Because methylxanthine alkaloids undergo enterohepatic cycling, activated charcoal administered every 3 to 4 hours may be helpful.

Tachyarrhythmia should be treated with metoprolol, $0.2-0.4$ mg/kg by slow IV injection. Propanol may be used if metoprolol is not available, but has the disadvantage that it may delay excretion of methylxanthine alkaloids. Lidocaine may be used for ventricular tachyarrhythmia in dogs but is contraindicated in cats. The suggested treatment regime is $1-2$ mg/kg IV, followed by infusion of 0.1% solution IV at a rate of 30 μg/kg/min.

Tremors or seizures may be treated with methocarbamol or diazepam, although severe seizure activity may require barbiturates.

Fluids should be administered to promote diuresis, and urinary acidification may be helpful. The animal should be catheterized because methylxanthine alkaloids can be reabsorbed from the urinary bladder if urine is held in the bladder.

The body temperature, acid−base balance, and electrolyte balance should be monitored and corrected as necessary.

Severe toxicosis may last for up to 3 days.

Prognosis

Prognosis is favorable with aggressive treatment of cardiac and neurological effects.

Necropsy

There are no characteristic lesions. Urine is the postmortem specimen of choice.

Prevention

Owners should be warned of the danger of baking chocolate and dark chocolate in particular.

MOTHBALLS

Mothballs may be composed of naphthalene or paradichlorobenzene. The latter chemical is most often used in cake deodorizers for use in bathrooms.

The acute oral LD_{50} of naphthalene in dogs is approximately 400 mg/kg. Naphthalene is more toxic to cats than to dogs.

The acute oral LD_{50} of paradichlorobenzene is approximately 500 mg/kg.

Clinical Signs

Naphthalene: vomiting, methemoglobinemia, hemolytic Heinz body anemia, hemoglobinuria, signs of liver damage, and possibly renal damage.

Paradichlorobenzene: vomiting, tremors, seizures, and signs of liver and kidney damage.

Treatment

Naphthalene: activated charcoal may be helpful. Methemoglobinemia should be treated with methylene blue at 4 mg/kg of 1% methylene blue in dogs and 1.5 mg/kg of 1% methylene blue in cats. Intravenous fluids containing bicarbonate should be used to minimize precipitation of hemoglobin in the kidneys.

Paradichlorobenzene is an organochlorine insecticide (q.v.). Treatment is symptomatic and supportive.

Prevention

Access to mothballs should be prevented.

PAINTBALLS

Paintballs contain a variety of chemicals of low to moderate toxicity. There have been cases of dogs ingesting paintballs and developing signs of toxicity, although it is not entirely clear which ingredient or ingredients are responsible. The commonest clinical signs reported are vomiting, diarrhea, tremors, and ataxia. Less commonly reported signs are weakness, hyperactivity, tachycardia, hyperthermia, apparent blindness, and seizures. Observed clinical pathology has included hypernatremia, hyperchloremia, hypokalemia, and acidosis. Given the known ingredients of paintballs, activated charcoal is unlikely to be beneficial. Electrolyte imbalances should be addressed, and treatment is otherwise symptomatic. Prognosis is good.

PERFUMES

In addition to alcohol, perfumes contain essential oils that may be hepatotoxic, nephrotoxic, or neurotoxic if ingested, and may contain volatile hydrocarbons. Pets are unlikely to find perfumes sufficiently palatable that a toxic dose is voluntarily ingested. Perfumes should not be applied to the coats of cats, which could be poisoned as a result of self-grooming.

PLAY DOUGH, HOMEMADE

Homemade play dough often contains a high salt content that may cause serious hypernatremia in dogs. Clinical signs have been reported in dogs following ingestion of as little as 1.6 g play dough/kg BW. Clinical signs include vomiting, polydipsia, polyuria, tremors, hyperthermia, and seizures. Animals should be treated for hypernatremia (see Section "Salt (Sodium Chloride)" in this chapter).

PROPYLENE GLYCOL

Propylene glycol toxicosis in domestic cats is of historical interest. Semimoist cat foods containing 3%−13% propylene glycol caused Heinz body anemia with reticulocytosis in cats and kittens. The mechanism of Heinz body formation by propylene glycol is uncertain. In comparison to other species, the feline spleen has large pores in the pulp venules, so that erythrocytes can pass through without being deformed. As a result, erythrocytes containing Heinz bodies are not sequestered by the spleen in cats as they are in other species. Nevertheless, feline erythrocytes containing Heinz bodies as a result of propylene glycol ingestion have been shown to have a shorter lifespan in circulation than unaffected erythrocytes. Chronic ingestion of propylene glycol caused splenic nodularity and mottled liver in cats. Histologically, the liver findings were those of periportal accumulation of glycogen droplets. Hemosiderin accumulation was increased in the liver and spleen, and hematopoietic foci developed in some spleens of cats fed high levels of propylene glycol.

Iatrogenic, sometimes fatal, propylene glycol toxicosis has occurred in horses when veterinarians mistook propylene glycol, intended for treatment of ketosis in ruminants, for mineral oil. Large animal practices that stock both liquids are advised to dye one or other liquid with a food coloring dye to prevent such errors.

ROAD SALTS

Road salts include sodium chloride, calcium chloride, or potassium chloride. The most common toxic effects in domestic pets are those of dermal irritation of feet. Pets should be prevented from access to road salts or salted roads, and if they have been exposed, the salts should be washed off promptly. Animals should be treated for hypernatremia or hyperkalemia as required. Other substances used for melting ice include urea, calcium carbonate, and calcium magnesium acetate, any of which may act as gastrointestinal irritants.

SALT (SODIUM CHLORIDE)

Synonyms

Sodium chloride may be called table salt to distinguish it from other chemical salts.

Circumstances of Poisoning

Direct sodium ion toxicosis results from excess salt in feed or water. Indirect sodium toxicosis results from inadequate water supply.

Sodium toxicosis is relatively rare in domestic pets, compared to livestock, but cases reported in dogs include those in which dogs ate homemade play dough, swallowed amounts of sea-water while playing in the ocean, swallowed fragments of rock salt, or were administered salt solutions in misguided attempts to induce emesis.

Mode(s) of Action

Hypernatremia occurs when the sodium ion content of the extracellular fluid increases or if the water content of the extracellular fluid decreases without a corresponding decrease in sodium ions.

Ingestion of salt causes gastrointestinal irritation. Very high ingestion of salt can cause acute gastroenteritis, dehydration, and death.

Hypernatremia is considered to be acute if the serum sodium increases above 160 mequiv./L within 48 hours. As plasma sodium increases, sodium ions passively diffuse into the cerebrospinal fluid, with toxic effects in the brain, including cellular shrinkage, hemorrhages, and infarcts. While sodium ions passively diffuse into cerebrospinal fluid respectively (CSF), the removal of sodium ions from the CSF requires active transport. One of the effects of increasing brain sodium is to inhibit glycolysis, decreasing the energy available for this active transport, and trapping sodium in the brain. Consumption of water at this stage results in an osmotic shift of water into the brain, causing cerebral edema.

If hypernatremia develops over 4−7 days, there is an increase in organic osmoles including taurine, myo-inositol, glycerophosphoryl-choline, betaine, glutamate, glutamine, and phosphocreatine.

Clinical Signs

Clinical signs may include vomiting, diarrhea, polydipsia, polyuria, fine muscle tremors particularly affecting the facial muscles, and clonic-tonic seizures.

Diagnostic Aids

Serum sodium in excess of 160 mequiv./L confirms hypernatremia. However if the animal has had access to water, the serum sodium may be in the normal range while the CSF sodium remains elevated.

Treatment

Hypernatremia must be corrected slowly. Serum sodium levels should be reduced by no more than 0.5 mequiv./hour. The initial sodium concentration in both parenteral and oral fluids should closely match the serum sodium level. If the serum sodium level is unknown, initial fluids should be 170 mequiv./L sodium.

If the animal has hypernatremia as the result of dehydration secondary to diarrhea, the animal may also be acidotic and/or hypoglycemic. Fluid should be 1.3% sodium bicarbonate, to which sodium and glucose can be added.

Cerebral edema should be treated with mannitol 25% at a dose of 1−2 g/kg, administered IV over 20−30 minutes. This treatment may be repeated at 4−6 hour intervals for up to 24 hours. However, mannitol is contraindicated if there is evidence of cerebral hemorrhage. It should be noted that mannitol facilitates the excretion of sodium and chloride and therefore these electrolytes must be monitored closely. Alternative treatments for cerebral hemorrhage are glycerin (1 mL/kg administered orally as a 50% solution), dexamethasone IV at 0.44−2 mg/kg, or dimethyl sulfoxide administered intravenously.

Prognosis

Prognosis is guarded. Mortality rate is in excess of 50%. Surviving animals may be left with permanent brain damage.

Necropsy

Lesions include cerebral and meningeal edema. The cerebellum may show "coning" because it has been forced toward the foramen magnum, or may be partially herniated through the foramen magnum. Hemorrhages and infarcts may be apparent in the brain.

There may be gastrointestinal irritation. Pulmonary edema has been reported in a dog.

Postmortem specimens of choice are CSF, fresh and fixed brain (transect the brain longitudinally and fix one half), and intact eyeball for measurement of sodium in the vitreous humor.

Although CSF is usually collected by dorsal approach in the living animal, it can be more easily aspirated from the cisterna magna after death, by ventral approach after the tongue, pharynx, and larynx have been detached from their normal positions and reflected back toward the thorax.

Prevention

Domestic pets should always have abundant fresh clean water available. Owners should be warned to never attempt to induce emesis by administering salt or saline solutions.

SOAPS AND SHAMPOOS

Soaps and shampoos are generally of minimal toxicity to pets. The exceptions are anti-dandruff shampoos which may contain selenium sulfide, zinc pyridinethione, coal tar derivatives, or salicylic acid. Ocular damage and blindness have been reported in domestic pets that consumed shampoo containing zinc pyridinethione. Findings included retinal detachment and exudative chorioretinitis.

Shampoos formulated for human use may have too much oil-removing function for use on domestic pets, resulting in dry pruritic skin. Anti-dandruff shampoos and other medicated shampoos formulated for human use should not be used on animals.

TEFLON (POLYTETRAFLUOROETHYLENE)

Toxicosis resulting from polytetrafluoroethylene (PTFE) is most commonly observed in domestic birds such as budgerigars and canaries. If heated above 280 °C PTFE can break down to release breakdown products including hydrogen fluoride, carbon fluoride, and carbon monoxide. These breakdown products cause caustic damage to the lungs, pulmonary edema, and pulmonary hemorrhage. Birds are often found dead.

TURPENTINE

Turpentine is an aliphatic hydrocarbon derived from pine trees.

Toxicokinetics

Turpentine is readily absorbed from the gastrointestinal tract or by inhalation, and some dermal absorption also occurs. Once absorbed it is widely distributed in the body with highest concentrations in the liver, spleen, kidneys, and brain. Excretion of turpentine and metabolites is principally renal.

Systemic toxicosis usually develops within 2−3 hours of exposure, and an animal that is asymptomatic after 6−12 hours is unlikely to develop clinical signs of toxicosis.

Mode(s) of Action

Turpentine dissolves lipids and thus disrupts and damages cell membranes. Pulmonary toxicity is attributed principally to destruction of surfactant, leading to alveolar collapse.

Clinical Signs

The most common manifestation of toxicity is aspiration pneumonia, although the risk of aspiration pneumonia is not as great as for the petroleum hydrocarbons (q.v.). Respiratory signs include coughing, dyspnea, and pulmonary edema.

Neurological signs observed in humans include weakness, ataxia, somnolence, agitation, or coma.

Turpentine is also irritant to the gastrointestinal tract if ingested, to the skin if applied dermally, and to the eye if ocular contact occurs. Dermal lesions include erythema, vesiculation, chemical burns, and necrosis.

Diagnostic Aids

If aspiration pneumonia develops, there may be decreased oxygen saturation and secondary leukocytosis.

Turpentine toxicosis can often be diagnosed by the distinctive odor. Serum can be analyzed for turpentine.

Treatment

Activated charcoal adsorbs turpentine *in vitro*, but should be used only in large ingestions and then only with a cuffed endotracheal tube in place.

Treatment is otherwise symptomatic. Respiratory support may be required. Although corticosteroids promote surfactant production in premature animals and humans, they have not been shown to be useful in alveolar collapse in turpentine toxicosis. In the event of aspiration pneumonia develops, antibiotics should be administered.

If turpentine has been spilled on the skin, the animal should be bathed with a mild hand-dishwashing detergent and copious water. Ocular exposure should be treated immediately with irrigation for at least 20 minutes, and the cornea should be checked for ulceration using fluorescein after irrigation.

Prognosis

Prognosis depends on the organs or systems affected.

Necropsy

There are no pathognomonic lesions. Findings may include dermal and/or gastrointestinal irritation, and lesions of aspiration pneumonia and/or alveolar collapse.

Public Health Considerations

Ingestion of turpentine of 2 mL/kg or more are potentially toxic in human beings, and fatal toxicosis occurred in a 2-year-old child who ingested 15 mL turpentine.

Prevention

Access to turpentine should be prevented.

XYLITOL

Circumstances of Poisoning

Xylitol is an artificial sweetener that has no toxic effects in human beings, but is toxic to dogs. Dogs may be fed xylitol-containing foods by owners unaware of the risk, or may help themselves to such foods.

Note: Other artificial sweeteners do not represent toxic hazards to dogs.

Toxicokinetics

Xylitol is rapidly absorbed and clinical signs may develop in as little as 30−60 minutes. However, some food products release xylitol only slowly, so that the toxic effects may last for 12 or 24 hours.

Mode(s) of Action

Xylitol stimulates release of insulin from the canine pancreas, resulting in hypoglycemia. Hypoglycemia may occur at a dosage of ∼75−100 mg/kg.

Xylitol ingestion may also cause liver failure in dogs, at dosage in excess of 500 mg/kg, but the mechanism is unknown.

Clinical Signs

The most common clinical signs are those of acute hypoglycemia and include weakness, vomiting, ataxia, collapse, and seizures.

Diagnostic Aids

Clinical pathological findings may include hypoglycemia.

Treatment

Activated charcoal is not effective for adsorbing xylitol.

Blood glucose should be monitored every 1−2 hours for at least 12 hours, while liver values should be evaluated every 24 hours for at least 72 hours.

Hypoglycemia should be treated with dextrose. Treatment for hepatotoxicity is symptomatic and supportive.

Prognosis

The prognosis for hypoglycemia, with or without mild hepatic toxicosis, is good, but severe liver injury carries a guarded to poor prognosis.

Necropsy

The hepatic lesion is acute hepatic necrosis, which is centrilobular to massive in distribution.

Prevention

Owners should be informed that foods containing xylitol may be toxic to dogs.

MISCELLANEOUS HOUSEHOLD ITEMS THAT MAY CONTAIN ACIDS OR BASES

Note: Toxicoses due to acids and bases are discussed elsewhere in this book.

Household Item	Acid or Base
Ant killer	Boric acid
Drain cleaner	Sodium hydroxide
Oven cleaner	Sodium hydroxide, hydrochloric, sulfuric, chromic, or phosphoric acids
Radiator cleaner	Oxalic acid
Rust remover	Hydrochloric, phosphoric, or hydrofluoric acid
Soldering flux	Hydrochloric, glutamic, boric, and salicylic acid
Styptic pencil	Breaks down to sulfuric acid

MISCELLANEOUS HOUSEHOLD ITEMS THAT MAY CONTAIN ALIPHATIC OR AROMATIC HYDROCARBONS

Note: Toxicoses due to hydrocarbons are discussed elsewhere in this book.

- Cooking fuel
- Solid firelighters
- Paint or varnish removers
- Furniture polish
- Lighter fluid
- Glues
- Fire extinguisher chemicals
- Oven cleaner

Chapter 14

Metals

INTRODUCTION

A number of metals are toxicants of importance in veterinary medicine. The following metals are covered in this chapter:

- Copper
- Iron
- Lead
- Mercury
- Molybdenum
- Zinc

As a general note, metals and their inorganic salts are not adsorbed by activated charcoal, being of too small atomic or molecular mass.

COPPER

Circumstances of Poisoning

Sources of excess copper include:

- use of copper-containing algicides and fungicides
- pasture treated with poultry manure or swine manure
- grazing of plants growing in soil that is high in copper and low in molybdenum
- use of copper sulfate footbaths for sheep
- feeding rations prepared for other species to sheep
- excessive supplementation of livestock in copper-deficient areas
- ingestion of copper-containing items by domestic pets

A dose of 25–50 mg copper/kg bodyweight is sufficient to cause acute toxicosis.

In ruminants, molybdenum deficiency or sulfate deficiency may result in excessive absorption and storage of copper. Liver damage secondary to hepatotoxins such as pyrrolizidine alkaloids (q.v.) predisposes to copper poisoning.

Chronic copper poisoning by grazing plants that have grown in copper-rich soil has been described in New South Wales and Victoria. Sheep breeds

Veterinary Toxicology for Australia and New Zealand
DOI: http://dx.doi.org/10.1016/B978-0-12-420227-6.00013-X

of English origin are much more susceptible to this form of copper poisoning than Merinos. Pastures in which subterranean clover is dominant are the most hazardous in the affected areas.

An inherited autosomal recessive disease characterized by excessive copper storage in liver has been found in some breeds of dogs. It is most well-known in Bedlington Terriers but has also been reported in other breeds including Doberman Pinschers and West Highland White Terriers.

Toxicokinetics

Elemental copper is absorbed in the stomach or rumen, and in the small intestine. Copper binds to albumin, ceruloplasmin, and transcuprein. Copper is stored in the liver, kidney, and brain. Copper is principally excreted in bile in a complex with molybdenum and sulfate, although small amounts are excreted in urine.

Mode(s) of Action

Acute intake of a high dose (25–50 mg/kg bodyweight) of copper salts causes acute gastroenteritis due to direct tissue irritation and necrosis.

Excess stored copper causes hepatocellular degeneration and necrosis. When the liver is unable to store sufficient copper to regulate circulating copper levels, copper is directly cytotoxic to erythrocytes, causing hemolysis. Excessive free copper accumulates in the kidneys.

Clinical Signs

Acute overdose of copper salts, such as that observed if thirsty sheep drink footbath solution containing copper sulfate, is characterized by hypersalivation, colic, fluid or hemorrhagic diarrhea, dehydration, shock, and death.

Animals, particularly sheep, may develop an acute crisis of liver necrosis and intravascular hemolysis after excess intake of copper, or normal intake of copper under circumstances of molybdenum or sulfate deficiency. Copper may accumulate to toxic levels over several weeks. The crisis may be precipitated by stress such as transport or acute starvation. Clinical signs in ruminants are those of hemoglobinuria, icterus, anoxia, and death.

Pigs with copper poisoning typically exhibit anorexia, depression, ill-thrift, icterus, hemoglobinuria, and melena.

Horses appear to be relatively resistant to copper toxicity, although experimentally, 50 mg/kg bodyweight may result in colic and be fatal in 2 weeks.

Dogs with inherited copper storage disease do not develop a hemolytic crisis, but exhibit signs of progressive liver failure including vomiting, weight loss, and anorexia. Dogs may develop ascites and/or hepatic encephalopathy.

Diagnostic Aids

In livestock with copper poisoning, liver enzymes are significantly elevated.

Normal values for copper vary from laboratory to laboratory, so the following values are presented only as a guide:

Species	Tissue	High Level of Cu (ppm Wet Weight)	Toxic Level of Cu (ppm Wet Weight)
Cattle	Liver	200–550	>250
	Kidney	5–7	>10
	Serum, no Se supplement	2.5–4	>4
	Serum, Se supplement	0.5–2.5	–
Sheep	Liver	100–500	>250
	Kidney	4–10	>18
	Serum	1–5	>3.3
	Muscle	1–1.6	–
	Brain	5–14	>17
	Spleen	1–1.5	>20
Goat	Liver	180–250	>230
	Kidney	–	>12
	Serum	0.9–1.8	>1.2
	Spleen	–	>40
Camelids	Liver	–	>250
	Serum	–	>2
Pigs	Liver	15–750	–
	Kidney	8–25	>30
	Serum	1.7–3	>4.5
Horses	Liver	1000–1500	–
	Kidney	30–40	–
	Serum	0.9–1.1	>7.7

Dogs with inherited copper storage disease have elevated liver enzymes, but serum copper levels and plasma ceruloplasmin levels are typically normal.

Treatment

Treatment of acute gastroenteritis due to ingestion of copper salts is symptomatic and supportive.

Treatment is often unsuccessful in ruminants with a hepatic/hemolytic crisis following hepatic storage of copper, but may be attempted with ammonium tetrathiomolybdate, 1.7–3.4 mg/day IV or SC, for three treatments on alternate days.

An alternative treatment is D-penicillamine, 50 mg/kg orally for up to 6 days.

Other animals in the flock or herd should be provided with a zinc supplement. Individual animals considered to be at risk can be dosed with 50 mg ammonium molybdate and 0.3–1.0 g thiosulfate daily for 3 weeks.

D-Penicillamine, 10−15 mg/kg orally twice daily, promotes urinary excretion of copper in dogs with inherited copper storage disease. Corticosteroids, up to 1.0 mg/day, may assist in reducing liver damage, and 500−1000 mg/day ascorbic acid increases copper excretion.

Necropsy

Gross lesions in sheep include icterus, enlarged spleen, and dark bluish-black kidneys, often referred to as "gunmetal kidneys." Histopathology reveals hepatocellular degeneration and necrosis, renal tubular necrosis, and excessive numbers of fragmented erythrocytes in the spleen. Evidence of chronic liver damage may be present in the form of periportal fibrosis and bile ductule proliferation.

In dogs with inherited copper storage disease, the liver may be swollen and necrotic, or shrunken with cirrhosis. Microscopic lesions are those of chronic active hepatitis and cirrhosis.

Prevention

Do not allow animals access to large volumes of copper salts. If it is necessary to treat sheep with a copper sulfate footbath, avoid having thirsty sheep in the footbath and monitor them to prevent drinking.

Ensure adequate molybdenum levels. Rations for sheep should have a maximum Cu:Mo ratio of 6:1.

Where possible, select dogs for breeding that do not have inherited copper storage disease. Affected dogs should be fed a diet with restricted copper.

IRON

Circumstances of Poisoning

Iron overdose may result from:

- Ingestion of preparations for oral supplementation of iron that contain ferrous salts. This may include overdose of veterinary medicines, or ingestion of preparations for human use such as multivitamins or iron tablets for use by pregnant women.
- Overdose with injectable iron preparations.
- Consumption of garden fertilizers that are rich in iron.

As a general rule, in excess of 20 mg/kg bodyweight of iron is likely to cause toxicosis, over 60 mg/kg is likely to cause severe toxicosis, and over 200 mg/kg is likely to be lethal.

Iron contents of various iron compounds are presented in the following table:

Chemical	Iron Content (% w/w)
Ferric ammonium citrate	15
Ferric chloride	34
Ferric hydroxide	63
Ferric phosphate	37
Ferric pyrophosphate	30
Ferricholinate	12
Ferroglycine sulfate	16
Ferrous carbonate (anhydrous)	48
Ferrous fumarate	33
Ferrous gluconate	12
Ferrous lactate	24
Ferrous sulfate (anhydrous)	37
Ferrous sulfate (hydrate)	20
Peptonized iron	16

Note that metallic iron and iron oxide (rust) are not of toxicological concern. Iron oxide gel in groundwater, such as that occurring in the sand country of the western Manawatu region in New Zealand, is a cosmetic issue and may impair water flow, but does not represent a source of iron toxicosis.

Toxicokinetics

Iron must be in ionized form to be absorbed from the intestinal lumen. Ferrous iron is more readily absorbed than ferric iron. Absorption is usually an active process, facilitated by a transferrin-like protein, but in acute overdose it appears that iron can be absorbed by a passive process. Iron is bound to transferrin in circulation or may be stored as ferritin in the liver. Most of the body's iron is in ferrous form and forms part of hemoglobin or myoglobin. Iron is also located in some enzymes including peroxidase, catalase, and cytochrome C. Iron in ferritin, hemosiderin, and transferrin is present in the ferric form. Iron is stored by the body in the liver, spleen, and bone marrow.

Iron absorption is facilitated by a high sugar level in the diet, but reduced by phosphate in the diet.

Iron is largely recycled by the body, with very little excretion. Some iron is lost by exfoliation of intestinal mucosal cells, and some iron is lost by carnivores through vaginal bleeding in proestrus.

Mode(s) of Action

In acute overdose, iron has a direct corrosive effect on the intestinal mucosa. When the capacity of iron-binding proteins are saturated, free iron is present in the circulation. Free iron acts as a strong oxidant, leading to membrane damage to organelles, of which mitochondrial damage appears to be the most toxicologically significant. Oxidative phosphorylation is disrupted, with a resultant increase in anerobic metabolism. Free iron also inhibits the Krebs citric acid cycle, interferes with the clotting of blood, and acts as a potent vasodilator. Toxic effects include hepatic necrosis, myocardial necrosis, impaired cardiac function, metabolic acidosis, and hemorrhagic diathesis.

Pigs may die suddenly after injections of iron, with clinical signs of anaphylactic shock.

Clinical Signs

Clinical signs of iron poisoning include vomiting, hematemesis, melena, hypotension, hypovolemia, metabolic acidosis, and shock. In massive overdose there may be acute liver failure. There may be CNS signs including depression, cerebral edema, tremors, seizures, or coma.

Iron poisoning tends to occur in phases. The first phase is that of gastrointestinal toxicosis, generally manifests within 6 hours of ingestion, and is followed by a second latent phase when the animal appears to recover. In mild to moderate iron toxicosis there may be no further clinical signs, but in severe iron toxicosis, a third stage develops 12−96 hours after iron ingestion. During this phase the gastrointestinal signs recur but are accompanied by systemic signs of shock, acidosis, hypotension, cardiovascular toxicity, hemorrhagic diathesis, and hepatic necrosis. If the animal survives the third stage, it may show a fourth stage 2−6 weeks after the initial exposure, when sequelae such as intestinal strictures, pyloric stenosis, cardiomyopathy, and hepatic insufficiency develop.

Diagnostic Aids

Clinical pathology findings include elevated liver enzymes, dehydration, anemia, hypoglycemia, bilirubinemia, delayed clotting times, and leucocytosis. Hemoglobinemia and or hemoglobinuria may be present.

Total serum iron levels are elevated at least 50% above normal.

Iron tablets may be apparent on radiographs.

Treatment

If ingestion is recent, administer milk of magnesia orally to precipitate iron in the gastrointestinal tract as insoluble iron hydroxide.

Administer deferoxamine intravenously to chelate iron, at 15 mg/kg/hour or at 40 mg/kg every 4−6 hours. Monitor for cardiac arrhythmia and/or evidence of histamine release when administering deferoxamine. Note that chelation of iron by deferoxamine will cause the urine to be reddish-brown.

Oral ascorbic acid enhances the action of deferoxamine.

Monitor serum iron levels and continue treatment until they are in the normal range.

Treatment is otherwise symptomatic and supportive.

Prognosis

Prognosis is guarded if the third stage of toxicosis develops, and is poor if the third stage develops and chelation with deferoxamine is not available.

Necropsy

Following oral poisoning, the gastrointestinal tract will show signs of enteritis and necrosis and may be ulcerated. The splanchnic vessels, liver, and kidneys are congested. Hepatic necrosis may be grossly evident, and there may be icterus and hemoglobinuria.

Normal values for iron vary from laboratory to laboratory, so the following values are presented only as a guide:

Species	Tissue	High Level of Fe (ppm Wet Weight, Except Otherwise Stated)	Toxic Level of Fe (ppm Wet Weight, Except Otherwise Stated)
Cattle	Liver, total iron	53–700	>9000
	Liver, ferritin	–	>250
	Kidney	49–300	>100
	Serum, total iron	400–600	>1800
	Serum, ferritin	>80	–
Dogs	Liver, total iron	>500	–
	Kidney	>120	–
	Serum, total iron	>200 µg/dL	–
	Serum, ferritin	>260 ng/mL	–
Pigs	Liver		>400
Horses	Liver	–	>600
	Kidney	–	>138
	Serum	–	>400 µg/dL

Prevention

Clients taking iron tablets should be warned that these are attractive to dogs but must be kept secure from dogs as well as from small children.

LEAD

Circumstances of Poisoning

Sources of lead include:

- Older paints and calking compounds. Paint flakes from older buildings are a major source of lead poisoning in domestic pets.
- Lead objects that may be retained in the stomach, such as lead fishing weights.
- Poorly glazed pottery.
- Lead plates in vehicle batteries.

- Old lead pipes.
- Old "lead head" nails.
- Solder.
- Old metal tubes (e.g., paint tubes), old toys, stained-glass window surrounds.
- Contaminated pasture near smelters.
- Sites where lead-rich materials, such as lead-painted timber, have been burnt.

Elemental lead is minimally absorbed and therefore of very low toxicity unless retained in the acid environment of the stomach. In animals that have been maliciously shot, bullets, or buckshot generally do not pose a risk of lead poisoning. However, systemic lead poisoning may result if the bullet is in contact with cerebrospinal fluid, pleural fluid, synovial fluid, or an intervertebral disk.

Toxicokinetics

Lead salts or organic lead compounds can be absorbed from the gastrointestinal tract. Fumes or very small particles (<0.5 μm) may reach the pulmonary alveoli and be absorbed from the lungs. Organic lead compounds may be absorbed dermally, but inorganic lead salts have negligible dermal absorption.

Generally $<10\%$ of ingested lead is absorbed, with the rest excreted in the feces.

Lead is highly bound to erythrocytes in the systemic circulation. Lead is distributed to, and accumulates in the liver, lungs, kidneys, brain, bones, and teeth. Lead most readily crosses the brain—blood barrier of young animals. Lead is able to cross the placenta and also enters milk.

Mode(s) of Action

Lead interferes with the biochemistry of the body in many ways. It binds sulfhydryl groups and interferes with the function of many enzymes that contain these groups. It competes with calcium ions, and also competes with or replaces zinc in many enzymes. Lead has multiple toxic effects in the CNS, including interfering with serotonergic pathways, GABA production and activity, dopamine uptake, cholinergic function, and calcium balance. In the PNS, lead causes demyelination and reduced conduction velocity. Lead interferes with normal synthesis of hemoglobin at multiple levels. Inhibition of δ-aminolevulinic acid dehydrase, heme synthase, and ferrochelatase results in reduced heme synthesis and accumulation of heme precursors aminolevulinic acid, coproporphyrins, and zinc protoporphyrin in the blood. In addition, inhibition of 5'-nucleotidase leads to retention of nucleic acid fragments and ribosomes in erythrocytes, leading to basophilic stippling and also making erythrocytes abnormally fragile. Lead causes alteration in vitamin D metabolism. In the fetus, neurological development may be delayed, or hyaline necrosis of the placenta may cause abortion or stillbirth.

Clinical Signs

Lead poisoning is generally associated with clinical signs affecting the gastrointestinal tract, hematological and neurological systems. Chronic lead poisoning can be insidious and difficult to diagnose.

Anorexia is typical in all species. Dogs and cats often exhibit vomiting. Constipation is common, particularly in dogs. Both constipation and diarrhea have been observed in cattle. Ruminants may exhibit rumen stasis. Horses may develop mild colic. Cats and dogs may exhibit signs of abdominal discomfort that are not made worse by palpation.

Anemia is also typical in chronic lead poisoning in all species. Basophillic stippling is most commonly seen in dogs, but is not pathognomonic for lead poisoning. Elevated free porphyrins may cause plasma to fluoresce under a UV lamp; this is most commonly seen in cattle.

Neurological signs vary with species, and are also variable between individual animals, so lead poisoning should always be considered in cases of neurological abnormality. Dogs may be depressed or agitated, exhibit behavioral changes and tremors, and develop seizures. Cats exhibit depression and may meow persistently, but seizures are quite rare in cats. Megaesophagus has been reported in cats. Cattle and horses may appear to be blind and may head-press. Cattle often show rhythmic bobbing of the head and twitching of the ears, circling and stumbling, hyperesthesia, tremors, but rarely have seizures. Cattle may become aggressive. Horses tend to exhibit depression, ataxia, and dysphagia, but may develop seizures in severe toxicosis. Peripheral nerve damage may affect the recurrent laryngeal nerve in horses, leading to "roaring."

Abortion is most often recognized in cattle.

Growing horses may exhibit epiphyseal enlargement.

Birds typically show anorexia and weight loss, and psitticines may regurgitate and develop diarrhea. Paresis of the wings is classical in waterfowl, whereas psitticines show ataxia, blindness, torticollis, circling, and seizures.

Diagnostic Aids

For determination of blood lead levels, whole blood is required because most lead in circulation is bound to erythrocytes. The laboratory to which the sample is to be sent should be contacted to determine what anticoagulant is preferred. In mammals, blood lead levels >0.3 ppm (30 µg/dL) support a diagnosis of lead poisoning, while levels >0.6 ppm (60 µg/dL) are diagnostic. In birds the equivalent values are 0.2 and 0.5 ppm, respectively.

Some laboratories may offer assays of erythrocyte ALAD activity, erythrocyte porphyrin assay, urinary ALA, and zinc protoporphyrin. However, normal and diagnostic values for these assays are not available for all domestic species. In cattle, erythrocyte ALAD activity <50 is considered diagnostic of lead poisoning, and urinary ALA levels >500 µg/dL are considered diagnostic of lead poisoning. Blood protoporphyrin levels >40 µg/dL are diagnostic of lead poisoning in waterfowl.

If the results of blood lead determination are equivocal, lead levels in 24-hour collections of urine can be tested before and after administering Ca-ethylenediaminetetraacetic acid (EDTA). An increase of 10-fold or greater in the urinary lead level as a result of Ca-EDTA administration is considered confirmatory of lead poisoning.

Radiography may reveal lead or lead-rich items, such as sinkers or paint flakes, in the gastrointestinal tract, or bullets in contact with synovial fluid. "Lead lines" within the epiphyseal plate of long bones are useful if present, but are not often seen. Puppies and foals may show metaphyseal sclerosis.

A number of hematological changes have been associated with lead poisoning, but none is pathognomonic. Contrary to popular belief, basophilic stippling is not pathognomonic to lead poisoning. It can occur with other conditions such as zinc poisoning (q.v.). Furthermore, ruminants normally have a small percentage of erythrocytes with basophilic stippling, and erythrocytic parasites such as *Mycoplasma haemofelis* (*Haemobartonella felis*) can be mistaken for basophilic stippling. Anemia is common but may be microcytic or normocytic, and hypochromic or normochromic. A high percentage of nucleated erythrocytes is suggestive of lead poisoning in dogs and cats. Other hematological changes reported in lead poisoning include anisocytosis, echinocytosis, poikilocytosis, polychromasia, and the presence of target cells.

There may be mature leucocytosis. Hematological changes associated with lead poisoning in birds include heterophilia, hyperchromic anemia, and vacuolation of erythrocytes.

Treatment

Chelating agents for removal of lead include calcium disodium EDTA, meso-2,3-dimercaptosuccinic acid (succimer), and D-penicillamine.

It is important that all lead-containing objects are removed from the gastrointestinal tract before administering calcium disodium EDTA or D-penicillamine, because both of these increase lead absorption from the gastrointestinal tract.

Calcium Disodium Ethylenediaminetetraacetic Acid

Lead may be chelated in calcium disodium EDTA (Ca-EDTA). It may be administered subcutaneously or intravenously. Ca-EDTA is toxic in its own right, with adverse effects including depression, anorexia, vomiting, and diarrhea. These adverse side effects may be partially ameliorated by zinc supplementation. Ca-EDTA should be administered for no more than five consecutive days or it may damage the proximal renal tubules, and renal function should be monitored when Ca-EDTA is used. Suggested treatment regimens for different species are as follows:

Horses and ruminants	73 mg Ca-EDTA/kg bodyweight/day, divided into two or three doses and administered by slow IV infusion, for 3−5 days. At least 2 days' rest before a repeat course. OR 110 mg/kg by slow IV infusion twice daily for 2 days, then 2 days' rest, then 2 more days of treatment.
Dogs	100 mg/kg/day, divided into four SC doses/day, for 2−5 days. Dilute to a final concentration of 10 mg Ca-EDTA/mL of 5% dextrose, and use different administration sites. Do not exceed a total of 2 g/day of Ca-EDTA, even in large dogs. At least 5 days' rest before a repeat course.
Cats	27.5 mg/kg/day in 15 mL of 5% dextrose SC, in four divided doses, for not more than 5 days.
Psitticines	Dimercaptosuccinic acid is preferred for pet birds, but if Ca-EDTA is the only chelating agent available, 35−40 mg/kg IM, twice daily for 5 days. At least 5 days' rest before a repeat course.

Administration of dimercaprol (BAL) in conjunction with Ca-EDTA may be considered, particularly if there are severe neurological signs, because it crosses the blood−brain barrier, absorbs lead from erythrocytes, and also enhances lead excretion. It can be nephrotoxic, and alkalinization of urine is recommended. It should not be used in animals with impaired hepatic function. Suggested doses are 3−6 mg/kg IM, three to four times daily, *or* 2−5 mg/kg IM every 4 hours for 2 days, then every 8 hours for 1 day, and every 12 hours thereafter. Side effects of dimercaprol include pain at the injection site, vomiting, tachycardia, hypertension, halitosis, and seizures.

Mobilization of lead by Ca-EDTA may result in a temporary worsening of clinical signs.

Note: It is critically important that calcium disodium EDTA, rather than sodium EDTA, is used. Sodium EDTA is likely to cause acute hypocalcemia.

Meso-2,3-Dimercaptosuccinic Acid (Succimer)

Succimer has emerged as a suitable chelating agent for lead toxicosis in dogs. It has a superior safety margin to Ca-EDTA, does not chelate zinc, and is more readily administered than Ca-EDTA. The recommended regimen is 10 mg/kg PO, three times daily for 10 days. Administration *per rectum* has been found to be effective in dogs with severe vomiting.

Succimer is also recommended for pet birds, at a dose regimen of 25−35 mg/kg PO, twice daily for 5 days.

D-*Penicillamine*

D-Penicillamine may be used on its own or following a course of Ca-EDTA. Side effects of D-penicillamine include anorexia, depression, and vomiting. Adverse effects of D-penicillamine may be ameliorated by administering diphenhydramine 30 minutes before administering D-penicillamine. As with Ca-EDTA, D-penicillamine can be nephrotoxic so renal function must be monitored.

D-Penicillamine is administered orally. The recommended dose regimen for dogs is 30−110 mg/kg/day, divided into four doses. Treatment should be suspended after 5−7 days and then resumed after a further 5−7 days. D-Penicillamine and Ca-EDTA can be cycled.

For cats, D-penicillamine may be administered as 125 mg/cat every 12 hours for 5 days.

For cage birds the dose regimen for D-penicillamine is 55 mg/kg PO every 12 hours, and it may be administered for up to 2 weeks before giving a 5 day rest.

Supportive Treatment

Seizures should be controlled with diazepam or barbiturates. It has been reported that thiamine supplementation (10−20 mg/kg/day) is beneficial in alleviating neurological signs of lead poisoning.

Zinc supplementation should be given if Ca-EDTA or D-penicillamine is used as chelating agents.

Cerebral edema may be present in lead poisoning and should be relieved with mannitol, corticosteroids, and diuretics as appropriate.

Cathartics may assist in clearing the gastrointestinal tract of small lead objects such as paint flakes. Sulfate cathartics are recommended because they will precipitate lead as insoluble lead sulfate.

Endoscopy or surgery may be necessary to remove lead objects in the gastrointestinal tract, or in contact with CSF, pleural fluid, synovial fluid, or an intervertebral disk.

Cats in particular should be bathed if the source of lead could be lead-rich dust or paint flakes.

Ruminal flora are often hypoactive in chronic lead poisoning, so reinoculation of the rumen with ruminal fluid from healthy ruminants, or with probiotics, may be beneficial.

Prognosis

Prognosis is usually good with timely treatment. Animals that suffer seizures may be left with permanent neurological damage.

Necropsy

Grossly, there are no specific lesions. Animals that die from chronic lead poisoning may be emaciated. Pale musculature has been described in cattle. Ruminants may have laminar cortical necrosis, which may be apparent grossly. Cerebral edema may result in flattening of cerebral gyri and coning of the cerebellum as it is forced into the foramen magnum. Meningeal vessels are often congested. Horses may have aspiration pneumonia, and cats may have megaesophagus.

Microscopically, intranuclear acid-fast inclusion bodies may be found in proximal renal tubule cells and, less commonly, in hepatocytes. Similar inclusion bodies may be present in the cytoplasm of osteoclasts.

Laminar cortical necrosis may be present in the brain of ruminants. Other CNS lesions in lead toxicosis include pale spongy neuropil, neuronal degeneration and necrosis, astrocytosis, and microgliosis. Astrocytosis may be found in the molecular layers of the cerebellum. Capillary endothelial cells are often swollen, and there may be proliferation of cerebral capillaries.

Tissues of choice for postmortem confirmation of the diagnosis are liver and kidney.

The following values are presented as a guide:

Species	Tissue	High Level of Pb (ppm Wet Weight Except Where Otherwise Stated)	Toxic Level of Pb (ppm Wet Weight Except Where Otherwise Stated)
Cattle	Liver	>2	>5
	Kidney	>3	>5
	Brain	>0.3	>0.7
	Milk	>0.05	>0.1
Cats	Liver		>10
Dogs	Liver	>3.6	>50
	Kidney	>5	>10
Goats	Liver	>3	>10
	Kidney	>3	>10
	Brain	>1.8	>5
Horses	Liver (chronic poisoning)	>3	>4
	Liver (acute poisoning)		>10
	Kidney (chronic poisoning)	>3	>5
	Kidney (acute poisoning)		>20
	Brain	>1	>3
	Milk	>0.05	>0.28
Pigs	Liver	>5	>37
	Kidney	>5	>25
Chickens	Liver	>5	>18
	Kidney	>5	>20
	Egg shell	>2	−
	Egg yolk	>0.4	−

(Continued)

(Continued)

Species	Tissue	High Level of Pb (ppm Wet Weight Except Where Otherwise Stated)	Toxic Level of Pb (ppm Wet Weight Except Where Otherwise Stated)
Rabbits	Liver	>3	>10
	kidney	–	>10
Sheep	Liver	>5	>10
	Kidney	–	>5
	Brain	>1.2	–
	Wool (ppm dry weight)	>12	>25
Waterfowl	Liver	>1	>6
	Kidney	>1	>8
	Brain	–	>3

MERCURY

General Remarks

The toxicity of mercury varies depending on the chemical form.

Circumstances of Poisoning

Inorganic mercury metal may be found in older thermometers, barometers, batteries, some fluorescent light bulbs, and some pressure-sensing devices.

Inorganic mercurial salts may be used as preservatives or fixatives, latex paints, some skin-lightening cosmetics, and older (obsolete) disinfectants (e.g., mercurochrome) and pesticides. Inorganic mercurials can be reduced in anerobic environments to methyl mercury.

Organic mercurials, including the alkyl mercurials, methyl mercury, and ethyl mercury, may be used as fungicides, and aryl mercurial may be found in anti-mildew paints. A diet very high in carnivorous fish could lead to excessive methylmercury intake. Methylmercury toxicosis has occurred in livestock that were fed seed grain that had been intended for sowing and treated with a methylmercury-based fungicide.

Toxicokinetics

Elemental mercury is the least toxic form by ingestion, but may release mercury vapor which can be inhaled. Gastrointestinal absorption of elemental mercury and inorganic mercurial salts is very slow. Ethyl and methyl mercury, on the other hand, are readily absorbed from the gastrointestinal tract.

Inorganic mercurial salts accumulate in lysosomes of the renal cortex, while alkyl mercury compounds accumulate in the brain. All forms of mercury can cross the placenta.

Elemental and alkyl mercurials are metabolized to divalent mercury, while aryl mercurial are rapidly metabolized to inorganic salts.

Inorganic mercury is primarily excreted in urine, while organic mercurials are excreted in bile.

Mode(s) of Action

Inorganic mercury salts cause tissue necrosis, including necrosis of the renal tubules.

Alkyl mercurial prevent synthesis of essential proteins, leading to cellular degeneration and necrosis. The most important target organ is the brain.

Clinical Signs

Signs of acute inorganic mercurial toxicosis are stomatitis, pharyngitis, vomiting, diarrhea, shock, and rapid death. Animals that survive the initial injury to the gastrointestinal tract may subsequently develop oliguria and azotemia.

Toxicosis due to alkyl mercurial develops slowly over 7 or more days, and may be delayed for weeks. Neurological signs include depression, ataxia, paresis and central blindness, intention tremor, proprioceptive deficits, seizures, slow respiration, coma, and death.

Early signs of dermal erythema and conjunctivitis have been reported in some cases of alkyl mercurial toxicosis. Dermatitis typically becomes progressively worse over the course of toxicosis. Some animals develop hematuria and malena.

Diagnostic Aids

Mercury levels in blood or urine may be elevated.

Treatment

In acute toxicosis due to an inorganic mercurial, egg white may be administered to provide an alternative substrate for protein denaturation. Alternatively, sodium thiosulfate, 0.5–1.0 g/kg bodyweight, may be administered orally to bind mercury. A saline cathartic should be administered to promote elimination of the toxicant from the gastrointestinal tract. Once the gastrointestinal tract has been cleared of mercury, administer D-penicillamine (15–50 mg/kg/day) or succimer (see lead poisoning) to increase elimination of mercury absorbed systemically.

Treatment is usually futile by the time poisoning due to an alkyl mercurial becomes apparent. Supplementation with selenium and vitamin E may ameliorate toxicosis.

Prognosis

Prognosis is guarded to poor.

Necropsy

Lesions of inorganic mercurial poisoning include ulceration and necrosis of the gastrointestinal tract, and pale swollen kidneys which microscopically have renal tubular necrosis.

Lesions in alkyl mercurial poisoning include degeneration of cerebral arterioles, perivascular cuffing in the CNS, laminar cortical necrosis, and, in kittens exposed prenatally, cerebellar hypoplasia.

The tissues of choice for postmortem diagnosis are liver and kidney. Brain may also be useful in alkyl mercurial toxicosis. Both fresh and fixed brain and kidney should be collected.

The following values are presented as a guide:

Species	Tissue	High Level of Hg (ppm Wet Weight Except Where Otherwise Stated)	Toxic Level of Hg (ppm Wet Weight Except Where Otherwise Stated)
Cats	Liver	> 5	> 30
	Kidney	> 5	> 20
	Blood	> 3	> 6
	Brain	> 7	> 10
	Urine	> 0.01	> 1.6
Cattle	Liver	–	> 2
	Kidney	> 14	> 40
	Blood	> 0.2	> 3
	Brain	> 0.2	> 0.5
Horses	Liver	–	> 5
	Kidney	–	> 5
	Blood	–	> 2
	Brain	–	> 3
	Urine	–	> 3
Pigs	Liver	> 1	> 5
	Kidney	> 1	> 10
	Brain	> 0.05	> 5
Chickens	Liver	> 1	> 3
	Kidney	> 2	> 5
	Brain	> 0.2	> 0.5
	Blood	–	> 0.2
	Muscle	> 1	> 5
	Feathers	> 0.4	> 6
	Egg white	> 5	> 10
	Egg yolk	> 0.5	> 0.9
Sheep	Liver	> 7	> 18
	Kidney	> 18	> 20
	Blood	> 0.2	–
	Wool (ppm dry weight)	> 0.2	–

MOLYBDENUM

Circumstances of Poisoning

Molybdenum toxicity has occurred in Australian and New Zealand livestock grazing on land where the soil molybdenum level is high and, less commonly, where there has been excessive use of fertilizer containing molybdenum. Molybdenum toxicosis has been observed secondary to use of sewage sludge as a fertilizer. Plants, particularly legume species, absorb water-soluble molybdates from soil and fertilizer.

Excess molybdenum in soil may be naturally occurring or may be a result of contamination from industries. Some industries that may cause molybdenum contamination include aluminum smelters, steel mills, and brick manufacturers that use clay high in molybdenum.

Toxicokinetics and Modes of Action

In ruminants, molybdates react with sulfides to produce thiomolybdates that then react with copper, resulting in a complex that is poorly absorbed. In addition, absorbed molybdenum forms a copper—molybdate complex in the liver, which is readily excreted. The net result in ruminants is clinical copper deficiency. Cattle are more susceptible than sheep. Monogastric species are far less susceptible to the adverse effects of excess molybdenum than ruminants, because intestinal bacteria in monogastric species form little thiomolybdate.

Excessive molybdenum also appears to impair a number of enzymes critical to stability of collagen and elastin, and may reduce the synthesis of phospholipids in nervous tissue.

High sulfur in the diet increases the risk of secondary copper deficiency due to excesss molybdenum.

Molybdenum is excreted in milk, so nursing calves and lambs may have an excessive molybdenum intake.

Clinical Signs

Clinical signs may become evident in as little as 2—3 weeks.

Clinical signs of molybdenum poisoning in cattle include persistent green bubbly diarrhea ("peat scours"), depigmentation of the hair, rough dull coat, epiphora and nasal discharge, decreased milk production, and anemia. Bulls may show decreased libido, and fertility of cows is decreased. Animals often show lameness and joint pain, and may suffer spontaneous fractures. For example, calving chains may fracture the legs of calves during assisted delivery. Cattle often show pica. In severe toxicosis, cattle may develop ascending ataxia.

In sheep, molybdenum toxicosis causes enzootic ataxia, or swayback, which is most often seen in lambs less than a month old. In adult sheep, the first clinical sign may be an outbreak of lameness, with evidence of joint pain. Sheep are anemic, and black or colored sheep lack color in the wool.

Abortions and signs of copper deficiency have been observed in horses grazing pastures severely contaminated with molybdenum.

Forage containing <3 mg Mo/kg dry matter are generally considered to be safe for ruminants, but the sulfur and copper levels must also be considered. Equine diets should contain <100 ppm Mo, and pig diets should contain <1000 ppm Mo.

Diagnostic Aids

Anemia is microcytic and hypochromic.

Clinical chemistry may reveal evidence of liver and kidney dysfunction, i.e., elevations in AST, GGT, bilirubin, BUN, and creatinine. Serum calcium may be electated.

Radiography of lame cattle may reveal osteoporosis, exostoses, and in growing animals, defects in the epiphyseal plates.

Blood Mo typically exceeds 0.1 ppm while blood Cu is <0.6 ppm. Blood copper levels are often normal even though there are clinical signs of copper deficiency.

Treatment

In severe toxicosis, subcutaneous copper glycinate may be administered (120 mg/adult cow; 60 mg/calf).

Animals should be removed from the source of molybdenum if possible, and appropriately supplemented with copper. The dietary ratio of Cu:Mo should be between 4:1 and 10:1. The S:Mo ratio should be less than 100:1.

Prognosis

Prognosis depends on the severity of toxicosis, but if the Mo:Cu ratio is corrected, excess Mo levels in the body usually fall rapidly.

Necropsy

Animals typically show loss of condition, and may be emaciated. Gross lesions may include swollen liver and pale kidneys, corresponding microscopically to periacinar to severe hepatic necrosis, hepatic hemosiderosis, and nephrosis. Sheep and lambs with enzootic ataxia have neuronal degeneration, demyelination, and lysis of white matter. Findings associated with lameness include exostoses and periosteal hemorrhages, and in sheep the greater trochanters may be loose. Microscopically, there is osteoporosis, and defects in epiphyseal plates of young animals.

The following values are presented as a guide:

Species·	Tissue	High Level of Mo (ppm Wet Weight Except Where Otherwise Stated)	Toxic Level of Mo (ppm Wet Weight Except Where Otherwise Stated)
Cattle	Liver	–	>2
	Kidney	–	>1.15
	Plasma	–	>0.08
	Milk (mg/L)	>0.2	>0.4
Chickens	Liver	>1	>6
Sheep	Liver	>2.6	>30
	Kidney	>7	>200
	Plasma (mg/L)	>1	>2
	Wool (ppm dry weight)	>1	–

ZINC

Circumstances of Poisoning

Zinc is found in a number of household items including automotive parts, storage batteries, galvanized items, some fungicides (e.g., zinc sulfate), zinc-rich (anti-rust) paints, and in zinc oxide sunscreen. Livestock may chew on galvanized items while domestic pets may swallow items containing zinc.

Cages and parts of cages are often galvanized. Small items such as nails, staples, and zipper pulls can also be a source of zinc.

Cats are much less commonly poisoned by zinc than dogs, because of their discriminating dietary habits.

Toxicokinetics

Zinc is an essential element, and is absorbed from the gastrointestinal tract by a carrier-mediated mechanism, for which calcium may compete. Systemic bioavailability is approximately 25%. Zinc is transported in the circulation bound to albumin and β2-macroglobulin, and accumulates in liver, kidney, pancreas, muscle, and prostate. Excretion of zinc is limited. Most zinc that is excreted is excreted in bile, with a smaller proportion excreted in urine.

Mode(s) of Action

The toxic mechanism(s) of zinc are not well understood. Zinc causes hemolytic anemia in most species. Some zinc compounds are directly corrosive to the gastrointestinal tract.

Clinical Signs

Clinical signs in small animals include anorexia, vomiting, lethargy, diarrhea, anemia, hemoglobinuria, pale mucous membranes, and icterus. Animals may show signs of hepatic, pancreatic, and/or renal failure. Disseminated intravascular coagulation has occurred in some cases.

Clinical signs in livestock are anorexia, diarrhea, lethargy, decreased milk production, anemia, and icterus. Polydipsia, exophthalmia, and seizures have been reported. Preruminants are much more susceptible to zinc toxicosis than adult ruminants. Ruminants may develop secondary copper deficiency.

In foals and pigs, there may be lameness and epiphyseal swelling. Foals develop a degenerative arthritis.

Diagnostic Aids

Clinical pathology in dogs and cats includes hemolytic anemia, uremia, hematuria, and proteinuria. Heinz bodies are often observed in blood. The anemia may be normocytic or macrocytic, and is commonly hypochromic. Evidence of a regenerative response is usually present, such as reticulocytes, basophilic stippling, variable RBC diameter, and polychromasia. Neutrophilia with a left shift is common. Alkaline phosphatase and alanine amonitransferase may be elevated.

Clinical pathology in ruminants, horses, and pigs has not been well characterized.

Zinc concentrations in the serum and urine are elevated. If collecting blood for serum zinc analysis, it is important to use syringes that do not contain rubber, and to prevent contact with the rubber bung of a vacuum tube, because rubber often contains zinc stearate.

Radiography may reveal the source of zinc in the gastrointestinal tract of small animals.

Treatment

The source of zinc should be removed.

Absorbed zinc may be chelated with Ca-EDTA or D-penicillamine (see Section "Lead" for dosages).

Treatment is otherwise symptomatic and supportive.

Prognosis

Prognosis is guarded. The patient should be assessed for damage to liver, kidneys, and/or pancreas.

Necropsy

Grossly apparent lesions in most species include gastroenteritis, icterus, hepato-megaly, splenomegaly, pale swollen kidneys, and nodular pancreas. Microscopic lesions include necrosis in the liver, hepatic hemosiderosis, necrosis in the renal tubules, and inflammation, necrosis, and fibrosis in the pancreas.

In pigs, there may be collapse of the bone under the cartilage of the proximal humerus. Excessive pericardial fluid and epicardial petechiae have also been described. There may be hemarthrosis in multiple joints.

Foals have severe generalized osteochondrosis in all four limbs. All limb joints may be affected but the pastern and fetlock joints are often the most severely affected.

In cattle, lesions may include pulmonary emphysema.

The following values are presented as a guide:

Species	Tissue	High Level of Zn (ppm Wet Weight Except Where Otherwise Stated)	Toxic Level of Zn (ppm Wet Weight Except Where Otherwise Stated)
Cats	Liver	–	> 80
	Kidney	–	> 25
	Serum	> 1.1	> 5
	Pancreas	–	> 60
Cattle	Liver	–	> 120
	Kidney	–	> 130
	Serum	–	> 3
	Milk (mg/L)	> 4	> 8
	Pancreas	–	> 180
Dogs	Liver	–	> 200
	Kidney	–	> 190
	Serum	> 2	> 10
	Urine	–	> 10
Horses	Liver	> 160	> 1000
	Kidney	> 65	> 295
	Serum	> 1.6	> 3.5
	Pancreas	> 90	> 600
Pigs	Liver	> 200	> 500
	Kidney	–	> 190
	Serum	–	> 1.4
	Pancreas	–	> 950
Chickens	Liver	> 90	> 200
	Kidney	> 60	> 300
	Feathers (dry weight)	> 400	–
	Pancreas	> 200	> 1000
Sheep	Liver	> 100	> 400
	Kidney	> 50	> 240
	Serum	> 4	> 30
	Pancreas	> 50	> 135
	Wool (ppm dry weight)	> 100	–

Chapter 15

Metalloids

Rhian Cope

A number of metalloids are toxicologically significant in veterinary medicine. Metalloids are chemical elements that have properties between those of metals and nonmetals. Important metalloids include boron, silicon, germanium, arsenic, antimony, and tellurium. Selenium, although less commonly included in the metalloid group, is included in this chapter. Polonium and astatine are inconsistently includes in the metalloid group.

The metalloids covered in this chapter are:

Antimony
Boron and borates
Inorganic arsenic compounds
Organoarsenicals (including arsine)
Polonium
Tellurium (included because of rare instances of poisoning by colors and glazing's used in amateur ceramic production).

Astatine is a radioactive metalloid and all of its isotopes are short-lived. The most stable is ^{220}At with a radioactive half-life of 8.5 hours. Astatine is extremely rare (with only about 1 g in existence at any given time), and it is exceedingly unlikely to be a veterinary toxicological issue.

Polonium and tellurium have been included primarily because of their biosecurity implications. Poisoning of domestic animals with these agents is exceedingly rare.

Germanium and silicon poisoning of domestic animals, while theoretically possible, is very unlikely to occur.

ANTIMONY (SB)

Alternative Names

Exists as oxides (antimony trioxide, antimony tetroxide, antimony pentoxide, sodium antimonite, antimonic acid), halides (SbX_3 and SbX_5), antimonides

Veterinary Toxicology for Australia and New Zealand
DOI: http://dx.doi.org/10.1016/B978-0-12-420227-6.00014-1

(combinations of Sb and various metals), stibine (SbH_3-gaseous), and organoantimony compounds.

Antimony compounds are used in homeopathy (antimonium metallalicum or antimony root, antimonium crudum, antimonium tartaricum, antimonite), particularly in the treatment of skin disorders.

Most antimony ores are sulfides (stibnite, pyrargyrite, zinkenite, hamesonite, boulangerite).

In Australia, antimony is mostly found in association with gold.

Circumstances of Poisoning

Trivalent (Sb^{3+}) and pentavalent (Sb^{5+}) antimony are the most common forms.

Typically poisoning occurs following acute ingestion or acute inhalation of stibine gas or chronic inhalation.

In Australia and New Zealand, occasional cases of poisoning due to use (including injection) of outmoded antimony pharmaceuticals still occur.

Notably the use of antimony compounds in homeopathy has increased, particularly for the treatment of skin diseases.

Pentavalent antimony compounds (e.g., stibogluconate) are still extensively used to treat leishmaniasis in Central America.

Most cases of veterinary poisoning involve the outmoded therapeutic use of antimony salts. Antimony salts were historically used to treat a variety of veterinary diseases, particularly in horses (antimony trisulfide, antimony potassium tartrate [tartarized antimony]). Antimony salts are still occasionally used in caustic dehorning products.

Other important sources of veterinary exposure are lead-acid batteries, lead alloys used for solders, flame retardants, ammunition primers, and feeds grown on antimony-contaminated soils.

Antimony salts are still used for the treatment schistosomiasis and leishmaniasis in humans.

Critically, environmental exposures to antimony are almost always accompanies by exposure to arsenic and it is often difficult, if not impossible, to separate between antimony and arsenic exposures.

Most antimony exposure occurs through water, particularly water discharges glass or metal processing operations, wastes and discharges from coal-fired power plants, refuse incineration and on firing ranges.

Occupational exposure used to be a significant problem in humans. Occupational antimony exposure almost always co-occurs with occupational arsenic exposures.

Stibine gas is used as a fumigating agent and is also generated when any metal containing antimony is exposed to acids. In domestic situations stibine exposure mostly occurs when lead-acid batteries are being charged or during welding, soldering, and etching zinc.

Toxicokinetics

Biologically antimony behaves like arsenic.

Absorption
- Most antimony compounds are absorbed from the gut. Gut absorption is influenced by solubility.
- Inhaled antimony particles and fumes can be absorbed through the respiratory system. Pulmonary clearance is relatively quick (in the order of days).

Distribution
- Sb^{3+} accumulates in erythrocytes.
- Sb^{5+} distributes in the plasma.

Metabolism
- There is very limited reduction of Sb^{5+} to Sb^{3+} (unlike arsenic where there is extensive reduction).
- There is negligible methylation of arsenic in mammals (unlike arsenic).
- Sb^{3+} is mostly conjugated to glutathione.

Excretion
- Sb^{3+} glutathione conjugates are mostly excreted in feces.
- Sb^{5+} is mostly excreted in urine.

Toxic Mode(s) of Action

The primary mode of action is postulated to be similar to arsenic, i.e., disruption of thiol proteins via binding to sulfhydryl ($-SH$) groups.

Acutely irritant in the upper respiratory tract and can cause delayed pulmonary edema/acute respiratory distress syndrome.

Chronic inhalation produces pneumoconiosis, emphysema, and perforation of the nasal septum in humans.

Chronic antimony exposure is associated with liver and kidney damage.

Antimony compounds are primary skin irritants. Exposure to antimony results in antimony spots. These resemble chicken pox lesions in humans.

Other skin effects include nodular ulceration in the axilla, groin, and other moist areas of the body and blistering of the lips.

Antimony compounds are usually gastrointestinal tract irritants (extreme), including the gums and mouth. Historically antimony compounds have been used as emetics and purgatives.

Antimony ions are potent disruptors of cardiac electrical activity and are myocardial toxins. This results in cardiac arrhythmias, myocardial damage, and cardiac arrest.

Sb^{5+} compounds, particularly those used to treat leishmaniasis, can induce pancreatitis, bone marrow hypoplasia, renal tubular damage, hepatocellular damage, uveitis, retinal hemorrhages, atrophy of the optic nerve, and blindness.

Antimony compounds are often locally irritant when injected.

Stibine behaves like arsine and is potent inducer of hemolysis.

Sb^{3+} compounds (particularly antimony trioxide and antimony trisulfide) are potential carcinogens.

Sb^{5+} compounds are not classical mutagens but act as carcinogens.

Antimony compounds are reproductive toxicants and disrupt conception and increase the risk of spontaneous abortion.

Clinical Signs

Acute oral poisoning by antimony compounds (excluding stibine).
- Typically violent gastrointestinal signs: violent intractable vomiting, continuous diarrhea with mucous.
- Evidence of liver and kidney damage may occur.
- Evidence of hypervolemia and shock may be present.
- Death may occur suddenly due to cardiac arrhythmias/cardiac arrest or may occur several hours following the onset of the toxidrome.

Chronic inhalation poisoning by antimony compounds (excluding stibine).
- Anorexia and other gastrointestinal signs such as nausea or constipation.
- Fatigue.
- Irritability.
- Joint and muscular pain.
- Upper respiratory irritation (laryngitis, tracheitis, nasal septal ulceration, or perforation).
- Chronic cough.
- Blistering of the lips and/or evidence of antimony spots.
- Gingivitis and/or stomatitis.
- Conjunctivitis and keratitis.
- Liver and/or kidney failure develops in the latter stages of the toxidrome.

Skin contact with antimony compounds is mostly associated with the appearance of antimony spots and other evidence of skin irritation. In veterinary medicine, this is most likely to occur as a side effect of the use of antimony compounds in homeopathy.

Stibine gas inhalation
- Primary feature is acute intravascular hemolysis and hemoglobinuria.

Diagnostic Aids

Samples of suspect homeopathic preparations should be analyzed.

Whole blood and urine antimony levels are diagnostic.

Stibine can be detected using the Marsh test or using an arsine/organic arsenic Dräger tube.

Electrocardiac effects include ST and T wave changes (particularly concave ST segment, decreased T wave height, T wave inversion), QT prolongation (followed by multiple ventricular ectopics, then ventricular tachycardia, torsade de pointes, ventricular fibrillation and arrest), atrial fibrillation, and various ventricular arrhythmias.

Clinical pathology studies may demonstrate evidence of liver or kidney damage.

Treatment

Treatment is largely supportive.

Acute oral poisoning.
- Treatment is primarily supportive and consists of fluid resuscitation. Patients are at risk of sepsis due to the degree of gastrointestinal damage.
- Chelation therapy may be required.
Chelation therapy.
- Chelation therapy may be warranted if elevated blood and/or urine antimony is present. This includes cases of acute ingestion, injection of antimony pharmaceuticals and chronic inhalation exposures.
- There has been little clinical experience with chelation therapy of antimony and most of the available data derives from experimental studies in animal models.
- The objective of chelation therapy is to provide additional sulfhydryl groups, to increase water solubility and to increase excretion.
- There is limited evidence that injected dimercaprol, DMSA and DMPS are helpful. DMSA is currently regarded as the chelator of choice.

Prognosis

Guarded, depending on the level of exposure.

Necropsy

In cases of acute oral poisoning, acute gastroenteritis and associated hypervolemia may be present. Acute hepatocellular, renal tubular, and myocardial damage may be present.

Chronic inflammation of the upper respiratory tract, mouth, lips, gums, conjunctivae, and corneas as well as evidence of pneumoconiosis, renal tubular damage, and chronic hepatocellular injury may be present following chronic inhalation. Antimony spots may be present on the skin (typically in moist areas of the body such as the axillae and groin).

Skin contact with antimony compounds is mostly associated with the appearance of antimony spots and other evidence of skin irritation.

Acute intravascular hemolysis is the primary necropsy picture with stibine gas exposure.

Public Health Considerations

Antimony exposure is a public health hazard. Significant antimony exposure of animals implies the possibility of heavy human co-exposures.

Prevention

There is currently no justification for the use of antimony-based pharmaceuticals or remedies in Australia. Adequate ventilation is required during charging of lead-acid batteries.

BORON AND BORATES (B)

Alternative Names

Elemental boron is rare and difficult to prepare. Most boron compounds are in the B (III) oxidation state and exist as oxides, nitrates, and sulfates. Organoboron compounds exist.

Borax (aka sodium borate, sodium tetraborate, or disodium tetraborate) is the most common mineral form and the most common household and industrial form. Borax has three common hydration states (anhydrous borax $[Na_2B_4O_7]$, borax pentahydrate $[Na_2B_4O_7 \cdot 5H_2O]$, and borax decahydrate $[Na_2B_4O_7 \cdot 10H_2O]$).

Boracic acid (H_3BO_3, sassolite when in solid form) is formed when borax is reacted with a mineral acid. Boracic acid has been extensively used as an antiseptic, insecticide, flame retardant, and neutron absorber. Boron neutron capture is used as a treatment of cancers of the head and neck in humans.

Borax and boracic acid are water-soluble.

Circumstances of Poisoning

Most poisonings have occurred due to boracic acid ant baits and borax household cleaners.

Poisoning in humans has been associated with the use of boracic acid impregnated dressings used on burns patients. Topical boracic acid solutions have been used as a treatment for vaginal infections in humans.

Boron preparations have been used in alternative medicine as a treatment for osteoarthritis and dementia.

Toxicokinetics

Boric acid is well absorbed through abraded or damaged skin (e.g., burns) but not absorbed through intact skin.

GI absorption of boric acid is rapid and complete.

Distribution is throughout the body, but higher levels occur in the brain, liver, and kidneys.

Most ingested boric acid is excreted unchanged in the urine.

Toxic Mode(s) of Action

Largely unknown, but assumed to be cytotoxic.

Boracic acid and borax are not caustic.

Toxicological targets are skin (topical), GI (ingestion) brain, kidney, and rarely liver.

There is some evidence that boron compounds have estrogenic effects.

Clinical Signs

Acute ingestion
- GI distress, excessive salivation.
- Feces are blue-green.
- Presence is not caustic to the GI.
- High doses can result in CNS effects (weakness, ataxia, seizure, coma), acute renal failure (proximal tubular nephrosis), metabolic acidosis, hypotension, and shock.

Chronic ingestion
- Growth suppression.
- Male infertility.
- GI disturbance.
- Skin rash.
- Alopecia.
- Microcytic hypochromic anemia.
- Cyanosis, hypotension.
- CNS depression.

Topical application
- Exfoliative dermatitis (particularly in humans; referred to as the "boiled lobster syndrome").
- Can produce systemic toxicity.

Teratogenic in birds.

Diagnostic Aids

The original sample container is the most useful diagnostic aid.

Systemically absorbed boron decreases the renal excretion of magnesium and hypermagnesemia can occur.

Metabolic acidosis, hypernatremia, hyperchloremia, evidence of hepatic damage may be present. Urinalysis may be consistent with proximal renal tubular damage, i.e., albuminuria, hematuria, proteinuria, and epithelial casts.

Blood, plasma, CSF, and urine boron levels are useful markers of exposure but are rarely available. Normal ranges have not been established in veterinary species. The concentrations of boric acid associated with toxicity are poorly established and may not correlate with clinical signs.

Rapid urine tests for boron are available but are unreliable.

Treatment

Treatment is largely supportive.
Activated charcoal is not effective.
Emesis is unlikely to be effective.

Prognosis

Cases of severe poisoning are uncommon.

Most veterinary cases consist of mild to moderate gastrointestinal upset that responds well to supportive care and fluid resuscitation.

Necropsy

Skin, GI, liver, kidneys, and CNS are the main target organs.

- Skin: in humans, exfoliative dermatitis is often present.
- GI: congestion, edema, mucosal exfoliation.
- Renal: gross pallor, proximal tubular nephrosis.
- CNS: congestion and edema.
- Liver: lesions are rare; fatty change, congestion.
- Pancreas: rarely—intracytoplasmic inclusion bodies in periacinar cells.

Public Health Considerations

With the decline in use of boracic acid impregnated dressings for the treatment of burns, poisoning of humans is now rare.

Prevention

Prevention of exposure is the most important measure (this includes appropriate care when using boron-based ant baits).

INORGANIC ARSENIC COMPOUNDS

Alternative Names

Inorganic arsenic compounds are primarily salts. There are two basic forms: trivalent (As^{3+}; arsenites) and pentavalent (As^{5+}; arsenates; AsO_4^{3-}).

Important trivalent arsenic salts:
- Arsenic trioxide
- Sodium arsenite
- Arsenic trichloride

Important pentavalent arsenic salts:
- Arsenic pentoxide
- Arsenic acid
- Arsenates

Historical materials of toxicological importance:
- Paris Green (copper(II) acetate triarsenite).
- Scheele's Green (cupric hydrogen arsenite).

Fowler's solution (Liquor Potassii Arenitis, Kali Arsenicosum, Kali arseniatum) is 1% potassium arsenite. It was originally marketed as a patent medicine and has historically been used as a treatment for malaria, chorea, syphilis, trypanosomiasis, and cancer (particularly leukemias) as well as a rodenticide. Fowler's solution is still used to treat psoriasis.

Tanalith is chromated copper arsenate. It is extensively used as a wood preservative because of its effectiveness against insects, bacteria, and fungi.

Arsenic salts are still very extensively used in some countries as pesticides, herbicides, fungicides, external parasiticides, and anthelmintics.

Various arsenic salts (notably arsenic trioxide) are still extensively used in some countries to control rats and mice.

Arsenic salts, notably arsenic trioxide, are still extensively used in some countries to control ants and termites.

Arsenic trioxide is still used in the treatment of leukemia, more than 140 years after its first use for this purpose.

[74]As is used as a radiotracer in Positron emission tomography (PET) imaging studies.

Circumstances of Poisoning

Inorganic arsenic compounds do not impart a taste or taint into water or foodstuffs; a fact that has been taken advantage by poisoners and assassins for millennia.

Arsenic and antimony poisoning commonly co-occur.

Historically arsenic trioxide mixed with vinegar and chalk was consumed as a skin whitener. Arsenic salts have also been administered to show animals (particularly horses) to lighten the coat color.

In small doses, arsenic salts are stimulants and have been extensively (and illegally) used as performance enhancing drugs in horses and racing dogs.

Inorganic arsenic pesticides, external parasiticides, and anthelmintics have now largely been phased out in Australia and New Zealand. However, poisoning from legacy products is an on going concern.

Historically, inorganic arsenic compounds were extensively used for the control of external parasites on sheep and the soils surrounding old sheep dipping facilities are often heavily contaminated with arsenic.

Acute arsenic poisoning in companion animals has been associated with liking psoriatic skin treated with Fowler's solution.

Acute arsenic poisoning has also been associated with arsenic trioxide ant/termite dusts and baits. These materials were extensively used in Australia. Approval for their use in Australia lapsed in 1999. However, illegal legacy stocks may still be available.

Arsenic is extensively used for bronzing, in pyrotechnics, in lead alloys used in ammunition, production of high-quality brass, and biological specimen preservation.

Contaminated water is the major source of human and animal exposure in some countries (including parts of Australia and New Zealand). In Australia, some groundwaters have become contaminated with arsenic due to historical mining activities. Acid mine drainage (AMD) is a major cause of groundwater contamination in Australia. AMD is a geochemical process that results in leaching of arsenite and arsenate from sulfide mineral ores. Arsenite released by AMD is oxidized to the less toxic arsenate form. However, the speed of this reaction depends on the redox potential and pH of the groundwater. Co-precipitation reactions with iron hydroxides and adsorption onto clay minerals also affects the level of available arsenic in groundwaters (iron hydroxide precipitation turns the groundwater yellow in color, referred to as "yellow boy." *Critically, leeching of phosphate and sulfate into groundwaters following soil fertilization operations can result in desorption of arsenite and arsenate from clay, increasing the level of available arsenic in ground waters*).

It is important to note that AMD is not only associated with mining activities. It can occur anywhere where the surface soil has been disturbed and sulfide minerals have been exposed or where mine overburden materials have been used for earthworks or other construction.

Toxicokinetics

Absorption
- Gastrointestinal absorption is dependent on solubility; soluble inorganic arsenic compounds are generally well absorbed from the gastrointestinal tract.

- Systemic toxicity can occur after dermal exposure indicating that skin absorption can be problematic under some circumstances.
- Inhaled arsenic is predominantly arsenic trioxide. Absorption following inhalation largely depends on particle size. Arsenic trioxide is relatively insoluble in water, thus pulmonary clearance of inhaled particles is likely to be relatively slow.

Distribution

- Most arsenic compounds are rapidly cleared from the blood.
- In some species (rats) arsenic concentrated in erythrocytes and bound to hemoglobin (predominantly as dimethyl arsenic acid, i.e., a metabolite).
- Inorganic arsenic initially accumulates in the liver, lung, and kidney. It subsequently distributes to keratin tissues (hair, skin), the upper gastrointestinal tract, teeth, and skeleton.
- In general, tissues rich in thiol (SH) groups usually concentrate arsenic (e.g., keratin, hair, nails).
- Within cells, arsenic tends to accumulate in mitochondria and binds to sulfhydryl compounds, particularly lipoic acid and α-ketooxidases.

Metabolism

- Metabolism primarily occurs in the liver and is efficient:

- The level of production of dimethylarsinous acid and trimethylarsenic oxide is species specific.
- The trivalent intermediates of the arsenic methylation process (methylarsenous acid and dimethylarsenous acid) are extremely toxic.

Excretion

- Methylarsenic and demethylarsenic are largely excreted in urine; proportions of MMA and DMA vary with species.
- As^{3+} is largely excreted in urine.
- As^{5+} is largely excreted in bile.

Toxic Mode(s) of Action

- Of the inorganic forms, As^{3+} (arsenites) are the predominant toxic forms; As^{5+} (arsenates) are 10 times less toxic.
- The renal proximal tubular epithelia reduce a small proportion of As^{5+} to As^{3+}. This results in redox damage and production of toxic methylated intermediates of metabolism. The end result is renal proximal tubular nephrosis.
- Accumulate in mitochondria and binds to sulfhydryl compounds, particularly lipoic acid and α-ketooxidases.
- Blocks mitochondrial ATP production. As^{3+} binds to lipoic acid, an important cofactor in pyruvate dehydrogenase (and other enzymes involved in the reduction of NAD to NADH). This reduces the amount of reduced electron carriers available for oxidative phosphorylation. As^{3+} also inhibits succinate dehydrogenase and blocks the citric acid cycle. This blocks the production of $FADH_2$, decreasing the amount of reduced electron carriers available for oxidative phosphorylation.

  As^{5+} uncouples oxidative phosphorylation because it competes with phosphate during conversion of ADP to ATP.

  The overall net result is the failure of cellular antioxidant systems + insufficient energy metabolism. *Tissues that have high dependence on oxidative metabolism are the most immediately affected, i.e., intestinal epithelium, epidermis, renal tubular epithelium, heaptocytes, and lung.*
- Inorganic arsenic induces capillary dilation and decreased capillary integrity by an unknown mechanism. This primarily affects the enterothelium and capillaries of the GI and results in transudation of plasma into the GU tract, submucosal congestion and edema, fluid volume shifts, acute hypovolemia, and shock.
- Inorganic arsenic exposure induces peripheral sensory and motor neuropathies (sensory is more sensitive and occurs earlier). The neuropathies have the classical stockings and gloves distribution pattern in humans.
- Inorganic arsenic exposure induces peripheral vascular disease in humans that results in: Raynaud's phenomenon, acrocyanosis, and eventually, peripheral arterial occlusive disease and gangrene (Blackfoot disease).
- Inorganic arsenic disrupts heme synthesis and increases urinary porphyrins. Arsenic exposure exacerbates porphyrias.
- Immunotoxicity.
- Chronic arsenic exposure is a carcinogen (particularly in the skin) although arsenic salts are generally not regarded as classical mutagens.

Clinical Signs

Important toxidromes include peracute/acute/subacute arsenic poisoning and chronic arsenic poisoning. Chronic arsenic poisoning is possible, but generally not found in domestic animals.

Peracute/acute/subacute arsenic poisoning
- In domestic animals it is typically due to ingestion of arsenites (commonly arsenic trioxide).
- The common cascade of events is summarized in the following diagram:

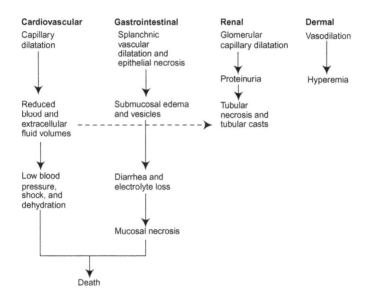

- Affected animals may have a garlic-like breath odor.

- High morbidity and mortality rates generally develop over a 2−3-day period.

- Initially gastrointestinal effects predominate, i.e., vomiting, intense thirst, intense abdominal pain, ruminal/gastrointestinal atony, and watery and/or bloody diarrhea.

- Cardiovascular shock due to hypervolemia secondary to systemic fluid shifts is common. Weakness, staggering, ataxia, and cardiovascular collapse are common.

- Cardiac arrhythmias are common due to direct effects on the myocardium (high peaked T-waves, conduction disorders, heart bloc, and asystole).

- Facial edema may develop.

- Acute cardiomyopathies can occur.

- Rhabdomyolysis may occur.

- Evidence of renal failure develop if the animals survive >3 days: proteinuria, oliguria, azotemia, dehydration, acidosis are often present.

- Individuals that survive the renal failure phase will often develop a reversible peripheral neuropathy 1−2 weeks postpoisoning as well as reversible anemia and leukopenia (particularly granulocytopenia). Pancytopenia with erythrocyte basophilic stippling can occur.

- Insoluble arsenic salts are radio-opaque and may be detectable in the gut using abdominal radiography.
- Mee's lines (leukonychia striata) may become evident in the nails/hooves of survivors.

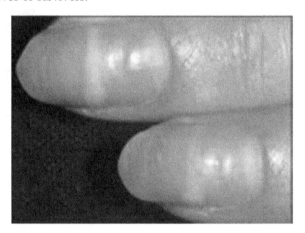

- Delayed dermatitis, skin hyperpigmentation, and skin vesiculation may occur in survivors.
- Survivors often develop sensorimotor peripheral axonopathies, autonomic neuropathies (unstable blood pressure, anhidrosis, sweating, and flushing), tremor, and encephalopathies.

Chronic arsenic poisoning

- Generally not found in domestic animals.
- Major targets: skin, liver, peripheral nervous system, peripheral vascular system.
- Results in skin, liver, bladder, lung, kidney, and prostate cancer.
- Effects on the skin include diffuse or spotted hyperpigmentation, palmar/plantar hyperkeratosis, and skin cancers (basal cell and squamous cell carcinomas).
- Effects on the liver include hepatomegaly, cirrhosis, icterus, and hepatic carcinomas.
- Effects on the peripheral nervous system include arsenic sensorimotor peripheral neuropathy, distal axonopathy, and demyelination. The sensory system is affected before the motor system. The sensory neuropathy has a stockings and gloves distribution. Notably the proximal muscle groups are affected before the distal muscle groups with the motor neuropathy (proximal to distal motor neuropathy).
- Produces Raynaud's phenomenon.

- Produces peripheral end arterial obstructive disease, acrocyanosis, and peripheral gangrene (Blackfoot disease).
- Carcinogenicity in humans.
- Chronic arsenic exposure in humans is associated with skin, bladder, and lung carcinogenesis. Chronic arsenic exposure has been implicated in liver, kidney, and prostate cancers in humans.
- *Animals generally do not develop skin cancers following chronic arsenic exposure.*

Diagnostic Aids

Samples of the baits/agent, urine, vomitus, feces, liver, kidney, surrounding soil, surrounding plants, and feed are often useful for arsenic testing.

Whole blood arsenic levels are generally less sensitive and less useful diagnostically than urine arsenic levels. Urinary arsenic levels are often reported in micrograms arsenic per gram creatinine to adjust for concentration or dilution of urine by variation in fluid intake.

False-positive tests for urine arsenic are possible if the animal has consumed seafood (i.e., fish meal) due to the consumption of asenobetaine (the nontoxic and predominant form of arsenic found in seafood).

Samples of keratin (hair, claws, and hooves) are useful in chronic arsenic poisoning and to determine past exposures. Specific techniques have to be used to rule out external contamination of the samples.

Treatment

Peracute and acute arsenic poisoning are difficult to treat, particularly if high doses of a soluble salt have been ingested.

The mainstay of treatment, apart from supportive care, has been chelation therapy.

- The objective of chelation therapy is to provide available thiol (SH) groups as alternative molecular targets and to enhance renal excretion.
- *Chelation therapy must commence as soon as possible following exposure. The effectiveness of chelation therapy rapidly declines as the exposure to treatment interval increases.*
- *Even if arsenic poisoning is only suspected, it is better to start chelation therapy rather than wait for a definitive diagnosis.*
- Dimercaprol (British anti-Lewisite, BAL) was the first arsenic chelator developed. It was developed in response to the development of Lewisite as a chemical weapon by the United States in the 1920s. *Dimercaprol is largely ineffective if it is administered after the appearance of clinical signs, i.e., it must be administered as soon as possible following exposure*

and before the appearance of clinical signs to be effective. Dimercaprol is the most toxic of the currently available arsenic chelators with hypertension being the most serious side effect.

- Thioctic acid has been successfully used as a chelating agent and may be cheaper than dimercaprol.
- Dimercaptosuccinic acid (DMSA, succimer), 2-3-dimercapto-1-propane-sulfonate (DMPS), or meso 2,3-dimer-captosuccinic acid are currently regarded as the chelators of choice. These are more water-soluble than BAL, and can be administered orally with lower toxicity.
- Combination treatment using BAL followed by DMSA has been suggested.

Prognosis

In general, trivalent arsenic poisoning has a poorer prognosis than pentavalent arsenic poisoning.

Peracute and acute arsenic poisonings are difficult to effectively treat and have a guarded to poor prognosis. Survivors often develop renal and/or neurological disease. Recovery, particularly from the neurological damage, is often incomplete.

Necropsy

Garlic odors may be present (body cavities, gut contents).

Peracute arsenic poisoning is characterized by severe damage to the gastrointestinal tract. Acute/subacute arsenic poisoning is associated with damage to the gastrointestinal tract, hepatic damage (fatty infiltration, congestion, centrilobular necrosis, cholangitis, and cholecystitis), renal tubular necrosis, renal cortical necrosis, bone marrow damage and rhabdomyolysis. Acute cardiomyopathies may occur.

Public Health Considerations

Soluble inorganic arsenic compounds are a substantial human health risk.

Prevention

Legacy arsenical pesticides and veterinary medicines should be disposed of correctly.

ORGANOARSENICALS

Alternative Names

Organoarsenicals have been extensively used as pharmaceuticals, disinfectants, pesticides, and growth promotants. Organoarsenicals are divided into pentavalent, trivalent, and univalent groups.

Pentavalent organoarsenicals include:

- Cacodylic acid.
- Phenylarsonic acid feed additives and pharmaceuticals such as 4-hydroxy-3-nitrobenzenearsonic acid (3-NHPAA, Roxarsone, 3-nitro), *p*-arsanilic acid (p-ASA, sodium arsanilate), 4-nitrophenylarsonic acid (4-NPAA), and *p*-ureidophenylarsonic acid (p-UPAA).
- Atoxyl (historically used to treat syphilis and to treat trypanosomiasis).
- Pentaphenyl arsenic pharmaceuticals, e.g., arsphenamine (salvarsan) is a mixture of a trivalent triphenyl and a pentavalent pentaphenyl organoarsenic compounds.
- Monosodium methylarsonate (methanearsonic acid; herbicide).
- Disodium methylarsonate (herbicide).
- Calcium acid methanearsonate (CAMA, herbicide).

Trivalent organoarsenicals include:

- Arsphenamine (first effective treatment for syphilis and used to treat trypanosomiasis).
- Lewisite (chemical weapon, vesicant, pulmonary agent, systemic toxicant).
- Phenyldichloroarsine (chemical weapon, vesicant, vomiting/incapacitating agent).
- Methyldichlorarsine (chemical weapon, MD, vesicant, hemolysis agent, pulmonary agent).
- Chlorodiphenylarsine (chemical weapon, Clark Agent 1, vomiting/incapacitating agent, pulmonary agent).
- Diphenylcyanoarsine (chemical weapon, Clark Agent 2, vomiting/incapacitating agent, pulmonary agent).
- Diphenylaminechlorarsine (chemical weapon, DM, Adamsite, vomiting/incapacitating agent, pulmonary agent).
- Arsphenamine (salvarsan) is a mixture of a trivalent triphenyl and a pentavalent pentaphenyl organoarsenic compounds.
- Neosalvarsan (pharmaceutical historically used for treating syphilis).
- Thiacetarsamide sodium (caparsolate, adulticide used in the treatment of heartworm).
- Melarsomine dihydrochloride (adulticide used in the treatment of heartworm).
- Trimethylarsine is produced by bacterial metabolism of inorganic arsenic (notably the historical use of arsenical pigments such as Paris

Green and Scheele's Green used in paints and wallpapers). It is a mutagen.

- Dimethylarsine is also a bacterial metabolite of inorganic arsenic. It is a mutagen.

Arsine

- Arsine is a nonirritating gas with a mild odor (odorless at low doses) that is used in the semiconductor and metals refining industries.
- Historically, poisoning from arsine occurred from degasing from pigments such as Paris Green and Scheele's Green.

Naturally occurring organoarsenicals include the arsenosugars (arsenic ribose derivatives), arsenobetaine, and arsenocholine. Arsenosugars are the predominant form of arsenic found in marine plants (particularly seaweeds) and are not acutely toxic. Arsenobetaine is the predominant form of arsenic found in fish and it has low toxicity. Trimethylarsine (Gosio's gas) is produced by bacterial metabolism of inorganic arsenic minerals. Although a wide variety of severe toxicoses have been ascribed to trimethylarsine exposure, the toxicity of this compound has been exaggerated.

Circumstances of Poisoning

Most cases of veterinary poisoning fall into the following categories:

- Overuse/overdose of arsenical feed additives/growth promotants in production animals (predominantly poultry and swine).
- Use of arsenical adulticides for the treatment of heartworm in dogs.
- Misuse of organoarsenical agrochemical products.
- Malicious poisonings.

Notably, poultry are relatively resistant to the effects of the pentavalent organoarsenical growth promotants compared with pigs.

The use of organoarsenical growth promotants is now no longer approved in Australia, New Zealand, and many other countries. Illegal use still occurs from time to time.

Arsine is produced when organoarsenical pesticides are accidentally mixed with acids. It is also produced during metal working, soldering, etching, and galvanizing. Arsine is also produced during recharging of lead-acid batteries. Arsine is 2.5 times denser than air, accumulates in low-lying areas and produces blanketing effect in the environment.

Toxicokinetics

As a general rule, organoarsenicals moderately well absorbed from the gastrointestinal tract. A number of organoarsenicals are absorbed through the skin. There are significant species differences in absorption from the gut and through the skin.

Organoarsenicals may distribute to both the plasma and erythrocyte, the relative amounts in each compartment depending on the individual compound and species.

Methylation and other biotransformations may occur. However, there is limited information available. Species differences in biotransformation occur.

Thiacetarsamide is metabolized in the liver and rapidly excreted ($T_{1/2} \approx$ 46 minutes).

The major route of excretion for most organoarsenicals is in urine with smaller amounts excreted in bile. However, there are substantial species differences.

Toxic Mode(s) of Action

Pentavalent organoarsenical feed additives can produce demyelination, axonal degeneration, and other CNS effects if feed for too long or if over fed. These problems mostly occur in swine and poultry. Poultry are less susceptible to these effects than swine.

Thiacetarsamide toxicity occurs in about 10%−15% of dogs that have received the normal therapeutic dose. It is a hepatic and renal toxicant. Melarsomine produces similar effects but is reputed to be less toxic than thiacetarsamide.

The organoarsenical chemical weapons are primarily vesicants and pulmonary agents. Several of them were developed specifically for their capacity to induce vomiting so as to defeat protective measures such as gas masks.

The organoarsenical herbicides produce effects that resemble inorganic arsenic poisoning. However, the organoarsenical herbicides are reputedly less toxic to humans than inorganic arsenic. Ruminants display an increases sensitivity compared with humans.

Arsine produces hemolysis.

Clinical Signs

Pentavalent organoarsenical feed additives.

- The toxidrome is typically acute or subacute.
- In pigs, signs may occur within 2−10 days of addition to the feed, depending upon the dose.
- It is predominantly a CNS syndrome characterized by ataxia, in coordination, torticollis, blindness. Affected animals assume a dog-sitting position and eventually become paralyzed in lateral recumbency. Most animals remain cognizant and their appetite remains normal.

Organoarsenical herbicide poisoning resembles inorganic arsenic poisoning.

Fulminant hepatorenal failure, cranial abdominal pain, vomiting, anorexia, respiratory distress, excessive salivation and diarrhea characterize thiacetarsamide and melarsamine poisoning.

Organoarsencial chemical weapons have vesicant and severe irritant effects on sites of first contact (skin, eyes) and act as pulmonary irritants (i.e., induce the acute adult respiratory distress syndrome). Several of them are designed to induce vomiting and sneezing.

Arsine

- Clinical signs can take several hours to become apparent.
- Nausea followed by evidence of hemolytic anemia, hemoglobinuria, and nephropathy are typical.
- Severe renal damage can occur.

Diagnostic Aids

As per inorganic arsenic.

Treatment

As per inorganic arsenic. Chelation therapy is reputedly helpful in thiacetarsamide and melarsamine poisoning. Chelation therapy should be instituted as soon as possible following organoarsenical herbicide poisoning.

Chelation therapy is ineffective in pentavalent organoarsenical feed additive poisoning.

Otherwise treatment is essentially supportive. The management of acute renal failure due to thiacetarsamide can be difficult and the use of intravenous crystalloids to maintain renal function is important. Patients are often started on intravenous crystalloids before thiacetarsamide is administered.

Prognosis

Guarded.

Necropsy

Pentavalent organoarsenical feed additive toxicity is characterized by:

- Edema of the CNS white matter.
- Neuronal degeneration in the medulla.
- Wallerian degeneration in optic and peripheral nerves.
- Wallerian degeneration in the dorsal proprioceptive and spinocerebellar tracts of the cervical spinal cord and damage to the lateral and ventral funiculi in the caudal cord.

Findings in organoarsenical herbicide poisoning resemble inorganic arsenic poisoning.

Organoarsenical chemical weapon exposure is characterized by acute and severe damage to the entire respiratory tract and severe pulmonary edema. Vesicant injuries at site of first contact (skin and eyes) are a hallmark of these weapons.

Arsine poisoning is characterized by intravascular hemolysis.

Public Health Considerations

Nonmarine organoarsenicals and arsine are a substantial public health concern.

Prevention

Organoarsenical herbicides, organoarsenical growth promotants, and organoarsenical pharmaceuticals are now largely outmoded and banned. They should not be used. Legacy stocks should be disposed of appropriately.

Lead-acid batteries should be recharged in adequately ventilated areas.

POLONIUM

Alternative Names

Thirty-three known isotopes occur. The most common are ^{210}Po (half-life 138.376 days; the most widely available). ^{209}Po (half-life 103 years) and ^{208}Po (half-life 2.9 years) are also available.

Various polonium salts and oxides have been synthesized.

A few curies of ^{210}Po in air emit a blue glow.

Circumstances of Poisoning

Primary concern is its use in terrorism as a weapon. Polonium is important mostly from a biosecurity perspective. The committed effective dose equivalent of ^{210}Po is 0.51 μSv/Bq if ingested, and 2.5 μSv/Bq if inhaled; thus a fatal 4.5 Sv dose can be caused by ingesting 8.8 MBq (240 μCi), about 50 ng, or inhaling 1.8 MBq (49 μCi), about 10 ng.

The most likely routine sources of exposure are exposure to radon daughters (^{214}Po and ^{218}Po are radon daughters), antistatic devices used in photographic printing and in textile mills, tobacco smoking and consumption of seafood.

Polonium−beryllium alloys are used as portable neutron sources in a variety of contexts (medical imaging, petroleum exploration, engineering, and research). The alpha particles emitted by polonium trigger the release of neutrons from beryllium.

Notably, background exposures to polonium are much higher in artic areas.

Toxicokinetics

Poorly described.

Absorption following transcutaneous diffusion is problematic during handling.

Accumulates in liver, kidneys, and testes.

May substitute for sulfur in sulfur-containing amino acids in biological tissues.

Toxic Mode(s) of Action

Polonium is extremely toxic, primarily because of its intense (alpha particle) radioactivity.

^{210}Pollonium appears to be especially damaging to the liver and spleen in humans.

^{214}Po and ^{218}Po radon daughters are the likely cause of most nontobacco-related cancer associated with radon daughter inhalation.

Clinical Signs

Systemic exposure resembles the acute and subacute radiation syndrome. The syndrome has three phases:

- Immediate phase: nausea and vomiting, diarrhea, fever and if there is sufficient exposure (> 2 Gy), cognitive impairment.
- Latent period of apparent recovery for 7−28 days if exposure is <8 Gy. The latent phase does not occur with exposures >8 Gy.
- Delayed phase: leukopenia, thrombocytopenia, pancytopenia, fatigue, weakness, clotting disorders and hemorrhage, opportunistic infections, hair loss, nausea, vomiting, high fever, fluid and electrolyte loss, and death.

Skin only exposure (remember that alpha particles do not penetrate through the epidermis) can result in the cutaneous radiation syndrome/radiation skin burns.

Diagnostic Aids

Alpha-particle spectrometry.

Treatment

BAL is helpful experimentally.

Prognosis

Poor.

Necropsy

Poorly described.

Public Health Considerations

Apart from lung cancer, the major concern is the use of polonium as a weapon.

Prevention

No information.

TELLURIUM

Most likely sources of veterinary exposure are colors used in ceramic production. Tellurite agar is used in the culture of *Corynebacterium* sp.

Tellurium alters the synthesis of myelin lipids (inhibits squalene epoxidase that blocks cholesterol synthesis) in Schwann cells and produces demyelination in the peripheral nervous system. Tellurium dioxide is a renal tubular toxicant.

Acute toxicity mostly follows inhalation during amateur ceramic production. Classical signs of poisoning include a pronounced garlic breath, sweating, nausea, cyanosis, stupor, and loss of consciousness.

Chapter 16

Site of First Contact Effects of Acids and Alkalis

Rhian Cope

This section covers the general toxicological effects of acids and alkalis. These effects may occur alone or may occur in conjunction with other toxicological effects. Thus mixed toxidromes may occur. Many toxic substances are acids and alkalis that are capable of producing a combination of site of first contact chemical burns and systemic effects (notably hydrofluoric acid, phenols [aka carbolic acid], cresols, formic acid, phosphoric acid, monochloroacetic acid, and oxalic acid).

The areas covered by this section include:

- General site of first contact effects of acids.
- General site of first contact effects of alkalis.

GENERAL SITE OF FIRST CONTACT EFFECTS OF ACIDS

Alternative Names

An acid is any chemical compound that, when dissolved in water, gives a solution with a pH <7.0.

Acids function as proton (H^+ donors).

Common acids encountered in veterinary practice include:

- Acetic acid (vinegar; glacial acetic acid is anhydrous, i.e., not diluted).
- Phenols and cresols (phenol-based disinfectants).
- Formic acid (used as a preservative and antibacterial agent in livestock feeds, applied to silage to promote fermentation, commonly used in lime-scale removers and toilet bowl cleaners, used as a miticide in bees).
- Oxalic acid (found in inks and ink solvents, rust removers, cleaning agents, and bleaching agents).
- Phosphoric acid (food additive, fertilizers, rust removers, solder fluxes, hydroponics).

Veterinary Toxicology for Australia and New Zealand
DOI: http://dx.doi.org/10.1016/B978-0-12-420227-6.00015-3
© 2017 Elsevier Inc. All rights reserved

- Hydrofluoric acid (chrome cleaners, aluminum cleaners, automotive cleaning products, car wheel cleaners).
- Nitric acid (etchants, cleaning agents, wood aging solutions; see also Silo Filler's Disease).

Circumstances of Poisoning

Poisoning typically occurs because of misuse. Deliberate ingestion of strong acids in animals is usually limited because of the immediate pain produced. Under such circumstances, lesions are usually limited to the face and mouth. However, esophageal burns can occur. Importantly, weak acids such as hydrofluoric acid may not initially induce pain following ingestion and phenols (i.e., carbolic acids) act as local anesthetics. Thus ingestions of these materials may be substantial.

Skin burns often occur on the feet following walking through acidic materials. Skin burns can also occur following ill-advised application of acidic material to the skin. Notably an occlusive dressing placed over the area of application will increase the amount of local damage. Again, phenols act as local anesthetics and pain on initial contact may not occur.

Toxicokinetics

Acids typically denature protein (i.e., loss of protein secondary, tertiary, and/ or quaternary structure). This results in localized coagulation necrosis that appears grossly as an eschar (i.e., a zone of dead tissue that eventually separates and detaches from the surrounding viable tissues). Eschar formation usually limits the depth of tissue penetration. However, an eschar can also act as a reservoir for the chemical involved, thus allowing for absorption.

Acid burns are not always immediate. There are noted examples (e.g., hydrofluoric acid), where delayed onset (up to 24 hours postexposure) is the norm.

Mode(s) of Action

The primary mode of action is protein denaturation.

Notably, for a given titratable acid or alkali reserve, acids tend to result in more superficial injuries than alkalis. However, the notable exception to this general rule is hydrofluoric acid.

While materials with a $pH \leq 2$ are often corrosive, pH is not the only determinant of the degree of injury. The degree of injury is often determined by other factors:

- Titratable acid reserve (how much base is required to neutralize the acid) is a better measure of tissue damage potential.
- The larger the volume, the larger the area of damage.
- The longer the contact time, the more severe the injury.

- The formation of crystals in the wound tends to make the injury worse.
- The more concentrated the solution, the more likely injury will occur.
- Solid pelleted materials tend to produce worse injuries than liquid materials. Pelleted materials tend to produce higher local tissue concentrations and remain in contact with the tissues longer.
- In the GI the volume of liquid and the material in stomach affect the degree of injury.

Clinical Signs

Moderate to severe skin burns can cause a loss of airway security due to laryngospasm and/or upper airway edema irrespective of the site of the injury.

Acid injuries to the eyes, while painful, are often less severe than alkali burns; however, they are genuine ophthalmic emergencies and specialist referral may be required following the initial treatment phase.

Acid injuries typically have three general phases:

- Acute inflammatory phase (first 4–7 days)—characterized by vascular thrombosis and necrosis; generally the level of injury peaks at 24 hours.
- Latent granulation phase—characterized by fibroplasia and collagen formation.
- Chronic cicatrization phase (2–4 weeks after injury)—characterized by excessive scar tissue and dense fibrous tissue. If the injury involves the GI, the risk of stricture is highest at this stage.

Ingestion injuries often result in:

- Potential for aspiration and damage to the trachea (including strictures) and lungs.
- Esophageal diverticula.
- GI strictures.
- Subcutaneous air (Hamman crunch).

Common long-term effects of skin burns include scarring. Scarring can be problematic.

Diagnostic Aids

Case history commonly provides the best diagnostic information. If possible, obtain the original product container and information about any dilution and methods of application.

Critical points in the case history include:

- Offending agent, concentration, physical form, and pH.
- Route of exposure.
- Time of exposure.

- Volume of exposure.
- Possibility of coexisting injury.
- The timing and extent of irrigation

Materials with pH < 4.5 turn litmus paper red. Other pH indicator papers may be useful if samples of the suspect agent are available.

Litmus paper other pH indicator papers can be used on body surfaces or on samples of wound irrigation fluids.

If the injury involves the eyes, a fluorescein uptake test should be performed.

Treatment

Appropriate personal protective equipment is usually required for the treatment team.

Under no circumstances should any attempt be made to neutralize the acid. Acid neutralization reactions are exothermic and increase the amount of tissue damage.

Do not induce emesis.

Active charcoal is not effective following acid ingestion and interferes with subsequent endoscopy.

Ice should not be applied to burns.

Airway security is paramount. It is always better to intubate if in doubt and to intubate sooner rather than later. Upper airway edema may occur even when the upper respiratory tract is not directly injured. If in doubt, intubate: many burns patients die from airway compromise.

Chemical eye injuries are commonly genuine ophthalmic emergencies and specialist evaluation as soon as possible is recommended.

Euthanasia is an important option: older patients with burns covering ≥ 80% of body surface area are unlikely to survive irrespective of treatment.

Renal failure can occur after burn injury.

The use of corticosteroids for chemical burn treatment is controversial. They may help airway inflammation. However, they may predispose to infection and may mask the clinical signs of gut perforations. Corticosteroid therapy does not reduce the risk of eschar contractures, cicatrization scarring or the formation of strictures in the gastrointestinal tract.

Skin acid burns

In cases of skin and eye acid burns, the most critical treatment is copious wound irrigation (note the situations were wound irrigation is contraindicated below). Both the time to irrigation and the volume of irrigation is critical. Wound irrigation within 10 minutes of exposure will decrease the depth of skin injury by a factor of 5.

A common error in treatment is not irrigating the affected area for long enough. Irrigation should continue for at least 30−60 minutes or until the pH of the irrigating solution is at least 7.3, but preferably 7.4.

The irrigating solution should be cool, but not cold. Cold water produces dermal vasoconstriction and worsens tissue ischemia and local edema.

Care is required during wound irrigation:

- The burn site can be irrigated with water or saline.
- Great care should be taken to avoid hypothermia.
- The contaminated irrigation solution should not be allowed to run onto unaffected tissues.
- One of the aims of the irrigation process should be to remove any particulate material present.
- Diphoterine is claimed to be more effective than water or saline; however, definitive veterinary data are lacking.

If there will be significant delay between the initial first response of wound irrigation and hospitalization, current recommendations are to either apply specialist burn dressings or to cover the burn with polyvinylidene chloride plastic (i.e., glad wrap, saran wrap, or similar kitchen plastic wraps). The purposes of placing a temporary dressing over the burn site are to protect the damaged tissues, prevent entry of foreign material into the burn and to reduce pain.

Circumferential dressings should be avoided as they can cause constriction.

It is particularly important not to apply occlusive dressings to chemical burns unless the area has been thoroughly irrigated. Dressings like polyvinylidene chloride plastic are meant to be temporary only.

Escharotomies may be required if circumferential burns are present as tissue constriction may interfere with breathing.

Water or irrigation is contraindicated if metallic lithium, metallic sodium, metallic potassium, or metallic magnesium is present because the resulting chemical reactions with water are exothermic, worsening the burn.

Polyethylene glycol 300 or 400 (diluted 50:50 in water) and isopropyl alcohol have been suggested by some authors for the removal of phenols and cresols. Isopropyl alcohol may be very irritating if skin damage has already occurred.

Hydrofluoric acid burns should be treated as soon as possible with calcium gluconate or magnesium salts (in methylcellulose). Deep hydrofluoric acid burns usually require subcutaneous injections of calcium gluconate. Burns to the feed can be especially difficult to manage.

Tetanus prophylaxis is recommended.

Hospital management of chemical skin burns not involving hydrofluoric acid, phenols, or cresols is essentially the same as for thermal burns:

- Euthanasia should be considered for animals with extensive skin burns.
- If the area of skin affected involves more than 10%−15% of the body surface area, fluid resuscitation is necessary. Current recommendations are 3−4 mL of Hartmann's solution/kg BW/% total body surface area affected. Half of the calculated volume is given in the first 8 hours, and the

remainder is given over the following 16 hours. Alternatively, the Parkland Formula can be used to calculate the volume of fluid needed in the first 24 hours: 4 × %body surface area affected × BW (in kg).

- Albumin should be administered to replace lost plasma protein.
- Pain relief is paramount. Opiods are often required. However, their use requires care because of the risk of cardiovascular-respiratory depression.
- Debridement of blisters is controversial. Blisters do not act as a protective barrier and blister fluid is a medium for bacterial growth, promotes inflammation and increase the level of pain. Blisters increase the risk of infection. Blistering may obscure more severe full-thickness wounds.
- Wound management is the same as for thermal burns. Either the occlusive dressing approach using a biosynthetic membrane or topical antimicrobial dressings (e.g., silver sulfadiazine or mafenidine or acticoat or poloxamer 188 or nitrofuazone). Fungal infections are relatively common in burns patients.
- Escharotomies are indicated if circumferential cicatrization scarring is present on the torso, around an extremity or is interfering with joint function.
- Infection management is critical. Many burns patients die from a combination of toxemia and fluid loss.
- Skin grafting will usually be required for large burns.

Ingestions

Traditionally, administration of milk has been recommended on the basis that it acts as a diluent and an alternative source of protein for acid action. Milk has the disadvantage that it may interfere with subsequent endoscopy.

Administration of water has also been recommended. However, sulfuric acid mixed with water generates a substantial amount of heat. To minimize the risk of local build up of heat in the stomach, moderate quantities of water are recommended (250−500 mL).

Early endoscopy is recommended to evaluate the degree of damage to the gastrointestinal tract and to determine if surgical interventions are required.

Aspiration and associated lung injuries should always be suspected until definitively disproven.

The formation of strictures in the upper digestive tract is the norm following significant acid ingestions.

Eye injuries

In general, acid injuries to the eye tend to be less severe than alkali injuries. However, they can be very painful.

Specialized equipment (e.g., a Morgan lens) may be required eye irrigation. The affected eye should be irrigated with 2 L of irrigation fluid over 30–60 minutes or until the pH of the irrigation solution is 7.4.

The cornea, sclera, and conjunctiva should be thoroughly examined for evidence of damage (including fluorescein uptake).

Chemical eye injuries are commonly genuine ophthalmic emergencies and specialist evaluation as soon as possible is recommended.

Prognosis

Dependent the degree of the body surface affected, the age of the patient, and the presence of any complications.

Necropsy

The characteristic initial injury is coagulation necrosis at the site of first contact. Scarring and contracture are common subsequent findings. Infection is very common. Fungal infections are common if antibiotic therapy has been used.

Public Health Considerations

Chemical burns are very common in humans, particularly children.

Prevention

Correct storage away from animals is the best strategy.

GENERAL SITE OF FIRST CONTACT EFFECTS OF ALKALIS AND BASES

Alternative Names

An alkali is a basic, ionic salt of an alkali metal or an alkaline earth metal; alternatively an alkali is a base that dissolves in water.

A base is a substance that, in aqueous solution, is slippery to the touch (soapy or slimy feel due to saponification of skin lipids), tastes bitter, changes the color of indicators (e.g., turns red litmus paper blue), reacts with acids to form salts, and promotes certain chemical reactions (base catalysis).

A soluble base has a pH > 7.0.

Bases turn red litmus paper blue, phenolphthalein pink, keep bromothymol blue in its natural color of blue, and turn methyl orange yellow.

Bases that are commonly encountered in veterinary practice include:

- Sodium hydroxide (drain cleaners, oven cleaners, lye).
- Potassium hydroxide (drain cleaners, oven cleaners, lye).

- Calcium or sodium hypochlorite (swimming pool/spa chlorine).
- Ammonium hydroxide (household ammonia or cloudy ammonia).
- Calcium hydroxide (cement).

Circumstances of Poisoning

Similar to acids.

Cement is a common and important cause of alkali burns in domestic animals.

Absorption, Distribution, Metabolism, and Excretion

Alkalis and bases produce tissue liquefactive necrosis. This allows for relatively deep tissue penetration and favors systemic absorption.

Mode(s) of Action

Dissolve protein and saponify lipids resulting in tissue liquefaction necrosis. For a given titratable acid or alkali reserve, alkalis and bases produce deeper injuries than acids.

Materials pH > 11 are generally corrosive; however, pH is not the sole determinant of the degree of tissue injury. In general, granular formulations are more damaging than liquid formulations because they result in longer contact time with the tissues and higher local tissue concentrations.

Clinical Signs

Similar to acids, however, liquefaction necrosis, rather than coagulation necrosis, predominates.

Diagnostic Aids

As per acids.

Treatment

As per acids.

The depth of injury tends to be deeper than with acid injuries. Eye injuries tend to be worse.

Prognosis

Dependent the degree of the body surface affected, the age of the patient, and the presence of any complications.

Necropsy

The characteristic initial injury is liquefaction necrosis at the site of first contact. Scarring and contracture are common subsequent findings. Infection is very common. Fungal infections are common if antibiotic therapy has been used.

Public Health Considerations

Alkali and base burns are very common in humans, particularly in children.

Prevention

Correct storage away from animals is the best strategy.

Chapter 17

Miscellaneous Inorganic Toxicants

Rhian Cope

This section covers toxicants that are not metals, metalloids, organics, or gases/vapors.

The miscellaneous inorganic toxicants covered include:

- Battery ingestion.
- Bleaches (hypochlorites, sodium peroxide, and sodium perborate).
- Bromides and bromates.
- Fertilizers (see also nitrite/nitrate poisoning, ammonia poisoning, and iron poisoning).
- Flour and food bleaches (nitrogen trichloride [agene] and methionine sulfoximine).
- Hydrogen peroxide.
- Acute fluoride poisoning.
- Chronic fluoride poisoning.
- Hydrogen fluoride, hydrofluoric acid, ammonium fluoride, and ammonium bifluoride.
- Acute iodine poisoning.
- Chronic iodine poisoning.
- White (yellow) phosphorus poisoning.
- Acute selenium poisoning.
- Subacute selenium poisoning and porcine focal symmetrical poliomyelomalacia.
- Chronic selenium poisoning (alkali disease).

Ingested ammonia poisoning is covered in the feed additives chapter. Nitrite/nitrate poisoning is covered in Chapter 24, Poisonous Plants. Salt poisoning and water intoxication is covered in Chapter 14, Metals.

Veterinary Toxicology for Australia and New Zealand
DOI: http://dx.doi.org/10.1016/B978-0-12-420227-6.00016-5

BATTERY INGESTION

Alternative Names

None.

Circumstances of Poisoning

Ingestion of disk-type batteries is the most common problem. Lithium disk batteries appear to be more damaging than alkaline types.

Batteries can also lodge in the trachea, ears, and nose, and cause localized injuries.

AA, AAA, C, and D cells can be problematic in dogs.

Ingestion of lead-acid car and machinery batteries by livestock is covered under lead poisoning in Chapter 14, Metals.

Toxicokinetics

Effects are primarily site of contact related.

Toxic Mode(s) of Action

Important modes of action include:

- Direct pressure necrosis at the site of lodgement.
- Contact of the battery terminals with tissues and tissue fluids causes a flow of electrical current that causes corrosive tissue injury. The level of injury is usually greatest at the positive terminal end of the battery. Tissue damage can be severe enough to result in a perforated viscus.
- When in contact with body fluids, the cathode side of a battery tends to produce alkali burns (i.e., liquefaction necrosis) and the anode side tends to produce acid burns (i.e., coagulation necrosis).
- Battery contents tend to be alkaline and alkaline burns can result if the battery ruptures.
- Gastrointestinal and respiratory obstructions can occur.

Clinical Signs

The clinical toxidrome largely depends on the site of lodgement. The site of lodgement in the gastrointestinal tract is most commonly in the esophagus (with risk of subsequent stenosis) or pyloric sphincter (with risk of gastric outlet obstruction or gastric outlet stenosis). Accordingly cranial abdominal pain, anorexia, dehydration, vomiting (with blood), and vomiting following food consumption are likely clinical signs. Patients with batteries lodged in the stomach are always at risk of gastric rupture, peritonitis, and sepsis.

Lodgement in the esophagus may be associated with regurgitation, pain on swallowing, anorexia, drooling, and chest pain. Perforation of the esophagus is always a potential risk.

Nasal discharges (may be bloody), pain, head shaking, sneezing, and stertorous sounds on auscultation of the upper respiratory tract often accompany lodgement of batteries in the upper respiratory tract.

Lodgement of batteries in the ears is usually associated with head shaking and pain. The presence of the battery in the external ear canal and ulceration at the site of lodgement can usually be detected on examination using an otoscope.

Diagnostic Aids

Endoscopy is the preferred and most useful method.

Radiography and other diagnostic imaging can be used.

Otoscopy.

Treatment

Endoscopic inspection and removal is the usually method of treatment. Surgical repair of a perforated viscous may be required.

Other treatment is generally supportive.

Prognosis

Good provided that tissue damage and stricture formation is not severe.

Necropsy

When in contact with body fluids, the cathode side of a battery tends to produce alkali burns (i.e., liquefaction necrosis) and the anode side tends to produce acid burns (i.e., coagulation necrosis).

Public Health Considerations

Disk batteries are a public health menace in small children.

Prevention

Batteries, particularly disk batteries and appliance remote controls that contain batteries, should be stored where animals cannot access them.

BLEACHES (HYPOCHLORITES, SODIUM PEROXIDE, SODIUM PERBORATE)

Alternative Names

Spa chlorine.

Swimming pool chlorine.

Bleach.

Sodium hypochlorite (typical household bleach).

Potassium hypochlorite.

Calcium hypochlorite.

Lithium hypochlorite.

Nonhalogenated bleaches (oxygen bleaches): sodium peroxide, sodium perborate.

Circumstances of Poisoning

Note: Chlorine and chloramine gas poisoning is covered in greater detail in Chapter 20, Smoke and Other Inhaled Toxicants.

Hypochlorite bleaches and oxygen bleaches are ubiquitous household products.

Ingestion is the usual route of exposure; however, skin and eye exposures can occur. The volume of ingestion of concentrated hypochlorites is often limited because of pain.

Contact between the skin and powder, granulated or tablet hypochlorite preparations can result in acid skin burns.

Mixing of hypochlorites with acids results in chlorine gas release. Mixing of hypochlorites with household ammonia products results in chloramine release. Both chlorine and chloramine are denser than air and will tend to accumulate in low-lying areas.

Chlorine and chloramine gases are unpleasant and irritant. This usually triggers escape behaviors. Most cases of serious poisoning with these gases occur when the animal is unable to escape (e.g., caged birds).

Toxicokinetics

Typically have site of contact effects (skin, eye, gastrointestinal tract, and respiratory tract).

Toxic Mode(s) of Action

Chlorine and chloramine gases are pulmonary irritants and bronchoconstrictors. Chlorine forms hydrochloric and hypochlorous acids as well as oxygen radicals in the respiratory tract. In the presence of water, chloramines decompose to ammonia and hypochlorous acid or hydrochloric acid. In both cases hypochlorous acid reputably accounts for most of the toxic effects. The chemical reactions associated with chloramines are more rapid than those of chlorine. Thus the adverse effects of chloramines tend to occur more quickly than those of chlorine gas. Both are capable of producing delayed noncardiogenic pulmonary edema due to loss of pulmonary capillary integrity and the acute respiratory distress syndrome following significant exposures.

Chlorine and chloramine gas are capable of producing significant damage to the cornea and associated ocular tissues. The effects are essentially the same as an acid burn.

In the acid environment of the stomach hypochlorites form hypochlorous acid resulting in gastric mucosal acid burns.

Sodium peroxide dissociates in the gastrointestinal tract, releasing oxygen. This produces gastritis and emesis.

Sodium perborate decomposes to peroxide and borate in the gastrointestinal tract. This produces gastritis due to the actions of peroxide. Systemic borate toxicity can occur.

Clinical Signs

The most commonly encountered scenario in veterinary medicine is limited ingestions and accompanying burns to the perioral regions, the oral mucosae and the tongue. Typically these are accompanied by excessive salivation, pain on eating and drinking, anorexia and visible ulceration.

Clinically significant ingestion of hypochlorites is typically associated gaging, pain on eating and drinking, anorexia, dyspnea, pain, cranial abdominal pain and vomiting (may contain blood) as well as burns to the perioral regions, the oral mucosae and the tongue. The vomitus may have a distinct chlorine-like smell. A perforated viscus, peritonitis, and sepsis may occur in severe cases. Strictures and stenosis are common sequelae.

Hypochlorite ocular burns are a genuine ophthalmic emergency that requires specialist treatment.

Hypochlorite-induced skin burns are most commonly encountered when solid hypochlorite preparations have had prolonged skin contact or if there is any form of occlusive skin exposure. Hypochlorite burns are acid burns, thus blistering and eschar formation may occur.

Sodium peroxide ingestion typically produces nausea and emesis. Cranial abdominal pain may be present due to the presence of mild gastritis.

Sodium perborate ingestion typically produces nausea and emesis. Cranial abdominal pain may be present due to the presence of mild gastritis. Systemic boron toxicity may occur (see relevant section in Chapter 8: Insecticides and Acaricides).

The effects of chlorine and chloramine gas exposures are usually limited provided that the animal can escape and avoid exposure. Most cases will display relatively mild effects such as evidence of bronchoconstriction (wheezing), sneezing, nasal discharges, excessive salivation, and eye irritation (excessive lachrymation, conjunctivitis, blepharospasm). In cases where animals are unable to escape from the exposure (e.g., caged birds), damage to the respiratory system can be severe and result in acute inflammation of the pharynx and larynx (stertor, stridor, laryngeal sensitivity), laryngospasm, aphonia or changed voice traits, tracheitis, dyspnea, tachypnea, coughing, pain associated with respiration and progressive respiratory distress. Delayed-onset pulmonary edema (rales and decreased breath sounds on auscultation) may occur. Death is typically due to respiratory failure.

Diagnostic Aids

Case history commonly provides the best diagnostic information. If possible, obtain the original product container and information about any dilution and methods of application.

Endoscopy is indicated in cases of significant ingestion.

Treatment

Under no circumstances should any attempt be made to neutralize hypochlorous acid. Acid neutralization reactions are exothermic and increase the amount of tissue damage.

Do not induce emesis.

Active charcoal is not effective following acid ingestion and interferes with subsequent endoscopy.

Ice should not be applied to burns.

Airway security is paramount. It is always better to intubate if in doubt and to intubate sooner rather than later. Upper airway edema may occur even when the upper respiratory tract is not directly injured. If in doubt, intubate: many burns patients die from airway compromise.

Chemical eye injuries are commonly genuine ophthalmic emergencies and specialist evaluation as soon as possible is recommended.

Euthanasia is an important option: older patients with burns covering ≥ 80% of body surface area are unlikely to survive irrespective of treatment.

Renal failure can occur after burn injury.

The use of corticosteroids for chemical burn treatment is controversial. They may help airway inflammation. However, they may predispose to infection and may mask the clinical signs of gut perforations. Corticosteroid therapy does not reduce the risk of eschar contractures, cicatrization scarring, or the formation of strictures in the gastrointestinal tract.

Skin burns

In cases of skin and eye burns, the most critical treatment is copious wound irrigation (note the situations were wound irrigation is contraindicated below). Both the time to irrigation and the volume of irrigation are critical. Wound irrigation within 10 minutes of exposure will decrease the depth of skin injury by a factor of 5.

A common error in treatment is not irrigating the affected area for long enough. Irrigation should continue for at least 30−60 minutes or until the pH of the irrigating solution is at least 7.3, but preferably 7.4.

The irrigating solution should be cool, but not cold. Cold water produces dermal vasoconstriction and worsens tissue ischemia and local edema.

Care is required during wound irrigation:

- The burn site can be irrigated with water or saline.
- Great care should be taken to avoid hypothermia.
- The contaminated irrigation solution should not be allowed to run onto unaffected tissues.
- One of the aims of the irrigation process should be to remove any particulate material present.
- Diphoterine is claimed to be more effective than water or saline; however, definitive veterinary data are lacking.

If there will be significant delay between the initial first response of wound irrigation and hospitalization, current recommendations are to either apply specialist burn dressings or to cover the burn with polyvinylidene chloride plastic (i.e., glad wrap, saran wrap, or similar kitchen plastic wraps). The purposes of placing a temporary dressing over the burn site are to protect the damaged tissues, prevent entry of foreign material into the burn and to reduce pain.

Circumferential dressings should be avoided as they can cause constriction.

It is particularly important not to apply occlusive dressings to chemical burns unless the area has been thoroughly irrigated. Dressings like polyvinylidene chloride plastic are meant to be temporary only.

Escharotomies may be required if circumferential burns are present as tissue constriction may interfere with breathing.

Tetanus prophylaxis is recommended if significant burns are present.

Hospital management of chemical skin burns is essentially the same as for thermal burns:

- Euthanasia should be considered for animals with extensive skin burns.
- If the area of skin affected involves more than 10%−15% of the body surface area, fluid resuscitation is necessary. Current recommendations are 3−4 mL of Hartmann's solution/kg BW/% total body surface area affected. Half of the calculated volume is given in the first 8 hours and the remainder is given over the following 16 hours. Alternatively, the Parkland Formula can be used to calculate the volume of fluid needed in the first 24 hours: 4 × %body surface area affected × BW (in kg).

- Albumin should be administered to replace lost plasma protein.
- Pain relief is paramount. Opiods are often required. However, their use requires care because of the risk of cardiovascular-respiratory depression.
- Debridement of blisters is controversial. Blisters do not act as a protective barrier and blister fluid is a medium for bacterial growth, promotes inflammation, and increase the level of pain. Blisters increase the risk of infection. Blistering may obscure more severe full-thickness wounds.
- Wound management is the same as for thermal burns: either the occlusive dressing approach using a biosynthetic membrane or topical antimicrobial dressings (e.g., silver sulfadiazine or mafenidine or acticoat or poloxamer 188 or nitrofuazone). Fungal infections are relatively common in burns patients.
- Escharotomies are indicated if circumferential cicatrization scarring is present on the torso, around an extremity or is interfering with joint function.
- Infection management is critical. Many burns patients die from a combination of toxemia and fluid loss.
- Skin grafting will usually be required for large burns.

Ingestions

Traditionally, administration of milk has been recommended on the basis that it acts as a diluent and an alternative source of protein for acid action. Milk has the disadvantage that it may interfere with subsequent endoscopy.

Administration of water has also been recommended. However, sulfuric acid mixed with water generates a substantial amount of heat. To minimize the risk of local build up of heat in the stomach, moderate quantities of water are recommended (250−500 mL).

Early endoscopy is recommended to evaluate the degree of damage to the gastrointestinal tract and to determine if surgical interventions are required.

Aspiration and associated lung injuries should always be suspected until definitively disproven.

The formation of strictures in the upper digestive tract is the norm following significant acid ingestions.

Eye injuries

In general, acid injuries to the eye tend to be less severe than alkali injuries. However, they can be very painful.

Specialized equipment (e.g., a Morgan lens) may be required eye irrigation. The affected eye should be irrigated with 2 L of irrigation fluid over 30−60 minutes or until the pH of the irrigation solution is 7.4.

The cornea, sclera, and conjunctiva should be thoroughly examined for evidence of damage (including fluorescein uptake).

Chemical eye injuries are commonly genuine ophthalmic emergencies and specialist evaluation as soon as possible is recommended.

Clinically significant exposures to chlorine and/or chloramine gas (particularly in enclosed spaces)

Patients exposed to large concentrations in an enclosed environment and patients with underlying respiratory or cardiovascular disease should be hospitalized and monitored for delayed respiratory effects irrespective of their initial condition. A common mistake is to discharge such patients too early in the course of the toxicoses.

Historical recommendations that patients be nebulized with sodium bicarbonate have been demonstrated to be ineffective, and at worse, may exacerbate respiratory damage by causing chemical pneumonitis.

Airway security is paramount due to the risk of laryngospasm and laryngeal edema. It is always better to intubate too early than too late during the clinical course.

Short-acting β_2-agonist bronchodilators (e.g., salbutamol, clenbuterol) plus supplemental oxygen may be required to counteract the broncho-constrictor effects.

Ventilation may be required, but is often not available in veterinary practice.

Conservative fluid management (i.e., avoidance of over-hydration) has been historically recommended in the treatment of the acute respiratory distress syndrome. Recent human data suggest that conservative fluid management does not decrease the death rate. However, conservative fluid management was associated with improved oxygenation and less severe nonpulmonary effects. It should be noted that conservative fluid management does not mean the induction of dehydration; rather it means the maintenance of an even fluid balance.

The use of anti-inflammatories such as corticosteroids, statins, and macrolide antibiotics for treatment of the acute respiratory distress syndrome is controversial. There is equivocal evidence that corticosteroids decrease mortality. However, there is limited evidence that corticosteroids may reduce lung and other organ injury, although the effects are small.

Antioxidants such as *n*-acetyl cysteine and nebulized surfactant (recombinant surfactant protein C, synthetic surfactants, reconstituted animal surfactants) are often administered for the treatment of the acute respiratory distress syndrome. Despite promising experimental data, the clinical effectiveness of these treatments is often limited.

Prognosis

Most veterinary cases involve low-level exposure either because the animal escapes from the noxious fumes or because of pain associated with ingestion.

The prognoses for clinically significant ingestions, burns involving large body areas and chlorine/chloramine gas exposures are guarded to poor.

Necropsy

Acid burns are classically characterized by coagulation necrosis at sites of contact. This may include the gastric mucosa.

Classical features of inhaled chlorine and inhaled chloramine poisoning include pulmonary edema, pneumonia, pneumonitis, hyaline membrane formation, multiple pulmonary thrombosis, and ulcerative tracheobronchitis.

Public Health Considerations

Burns due to bleach spills, chlorine gas, and chloramine gas exposures are common household events.

Prevention

Safe storage is paramount. Household products containing hypochlorites and ammonia should never be mixed or co-applied.

BROMIDE

Alternative Names

Bromide (Br^-) is the anion of bromine (Br_2).

1-Bromo-3-chloro-5,5-dimethylhydantoin is used as a sanitizer in swimming pools and spas. It forms hypobromite and hypobromous acid when dissolved in water. Bromine products are superior water sanitizers than chlorine/hypochlorite-based products. Bromide hydantoins do not produce bromide poisoning.

Methyl bromide (bromomethane) has historically been extensively used as a fumigant (including soil fumigation). However, its use has been progressively curtailed. Methyl bromide does not produce bromide/bromate poisoning.

Bromates (BrO_3^-) are a bromine-based oxoanions. They are suspected carcinogens.

Bromide utilized by eosinophils to generate antiparasitic brominating compounds such as hypobromite, via metabolism by eosinophil peroxidase (eosinophil haloperoxidase). Eosinophil peroxidase preferentially utilizes bromide over chloride if it is available. However, bromide is not essential for animal life.

Despite the name, theobromine does not contain bromine or bromide.

Circumstances of Poisoning

Bromide salts (usually potassium bromide) are still used in veterinary medicine to control seizure disorders in dogs. *Bromides should not be used to control epilepsy in cats.*

Lithium and sodium bromide had extensive historical use as a sedative and as a treatment for bipolar disorders.

Bromide salts are drugs of addiction.

Bromide salts are used in black and white photographic processing.

The sedative effects of bromide are at least additive to those of the barbiturates and other central nervous system (CNS) sedatives.

There are cases of bromism in humans associated with the excessive consumption of soft drinks that contain high levels of brominated vegetable oils.

Toxicokinetics

Bromide is isostructural with chloride and its toxicokentics essentially resembles that of chloride.

Bromide is well absorbed from the gastrointestinal tract.

Bromide is largely eliminated in the urine. However, it undergoes active reabsorption in the renal proximal tubules and is resorbed in preference to chloride. Because of this, bromide has a very long elimination half-life and it takes weeks to months of continuous exposure to achieve plasma steady state levels. These effects increase the risks associated with the therapeutic use of bromides and make dose determination/dose titration difficult. With therapeutic use of bromides in dogs, it typically takes 4 months for blood levels to stabilize.

Toxic Mode(s) of Action

Bromide substitutes for chloride in excitable tissues and stabilizes excitable membranes, particularly those of the CNS.

Bromide salts are emetic when ingested in large amounts.

The use of bromide to control seizures in dogs is associated with diuresis and increased water requirement.

Chronic bromide use in cats is associated with inflammatory lower airway disease and endogenous lipid pneumonia. *Bromides should not be used to control epilepsy in cats.*

Clinical Signs

Acute bromide poisoning

- Typically occurs following ingestion.

- Episodes of acute renal failure and severe dehydration in dogs being treated with bromide salts can trigger acute bromide poisoning.
- Ingestion of clinically significant amounts of bromide salts typically induces emesis that often reduces the absorbed dose (a useful safety feature of bromide sedatives).
- Classically the syndrome is characterized by initial muscular pain, generalized weakness, ataxia, hyporeflexia, and CNS sedation. Death is typically due to central cardiovascular-respiratory depression combined.
- The effects of bromide salts are at least additive with those of other CNS sedatives.

Bromism (chronic bromide poisoning)

- The toxidrome is most likely to occur in patients using long-term bromide therapy to control epilepsy and amongst human addicts.
- The toxidrome is characterized by cognitive changes (e.g., hallucinations such as biting at imaginary flies), irritability/agitation or depression, ataxia, and hyperreflexia.
- Psychotic states and dementia have been associated with bromism in humans.
- Patients with bromism characteristically develop bromoderma (synonym: bromaderma tuburosum): a pustular bromide skin rash, skin granulomas, skin hyperpigmentation, and skin bullae formation.
- Renal disease and changes in salt intake

Bromide withdrawal seizures

- Sudden decreases in systemic bromide levels can induce seizures.
- Withdrawal seizures are most likely to happen if there is a sudden increase in dietary chloride (i.e., being placed on a high salt diet) or during the withdrawal of bromide treatment for epilepsy.

Diagnostic Aids

Serum bromine levels are helpful. Typically serum bromine should be <1000 mg/L (15 mmol/L) provided that the animal is not being treated with bromides for epilepsy.

For animals undergoing treatment for epilepsy, serum bromine levels should be maintained between 1000 mg/L (15 mmol/L) and 2000 mg/L (25 mmol/L).

Treatment

Gastrointestinal decontamination techniques are of no value.

Intravenous infusions of crystalloids that contain chloride and diuresis have been historically used. However, the effectiveness of this technique has not been systematically evaluated.

It should be noted that sudden changes systemic bromide levels causes withdrawal seizures. Withdrawal seizures can usually be controlled with benzodiazepines. However, barbiturates and possibly general anesthesia may be required to control the seizures.

Prognosis

Acute bromide poisoning: good to guarded depending on the level of sedation.

Chronic bromide poisoning: good to guarded.

Necropsy

Nonspecific.

Public Health Considerations

Bromides are drugs of addiction.

Prevention

The use of bromide salts to control epilepsy requires careful monitoring. Blood bromide levels should be ideally assessed 16 weeks following the start of treatment. Ideally serum bromide levels should be maintained between 1000 mg/L (15 mmol/L) and 2000 mg/L (25 mmol/L) provided, there is no sedation. Inadequate control of seizures with serum bromide levels of >1500 mg/L (20 mmol/L) suggest that a change in medication is required. Serum bromide levels should be assessed every 6–12 months or 8–16 weeks if there is a change in dose or if there is a breakdown in seizure control.

Dehydration should be avoided in dogs being treated with bromides to control epilepsy.

FERTILIZERS

See also nitrite/nitrate poisoning, ammonia poisoning, and iron poisoning.

Alternative Names

Fertilizers are a diverse group of products that typically contain nitrogen, phosphorus, potassium, and other trace minerals in various chemical forms.

Other common toxicants of concern in fertilizers are nitrate, iron, urea, and calcium cyanamide.

Circumstances of Poisoning

Typically involves ingestion by dogs.

Ingestion by livestock may occur, particularly in circumstances involving dietary mineral deficiencies and pica.

High phosphate and high potassium fertilizers are generally of low toxicity. The most common effects are gastrointestinal irritation and distress that is usually mild and self-limiting.

Urea in fertilizers is converted to ammonia in the rumen. This may result in ammonia poisoning in ruminants (see section on ammonia poisoning).

Nitrate ingestion by ruminants can result in nitrite poisoning (see nitrite poisoning section).

Ingestion of iron at levels can result in acute iron toxicity (see iron toxicity in Chapter 14: Metals).

Calcium cyanamide is a skin irritant. Systemic effects can include hypotension, shock, pulmonary edema, and ataxia.

Ingestion of fertilizers of biological origin (e.g., blood and bone meal, composts) can be a cause of botulism.

FLOUR AND FOOD BLEACHES (NITROGEN TRICHLORIDE, METHIONINE SULFOXIMINE)

Alternative Names

Synonyms for nitrogen trichloride include: trichloramine and agene. Bleaching of flower using nitrogen trichloride is referred to as the agene process. This process produces "agenized" flour.

Methionine sulfoximine is a rare amino acid that is formed as a byproduct of nitrogen trichloride treatment of flour.

Circumstances of Poisoning

Agenized flour was extensively used in bread production and cooking for more than 50 years. Agenization is occasionally still used (inappropriately) in pet food manufacturing.

Methionine sulfoximine is marketed as an alternative medicine/natural medicine for the treatment of neurological problems.

Methionine sulfoximine is extensively used as a research agent in animal models of epilepsy and other brain disorders.

Methionine sulfoximine and related derivative have been proposed as pharmaceutical candidates. Subconvulsive doses of methionine sulfoximine are neuroprotective in rodent models of hyperammonemia, acute liver disease, and amyotrophic lateral sclerosis.

Toxicokinetics

Nitrogen trichloride reacts with methionine in protein to form methionine sulfoximine. On hydrolysis of the proteins in the gut, this amino acid derivative is released and absorbed.

Toxic Mode(s) of Action

Methionine sulfoximine is highly toxic to dogs, ferrets, cats, and rabbits. Primates and rodents are relatively resistant to the effects.

Methionine sulfoxamine produces irreversible inhibition of astrocyte glutamine synthetase in brain. This results in a decrease in brain GABA synthesis and loss of central GABA inhibition.

Methionine sulfoxamine also triggers brain cortical glutamate release, increasing cortical activity via glutamate activation of cortical NMDA receptors. This triggers neuronal excitotoxicity and neuronal death.

Clinical Signs

The toxidrome is classically referred to as "canine hysteria."

Characterized by irregular "grand mal" seizures, "running fits," ataxia, and "hysterical" states, with apparent recovery between attacks. Attacks are not triggered by external stimuli.

Diagnostic Aids

Detection and measurement of methionine sulfoxamine levels in food samples is helpful.

Treatment

GABA agonists/allosteric modulators are the mainstay of treatment. Benzodiazepines and barbiturates are the agents most commonly used. Other sedative-hypnotic allosteric GABA modulators such as zaleplon, zolpidem, or zopiclone may be helpful.

Other treatment is supportive. Prevention of misadventure and self-harm is important.

Prognosis

Good provided exposure is discontinued and seizures can be controlled.

Necropsy

No specific findings.

Public Health Considerations

Nitrogen trichloride food bleaching is no longer approved in most countries.

Prevention

Nitrogen trichloride should not be used in pet food manufacturing.

HYDROGEN PEROXIDE

Alternative Names

Dihydrogen dioxide.

Domestically available and medical/veterinary hydrogen peroxide solutions typically contain about 35% hydrogen peroxide in water.

Higher concentrations are used in industrial and laboratory settings.

Circumstances of Poisoning

Hydrogen peroxide is extensively used in industrial processes.

Typically adverse events in veterinary practice are associated with its use as a disinfectant, its use during wound debridement and its use as an emetic.

Other potential causes of veterinary poisoning include consumption of hair dye and hair bleach products.

Toxicokinetics

Effects are most commonly at the site of first contact. Rarely, gas emboli can result from ingestion or wound treatment with hydrogen peroxide.

Toxic Mode(s) of Action

Oxidizer.

Clinical Signs

The most commonly encountered scenario in veterinary practice is nausea and emesis with or without mild gastritis.

Ingestion of very concentrated solutions of hydrogen peroxide can produce severe gastritis.

Very rarely, gas emboli have occurred following the use of hydrogen peroxide for wound debridement/wound cleansing.

Diagnostic Aids

The package and/or container are the best source of diagnostic information.

Treatment

Treatment is usually supportive.

Antacids, proton pump inhibitors, H_2 histamine antagonists, and gastric protectants may be required under some circumstances.

Vomiting is rarely protracted, thus antiemetics are usually not required.

Prognosis

Generally good.

Necropsy

Gastritis is the predominant finding.

Public Health Considerations

None.

Prevention

Adequate storage of hydrogen peroxide-containing products.

Concentrated hydrogen peroxide solutions should not be used in veterinary practice or should be diluted before use.

ACUTE FLUORIDE POISONING

Alternative Names

Floride (F^-) is the anion of fluorine (F).

Fluorite is calcium fluoride (CaF_2).

Sodium fluoride and fluorite were historically used to fluoridate water. In current times hexafluorosilicic acid (H_2SiF_6) and its salt sodium hexafluorosilicate (Na_2SiF_6) are more commonly used.

In some countries, table salt is fluoridated.

Sodium fluoride, acidulated fluoride phosphate, sodium monofluorophosphate (MFP) are typically used in toothpaste. Fluoride toothpaste usually contains around 0.22% (1000 ppm) and 0.312% (1450 ppm) fluoride. A 0.76 g MFP is equivalent to 0.1 g fluoride.

Mouth rinses and mouth washes typically contain about 0.05% sodium fluoride (225 ppm fluoride).

Dental products containing higher levels of fluoride are available. However, they may require a prescription.

Circumstances of Poisoning

The toxidrome occurs when high doses of soluble fluorides are ingested. The acutely lethal dose is about 32–64 mg/kg elemental fluoride/kg BW. Ingestion of fluoride can produce gastrointestinal discomfort at doses at least 15–20 times lower (0.2–0.3 mg/kg) than lethal doses.

Classically the toxidrome is associated with large ingestions of sodium fluoride or fluoride-containing mouth washes.

Sodium fluorosilicate was historically used as a rodenticide. When dissolved in water at neutral pH it forms fluoride, hydrofluoric acid, and silicic acid. It causes acute fluoride poisoning.

Sodium fluoride was historically used as an ascaricide in pigs.

Toxicokinetics

Soluble forms of fluoride are rapidly and efficiently absorbed from the gastrointestinal tract. Increasing the pH of the stomach favors the ionized form, thus reducing absorption. Increasing the aluminum, calcium, and magnesium levels in the diet or in the gut contents decreases absorption because fluoride forms relatively insoluble salts with these metals. Water hardness does not affect fluoride bioavailability in a toxicologically significant manner.

Fluoride distributes to the total body water. Fluoride accumulates in calcifying organs, i.e., bone and the pineal gland. The blood–brain barrier appears to be a barrier to fluoride, at least in the short term.

Fluoride is cleared from the plasma by two mechanisms: sequestration in mineralized tissues and excretion in urine. Renal excretion is influenced by pH and glomerular filtration rate. At low pH more hydrogen fluoride is formed which promotes reabsorption by the renal tubules. Renal excretion is relatively rapid. The half-life of fluoride in bone is about 20 years.

Toxic Mode(s) of Action

Fluoride combines with calcium in blood and tissues forming insoluble calcium fluoride. This results in acute hypocalcemia.

Clinical Signs

The onset of clinical signs is usually rapid: within 5–60 minutes postingestion.

The toxidrome is followed by evidence of CNS excitation followed by seizures. CNS depression occurs in the terminal phase.

Signs of gastrointestinal upset such as excessive salivation, vomiting, and defecation are common.

Severe cardiac arrhythmias and sudden cardiac function related deaths occur due to the presence of hypocalcemia.

Diagnostic Aids

The original product container is often the most important diagnostic aid.

The patient's ECG often reflects hypocalcemia, i.e., narrowing of the QRS complex, reduced PR interval, T wave flattening and inversion, prolongation of the QT-interval, prominent U-wave, prolonged ST and ST-depression.

Treatment

At least in theory and if the patient presents very soon after ingestion or if delayed-release preparations have been swallowed, a dilute solution of calcium hydroxide or calcium chloride can be orally administered to precipitate the fluoride, thus reducing its bioavailability. In reality, patients are rarely presented for treatment early enough for this to be effective.

The mainstay of treatment is reversal of the hypocalcemia using intravenous calcium gluconate. Care must be taken not to overdose. Calcium should be administered slowly, preferably while monitoring cardiac electrical activity. Mild hypercalcemia is characterized by broad-based tall peaking T waves; severe hypercalcemia is extremely wide QRS, low R wave, disappearance of p waves, and tall peaking T waves.

Prognosis

Guarded. Depends on the dose and how quickly the hypocalcemia can be reversed.

Necropsy

None.

Public Health Considerations

None.

Prevention

Fluoride dental products should be correctly stored where animals cannot access them.

CHRONIC FLUORIDE POISONING (FLUOROSIS)

Alternative Names

See acute fluoride poisoning.

Circumstances of Poisoning

Fluorosis in Australia is most commonly associated with the use of artesian water with a high concentration of natural bioavailable fluoride. This problem occurs mostly in Queensland. A hot climate, high levels of water consumption, surface evaporation from long open bore-drains, and drought-induced grazing patterns exacerbate the problem. Evaporation is a significant concern, e.g., a 1 ppm fluoride concentration at the bore-head can increase substantially as water moves down a 100 mile-long bore drain in a climate with evaporation rates exceeding 250 cm per year.

Problems with fluorosis have also occurred with geothermal water sources.

Fluorosis can also result from the use of poor quality rock phosphate-derived fertilizers and dietary phosphorus supplements. Rock phosphate-derived fertilizers include single super phosphate, triple super phosphate, partially acidulated rock phosphate, and diamonium phosphate. Phosphate fertilizers that have not been adequately de-fluoridated represent a substantial risk because the fluoride they add to the soil remains and concentrates in the biologically active topsoil due to strong adsorption to soil constituents. Fluoride derived from poor quality fertilizers.

The major route of exposure of livestock is by drinking water and by soil consumption. Soil consumption is problematic particularly during droughts and if mineral deficiency-related pica is present.

Fluoride uptake by mineralized tissues is cumulative, i.e., chronic consumption of excessive levels will result in toxicity. Because fluorides accumulate when dietary intake is constant, exposure time is often a major factor in toxicity. Animals that have a long productive lifespan (e.g., dairy cows) are at greater risk.

Notably, intermittent high exposures may result in increased severity of toxicosis even when the overall annual intake is within the acceptable range.

Younger animals are at greater risk because of active bone growth and tooth formation.

Animals with higher skeletal turnover are at greater risk, e.g., lactating animals, dairy cattle.

Chickens relatively resistant, mink are amongst the most susceptible species.

Calcium deficient diets promote fluoride accumulation.

High levels of dietary fat in poultry increase fluoride accumulation.

Toxicokinetics

See acute fluoride poisoning.

Toxic Mode(s) of Action

Effects on teeth

- Teeth are most seriously affected during their development, i.e., erupted teeth with already formed enamel and dentine are not damaged.
- In fully formed teeth, ameloblasts cannot repair enamel, but odontoblasts can produce secondary dentine to compensate to some degree.
- Changes in teeth can extend from simple white mottled areas in teeth that are purely cosmetic differences through to soft teeth and excessive wear.
- Damage to ameloblasts and odontoblasts results in abnormal mineralization of enamel, dentine, and cementum. This results in softer and weaker teeth, which in turn results in excessive pitting and excessive and/or uneven dental ware (pits appear as brown or black spots on the teeth).
- Defects in enamel and dentine result in teeth that are mottled and pitted (pitted areas usually stain black due to accumulation of oxidized debris).
- Exposure of the pulp cavity results in pain. This decreases mastication and food intake, which results in reduced growth/performance.

Effects on the skeleton

- F^- replaces OH^- in hydroxyapatite. This results in a change in the crystalline structure of hydroxyapatite.
- Disruption of bone matrix formation and mineralization due to effects on osteoblasts resulting in accelerated bone remodeling, subperiosteal hyperostosis. The end result is long bones with thickened and irregular surfaces, exostoses, and sclerosis, particularly on the metatarsals, metacarpals, and ribs. The effects are characteristically bilateral.
- Classically, initial occurrence of bone lesions is on the medial surfaces of the proximal 1/3 of the metatarsals.
- Periosteal hyperostosis results in spurring and bridging near joints. This results in intermittent joint associated/appendicular lameness

Thyroid effects

- High levels of fluoride intake are associated with hypothyroidism. Fluorotyrosine has been historically used to treat hyperthyroidism.
- The mode of action of these effects is poorly understood. Fluoride decreases iodine uptake by the thyroid glands.
- High-fluoride intake in association with low iodine intake exacerbates the problem.
- In general the effects are regarded as being relatively mild and clinically overt hypothyroidism is usually not predominant feature of fluorosis.

Clinical Signs

Effects on general condition and growth
- Lowered growth and performance despite adequate feed availability.
- Poor body condition, cachexia, and weight loss.
- Anorexia or lowered food consumption.
- Typically have a dry hair coat and roughened skin.
- Typically only a few animals are obviously affected in a herd at any given time.
- Anemia, hypothyroidism, stunted growth, delayed estrus, poor breeding performance may be present.

Dental effects
- Affects the incisors, premolars, and molars.
- Excessive dental wear.
- Uneven dental wear.
- White mottling of teeth.
- Defects in enamel and dentine result in teeth that are mottled and pitted (pitted areas usually stain black due to accumulation of oxidized debris).
- Characteristic feature in cattle is that they lap water (presumably ↓ pain associated with contact of cold water on exposed pulp cavities).

Skeletal effects
- Abnormal postures, arched backs.
- Intermittent joint associated/appendicular lameness.
- Abnormal exostoses, particularly on the metatarsals, metacarpals, and ribs.
- Abnormal hoof ware, particularly in the hind legs (elongated toes).

Diagnostic Aids

Water fluoride determination: samples must be taken where stock are actually drinking as well as at the bore-head in order to account for evaporation.

Increased urinary fluorine indicates relatively recent exposure (1—3 weeks) or evidence of continuing release from bone.

Radiographic examination of skeleton/teeth (radiolucent irregularities will be present).

Transillumination examination of the skeleton can be helpful.

Bone biopsy
- Preferable sites are the rib or coccygeal vertebrae. However, samples from the mandible, metacarpus, pelvis, and metatarsals can be used.
- *Note*: levels vary for different bones, i.e., need to know what is normal; thus control samples from nonfluoride exposed animals of similar breed and age are needed.
- Cancellous bone generally contains higher fluoride than cortical bone.

Feed analysis

Treatment

Treatment is supportive. Removal from the source of fluoride is essential. Easily masticated foods should be supplied.

Prognosis

Poor, particularly if significant dental and skeletal damage, is present. Mild forms of chronic fluorosis have an adequate prognosis provided that effecting grazing/feeding is not disrupted and exposure is stopped.

Necropsy

Dental effects
- Affects the incisors, premolars, and molars.
- Excessive dental wear.
- Uneven dental wear.
- White mottling of teeth.
- Defects in enamel and dentine result in teeth that are mottled and pitted (pitted areas usually stain black due to accumulation of oxidized debris).

Skeletal effects
- Hyperostosis of the proximal 1/3 of the metatarsals, hyperostosis of ribs, mandible, metacarpal, joint spurs, and bridges.
- Note: articular surfaces per se are not affected.
- Periosteal hyperostosis.
- Thickened bone cortex.
- Irregular or intermittent mineralization.
- Endosteal bone reabsorption.
- Abnormal size and shape of the Haversian system of compact bone due to dysfunctional bone remodeling.
- Abnormal development of osteoclasts and osteoblasts.

Public Health Considerations

In Queensland livestock fluorosis has often been accompanied by fluorosis in humans using the same artesian waters for drinking.

Fluoride accumulation in animals is generally not considered to be a risk to the human food supply since high-fluoride tissues are usually not eaten.

Prevention

Phosphate dietary supplements must be de-fluoridated and contain a P:F ratio of >100:1.

Livestock feeds must contain a P:F ratio of $>100{:}1$ and the fluoride level should not exceed 50 m/kg. Levels greater than 50 mg/kg are associated with growth retardation. Dietary calcium intake should be adequate.

Livestock drinking water should not exceed 2 mg/L. Cattle develop mottled teeth when given water with fluoride at $0.5{-}0.6$ mg/L, and teeth become eroded at $3.3{-}5$ mg/L. If the feed contains significant amounts of fluorides, the acceptable water level should be reduced to 1 mg/L.

The risk of fluorosis in either sheep or cattle may be reduced stock of ≤ 3 years of age is only provided with low-fluoride water (e.g., surface water and rainwater).

If only limited quantities of low-fluoride water are available, the damage from fluorosis will be minimal if young stock are supplied with high-fluoride water for no more than 3 months at a time and are then maintained for at least 3 months on low-fluoride water.

Lactating animals should be maintained on low-fluoride water over the lactation period because of the higher skeletal turnover and increased skeletal uptake of fluoride.

When bore-drains are used, it is critical that young stock are watered as close to the bore-head as possible because of concentration of fluoride in bore waters due to evaporation.

Water filtration is possible, but is typically expensive and impractical for livestock.

The addition of aluminum sulfate, aluminum chloride, calcium aluminate, and calcium carbonate to the diet reduces the absorption of dietary fluorides.

Supplemental feeding with low-fluoride feed will help to reduce the total fluoride intake.

Early detection of dental lesions in young animals combined with feed/water monitoring may allow for relocation of stock to safer areas.

HYDROGEN FLUORIDE, HYDROFLUORIC ACID, AMMONIUM FLUORIDE, AND AMMONIUM BIFLUORIDE

Alternative Names

HF

HF is a water-soluble gas that forms hydrofluoric acid when dissolved in water.

Circumstances of Poisoning

Hydrogen fluoride
- Spontaneously forms fumes at concentrations $>48\%$. The inhalation of fumes is highly dangerous.

- Used as a rust remover (2−12% concentration) and in various industrial processes.
- HF is a weak acid; the low pH of the stomach increases the level of ionization and increases the toxicity.

Ammonium fluoride and ammonium bifluoride
- Used as aluminum cleaners.
- Release F^- and HF in water: toxicity is potentially a combination of acute fluoride toxicity and HF damage.
- Ammonium bifluoride is potentially more toxic than ammonium fluoride.

Hydrofluoric acid solutions are domestically available as metal cleaners and wheel cleaners. It acts as a metal pickling agent and etchant by removing oxides and other impurities from stainless and carbon steels.

Hydrogen fluoride is generated upon combustion of viton and polytetrafluoroethylene (PTFE) (Teflon).

Hydrofluorocarbons in automatic fire suppression systems can release hydrogen fluoride at high temperatures.

Toxicokinetics

Absorption occurs through intact skin, mucous membranes, gastrointestinal, and respiratory tracts. Minor skin damage (e.g., washing with detergents) increases absorption.

Toxic Mode(s) of Action

Local effects
- Produce acid burns (coagulation necrosis) at the site of first contact.
- The onset of burns depends on the concentration of the solution; varies from immediate (high concentrations) to delayed up to 24 hours (dilute solutions). *Critically, domestically available hydrofluoric acid solutions are likely to cause delayed burns, i.e., burns that are not evident until 24 hours or so after exposure.*
- Because HF is a relatively weak acid, the depth of dermal penetration is often much greater than with the strong acids; result is severe dermal burns.
- Disrupts local membrane potentials in nerves → severe pain out of all proportion to the physical findings.
- Inhalation usually rapidly results in pulmonary edema that can be due to primarily chemical damage or cardiogenic due to systemic toxicity.
- Ocular exposure to dilute solutions usually results in severe, delayed corneal injury and other more severe damage to the globe.

- Ingestion of HF concentrations >20% usually result in immediate upper GI injury and emesis.

Systemic effects

- *Systemic toxicity should always be suspected until proven otherwise.*
- Systemic toxicity commonly occurs following skin exposures.
- Systemic toxicity almost always occurs following exposure of >10% body surface area to dilute solutions. However, systemic toxicity has been associated with exposures of <1% of the body surface area to concentrated solutions.
- Systemic toxicity generally always occurs after ingestion of dilute solutions or inhalation.
- *Be aware: GI and respiratory signs may be relatively mild and there may be a latency period of several hours before systemic toxicity occurs.*
- F^- forms calcium and magnesium complexes leading to hypocalcemia and hypomagnesemia; hyperkalemia also develops.
- Most deaths are due to cardiac effects of hypocalcemia.
- Cardiogenic pulmonary edema and hypoxia are common.

Clinical Signs

Be aware: there is almost always a latency for local effects of several hours to 24 hours following exposure except if concentrated fumes have been inhaled.

The initial skin, gastrointestinal, and respiratory effects may be comparatively mild.

Always suspect systemic toxicity until proven otherwise.

Regular monitoring of the ECG is highly advised irrespective of the current state of the patient.

Ingestion of concentrated materials usually results in immediate upper gastrointestinal injury and emesis.

Ingestion, eye contact, and skin contact resemble typical acid burns (see Chapter 16: Site of First Contact Effects of Acids and Alkalis). Delayed-onset burns are common. For a given pH level, HF burns are much more severe than other acids because eschar formation is typically less.

Pain at the sites of contact is often disproportionate to the apparent injury, particularly in the early stages of the toxidrome.

Dsypnea, tachypnea, cyanosis, and rales on auscultation may develop and are associated with cardiogenic edema.

Diagnostic Aids

The original product container is often the best source of diagnostic information.

Hydrofluoric acid is a weak acid. This reduces the value and usefulness of litmus papers and pH indicator papers as diagnostic aids.

The patient's ECG often reflects hypocalcemia, i.e., narrowing of the QRS complex, reduced PR interval, T wave flattening and inversion, prolongation of the QT-interval, prominent U-wave, prolonged ST and ST-depression.

Treatment

The use of personal protective equipment is paramount.

Remember: death can occur following ingestion of small volumes of dilute HF solutions with few premonitory signs.

Do not induce emesis.

Do not administer activated charcoal—it is ineffective following HF ingestions.

Do not use detergents or soap for dermal decontamination since these will potentially increase systemic absorption. Immediate vigorous flushing with copious volumes of water is recommended. Flushing should continue for at least 30 minutes. Hypothermia should be avoided during the procedure.

Exposed eyes should be flushed with water or saline for at least 30 minutes. Flushing using a Morgan lens may be helpful. Remember that delayed and/or on going eye injuries are common following HF exposure.

Diphoterine has been recommended for dermal decontamination. However, there is limited data regarding effectiveness and its safety properties have not been evaluated in companion animals.

Flushing the affected area with hexafluorine solutions has been recommended. However, this is rarely available in veterinary practice.

Cations that bind F^- reduce penetration, tissue injury, and pain. Typically topical 2.5% calcium gluconate gels (calcium gluconate dissolved in methylcellulose) are used. Nebulized 2.5% calcium gluconate solutions are recommended following inhalation exposures.

Intra-arterial infusion and regional perfusion with 5% calcium gluconate solutions may be of value.

Regular ECG monitoring is critical. HF effects of cardiac electrical function are unpredictable and often difficult to reverse. Early recognition and treatment of arrhythmias is essential.

Intravenous calcium gluconate should be administered as soon as possible taking care not to administer too quickly and avoiding overdosing. Ideally the ECG should be monitored during the procedure (mild hypercalcemia is characterized by broad-based tall peaking T waves; severe hypercalcemia is extremely wide QRS, low R wave, disappearance of p waves, and tall peaking T waves).

Prognosis

Guarded to poor.

Necropsy

Findings reflect acid burns (i.e., coagulation necrosis). Often eschar formation is minimal.

Public Health Considerations

Even dilute HF solutions are a significant hazard.

Significant amounts of HF gas can be released when PTFE (Teflon) coated cookware is burnt (see polymer fume toxicity).

Prevention

Correct storage and use is paramount.

ACUTE IODINE POISONING

The toxidrome occurs following exposure to concentrated solutions of iodine. Concentrated iodine solutions precipitate protein and behave as corrosives.

Ingestion of concentrated iodine solutions produces corrosive effects on the entire gastrointestinal tract and shock. Edema of the glottis and pulmonary edema have also resulted from oral ingestion. Gastrointestinal perforations are common. Stenoses and strictures are common outcomes in survivors.

In general, household iodine preparations are not concentrated enough to produce severe effects; however, their ingestion can cause severe vomiting if ingested.

Eye exposure may result in severe ocular burns.

Inhalation of iodine vapor may result in severe pulmonary irritation leading to pulmonary edema.

Dermal application of strong iodine solutions may result in burns.

CHRONIC IODINE POISONING

Alternative Names

Iodine toxicosis.
   Iodism.
   Iodinism.

Circumstances of Poisoning

Plant levels are directly related to soil levels and areas with high soil iodine levels will result in feeds that are high in iodine. This is generally not a problem in Australia and New Zealand since soils in these regions are more likely to be iodine deficient.

The use of seaweed and seaweed products results in high dietary iodine levels.

Iodine is usually added as part of the mineral mix in stock feeds and salt licks. Ethylene diamine dihydroiodide (EDDI) and calcium iodate are commonly used for this purpose.

Excessive EDDI interferes with vitamin A metabolism and may produce vitamin A deficiency.

High dietary calcium nitrate, thiocyanate (*Brassica* sp., i.e., rape, kale, cabbage), chronic low-level cyanogenic glycoside ingestion, glucosinolate, perchlorate, rubidium, and cobalt interfere with iodine metabolism and can increase iodine requirements.

Supplemental iron reduces iodine toxicity, but can increase iodine requirements.

Iodine and iodine salts are widely used disinfectants.

Toxicokinetics

Absorption
- Readily absorbed from GI tract.
- Readily oxidizes from iodine to iodide.
- Absorbed through abraded skin and through wounds: excessive use for wound irrigation can result in systemic toxicity.
- Well absorbed through the mucous membranes of the eye (iodine eye drops can cause systemic toxicity).

Distribution
- Freely distributed to the extracellular fluids and glandular secretions.
- Concentrates in thyroid (thyroglobulin), salivary glands, and tracheobronchial glands.

Excretion
- Excreted primarily in urine, but also excreted through salivary glands and thus recycled through the intestinal tract.
- Elimination half-life is $6 - 10$ hours, i.e., toxicity rapidly diminishes once the source of iodine is removed

Toxic Mode(s) of Action

High blood iodine levels result in disruption of thyroid function resulting in clinical hypothyroidism. Elevated blood iodine has the following effects:

- Decreases thyroid stimulating hormone (TSH) production with associated decreases in T_3 and T_4.
- Decreases follicular thyroid epithelial proliferation.
- Inhibits practically all thyroid functions.

Contact sensitization to povidone iodine can occur.

Clinical Signs

The predominant effect is hypothyroidism:

- Dry flaky skin, especially around head, neck, and back.
- ± Goiter (thyroid gland 2– 3 × normal size) if exposure is chronic.
- Excessive lachrymal, nasal, and respiratory secretions.
- Decreased appetite, reduced growth, developmental delay.
- Tachycardia.
- Hypotension.
- Abortion/infertility.
- Cardiomyopathy has been reported in cats.
- Decreased cellular and humoral immunity resulting in an increased frequency and severity of opportunistic infections. Bronchopneumonia is common.

Diagnostic Aids

- Affected animals have abnormally low serum TSH, T_3, and T_4.
- Iodine levels in feed, serum, milk, liver, muscle, thyroid gland, eggs, and hair can be determined. Outside of the thyroid and hair, iodine levels reflect recent consumption because of the short elimination half-life.

Treatment

Because of the short half-life, elimination of exposure is usually rapidly effective provided secondary complications (e.g., infections, bronchopneumonia) are controlled.

Prognosis

Depends upon age, pregnancy, and duration of exposure. Many of the clinical signs are reversible.

Necropsy

Gross findings
- Dry flaky skin.
- ± Goiter.
- Serous to mucopurrulent nasal discharge and congestion of upper respiratory tract and conjunctival mucosa.
- Variable degrees of bronchopneumonia.

Microscopic findings
- Squamous metaplasia of the tracheal mucosa.

- Necrosis of the tracheal mucosa and inflammatory infiltrates in the mucosa.
- Various degrees of bronchopneumonia.
- Thyroid gland: epithelium is flattened, excessive pale or granular colloid.

Public Health Considerations

Rarely of concern for humans.

Prevention

The most common cause is over supplementation. Iodine supplements should only be used in areas where the soils are known to be iodine deficient or in proven cases of iodine deficiency due to other causes (e.g., using of brassica feed sources, diets high in glucosinolates, low-level cyanogenic glycoside consumption).

WHITE (YELLOW) PHOSPHORUS POISONING

Alternative Names

Important chemical definitions.

- White (yellow) phosphorus is a tetrahedral P4 compound:

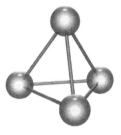

- Red phosphorus (the type used on matches) is a polymer of white phosphorus:

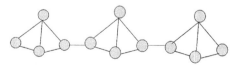

- Red phosphorus does not ignite in air at temperatures below 240°C. Red phosphorus can be converted to white phosphorus upon heating to 260°C, which is what happens when you strike a modern "safety" match.

- Black phosphorus and violet phosphorus are other thermodynamically stable phosphorus polymers. Red, violet, and black phosphorus are relatively nontoxic.
- White phosphorous is a strong oxidizer and spontaneously combusts on exposure to air. Usually stored in oil to prevent exposure to air and baits are typically oil based.
- White phosphorus has a distinctive odor of garlic when exposed to air and, when exposed to moisture, emits a greenish light and white fumes (literally glows in the dark).
- White phosphorus is still extensively used for smoke munitions, tracer munitions, and illumination munitions.
- Burning white phosphorus produces a hot, dense, white smoke consisting mostly of phosphorus pentoxide. Phosphorus pentoxide is an eye, mucous membrane, and respiratory irritant.
- Contact with white phosphorus produces extremely severe burns.

Circumstances of Poisoning

Historically white phosphorus exposure was a major occupational disease of humans, particularly in the white phosphorus match production industry. The disease consisted of progressive erosion of the teeth, mandible, and maxilla due to inhalation of white phosphorus fumes.

White phosphorus is still used as a rodenticide in some areas. Phosphorus rodenticides typically contain 2%−5% white (yellow) phosphorus in some form of oil-based preparation. White phosphorus rodenticides are still approved under some very limited and well-controlled circumstances because:

- They are considered environmentally friendly because the phosphorus readily oxidizes in the environment to materials that are relatively nontoxic.
- There is no genetic resistance to these products in rodents. White phosphorus is often the rodenticide of last resort when rodent populations with high levels of resistance to the vitamin K antagonist rodenticides are present.

Toxicokinetics

Absorbed through GI and respiratory tracts and through damaged epithelia.
Excreted in urine and expired air.

Toxic Mode(s) of Action

Described as a "general protoplasmic poison." Important effects include:

- Impairs ribosomal function and protein synthesis, inhibits blood glucose regulation, causes free radical injury.
- Impairs lipoprotein synthesis and triglyceride secretion lead to fatty degeneration in a variety of tissues.
- Directly impairs myocardial contractility and causes vasodilatation, hypotension, shock, and cardiovascular collapse.
- Hepatic injury develops in those that survive the initial cardiovascular events. This generally develops over several days but histopathological changes occur within hours of exposure. The predominant lesion is hepatic fatty infiltration followed by acute parenchymal inflammation and necrosis. The damage is typically periportal, but centrilobular or panlobular damage occurs in some patients.
- Renal toxicity is common. It is unknown if this is a primary effect or secondary to hemodynamic changes.
- Triggers hypocalcemia.
- Strong irritant and causes direct necrosis to the gastric mucosa when ingested.

Clinical Signs

Site of contact effects.
- Severe, deep, and painful chemical burns.
- Wounds typically have a distinct garlic odor and may emit a white smoke (phosphorus pentoxide).
- Wound healing is prolonged and often heavy scarring occurs.
- Systemic hypocalcemia and hyperphosphatemia may occur.
The oral ingestion toxidrome is typically biphasic. The early phase consists of:
- Violent vomiting and diarrhea followed by apparent recovery 24−48 hours later.
- This phase is often confused with acute viral gastroenteritis syndromes.
- Breath (and stomach contents) often has a distinct garlic smell.
- Animals may show signs of recovery before recrudescence of the late toxidrome.
The late phase of the oral ingestion toxidrome is dominated by signs of fulminant hepatic failure:
- Animal relapses into profound depression.
- Severe shock and icterus are prominent.
- Vomiting, hemorrhagic diarrhea often reappears.
- Death is most commonly due to fulminant hepatic failure.

The oral ingestion toxidrome is easily confused with death cap mushroom (Amanita phalloides) poisoning because of the similarities of the biphasic toxidromes (initial phase—GI syndrome; late phase—hepatic syndrome).

Diagnostic Aids

The product packaging is the single most valuable piece of diagnostic information.

Clinical pathology findings typically reflect severe hepatic injury, i.e., elevated AST, ALT, GGT, and total bilirubin. Disorders of clotting are commonly present, particularly in the late phase. Hypoglycemia is common. Evidence of fulminant renal failure (increased BUN and creatinine) may also be present.

Stomach contents and baits have a distinct garlic smell.

Stomach contents for analysis should be collected in airtight containers and analyzed as soon as possible.

An analysis of baits usually confirms the diagnosis.

Treatment

The use of personal protective equipment is critical.

White phosphorus burns
- Do not flush with water if large particles are present since this ignites white phosphorus.
- Manually remove large particles and then flush.
- Flushing with a silver nitrate solution has been suggested, but this is rarely available. There is little information that demonstrates that silver nitrate flushing is of significant clinical benefit.
- Serum calcium and phosphorus should be monitored and corrected using intravenous crystalloids and calcium gluconate if needed.

White phosphorus ingestion
- Do not induce emesis.
- A nonabsorbable oil (mineral oil) should be administered to solubilize the phosphorus and reduce absorption. Single dose activated charcoal may be of some benefit. However, gastric perforation is always a risk following white phosphorus ingestion. Administering mineral oil and/ or activated charcoal may increase the difficulties associated with managing a gastric perforation.
- Management is largely supportive.

Prognosis

Guarded. In general the outcome is mostly associated with the dose ingested. White phosphorus burns are generally very deep, severe, and take a long time to heal.

Necropsy

The use of personal protective equipment is critical.

Burns are usually very severe.

Hepatic injury develops in those that survive the initial cardiovascular events. This generally develops over several days but histopathological changes occur within hours of exposure. The predominant lesion is hepatic fatty infiltration followed by acute parenchymal inflammation and necrosis. The damage is typically periportal, but centrilobular or panlobular damage occurs in some patients.

Renal tubular injuries are common.

Public Health Considerations

White phosphorus is a public health menace. In modern times its availability and use is very strictly controlled.

Even very old rodenticide products can be hazardous.

In many countries, munitions continue to be an important source of white phosphorus exposure.

Prevention

White phosphorus rodenticides should only be used under very strictly controlled circumstances and by personnel trained and experienced in their use.

Phosphorus munitions should not be available to the general public.

ACUTE SELENIUM POISONING

Alternative Names

There are three toxicologically important chemical classes:

- Selenites (Se^{4+}). Selenites are extremely toxic and undergo reduction to elemental selenium. Damp heavy soils favor reduction of naturally occurring selenites.
- Selenates (Se^{6+}). Selenates are water soluble and toxic. Alkaline and oxidizing conditions promote the formation of selenates in soils.
- Arid, alkaline soils maintain selenium near the surface where it is available to plants; plants convert mineral Se to organoselenium compounds, particularly selenomethionine. This increases selenium bioavailability.

Circumstances of Poisoning

Many soils in Australia and New Zealand are selenium deficient. The selenium that is present is usually in an insoluble, nonbioavailable form. This reduces the amount of bioavailable selenium in plants. Se deficiency in Australia usually occurs on acidic soils with more than 500 mm rain per year, such as the Central and Southern Tablelands and Slopes and the Northern Tablelands of New South Wales, the south-eastern coast of Queensland, southwest Western Australia; coastal and central regions of Victoria, much of Tasmania, and South Australia's Mount Lofty Ranges and Kangaroo Island. Accordingly selenium supplementation and selenium fertilization have been extensively used in many areas of Australia.

Acute selenium poisoning has mostly been associated with selenium supplementation, particularly with injectable products. Other forms of selenium supplementation are more likely to cause subacute or chronic poisoning. However, cases of acute selenium poisoning associated with oral selenite supplements have occurred.

Very rarely, selenium solutions and products used in gun-smithing and ceramic production have been a cause of acute selenium poisoning. Acute selenium toxicosis after ingestion of selenium-containing shampoos or selenium supplement tablets can also occur, but is rare.

Selenium supplements are popular in alternative medicine.

Toxicokinetics

See chronic selenium poisoning (alkali disease).

Toxic Mode(s) of Action

Poorly described for acute poisoning.

Clinical Signs

Oral selenite supplements
- Horses: associated with depression and anorexia.
- Cattle: associated with respiratory distress, cyanosis, dyspnea, and evidence of pulmonary edema (rales on auscultation).
- Swine: colic and diarrhea.
- Animals may have a garlic-like breath smell.

Parenteral supplements
- Occurs in horses, cattle, swine, and sheep.
- Typically an acute neurological syndrome with trismus, mydriasis, and incoordination.
- Sudden deaths can occur.

Diagnostic Aids

The original product container is the best diagnostic aid.

Supplement selenium content and the administered dose are important. Toxicity has been associated with oral selenite supplements at the following dose rates:

- Horses: 3.3 mg/kg.
- Cattle: 10 mg/kg.
- Swine: 17 mg/kg.

Parenteral supplements are known to produce toxicity at doses of 0.2−0.4 mg/kg.

Blood selenium levels >2 ppm are generally associated with toxicity.

Liver selenium levels are usually >3−5 ppm selenium in acute cases.

Treatment

In advanced cases treatment is of limited value. Euthanasia should be considered.

N-Acetyl cysteine is claimed to be effective based on the rationale that glutathione depletion is toxicologically important. However, there is limited data on its effectiveness. Vitamin E is of unproven benefit, but is commonly administered.

Prognosis

Generally poor.

Necropsy

Common findings include:

- Vascular congestion.
- Gastroenteritis.
- Renal necrosis and hemorrhage.
- Hydrothorax.
- Pulmonary edema.
- Pale cardiac muscle.
- Stomach contents have a garlic-like odor.

Public Health Considerations

Acute selenium poisoning in humans is rare and has mostly been associated with gun-smithing products (metal bluing) and selenium dietary supplements.

Prevention

Most veterinary problems are associated with the overuse of selenium supplements, particularly injectable supplements. Overdosing with these products and errors in mixing of selenium-fortified foods should be avoided. Selenium supplementation is generally only of benefit to animals with dietary selenium intakes of ≤ 0.1 mg/kg.

There is a significant advantage of using selnomethionine fortified grains and feeds as dietary selenium supplements since selenium in this form is more bioavailable and less likely to produce acute toxicity. Selenium deficiency can also be addressed by selenium fertilization of deficient soils since the selenium is incorporated into plants and thus into the food chain.

SUBACUTE SELENIUM POISONING AND PORCINE FOCAL SYMMETRICAL POLIOMYELOMALACIA

Alternative Names

See chronic selenium poisoning (alkali disease).

Circumstances of Poisoning

Mostly associated with errors in selenium supplementation or feeding high selenium grains to pigs and poultry.

High selenium grains typically derive from growing areas with high selenium soils or excessive selenium fertilization.

Alkaline and oxidizing soil conditions favor the formation and accumulation of selenates in the biologically active areas of soil.

Wheat grown on high selenium soils is noted for its high selenium content. In Australia, high selenium soils are only reported from central Queensland and Cape York.

In Australia and New Zealand, the disease is most likely to be associated with over supplementation and ration formulation errors.

Pigs fed diets with diet $>20-50$ ppm for more than 3 days are at risk.

Toxicokinetics

See chronic selenium poisoning (alkali disease).

Toxic Mode(s) of Action

See chronic selenium poisoning (alkali disease).

The disease resembles nicotinamide/niacin deficiency.

However, supplementation with niacin only partially prevents the disease.

The toxidrome primarily affects the cervical and thoracic spinal cord, particularly the ventral horns.

Clinical Signs

Subacute selenium poisoning in pigs is primarily a neurological syndrome characterized by:

- Incoordination.
- Lameness.
- Anterior paresis and paralysis. Pigs will often walk on the dorsal surface of the manus and will often support themselves with their nose while walking due to the front limb paresis.
- The paresis progresses to full quadriplegia and permanent paralysis.
- Alopecia is common.
- Swelling and separation of the coronary hoof bands and impaired hoof growth is common (resembles hoof lesions in alkali disease).

Diagnostic Aids

Feeds containing >20 ppm of selenium are suspect.

Blood selenium levels >2 ppm are generally associated with toxicity.

Liver selenium is usually >1.5 ppm. Kidney is usually >1 ppm. Hair and hoof wall may have >1.5−5 ppm selenium if the animals survive long enough (*note*: in swine, hair color affects the selenium content. Appropriate control samples are required).

Treatment

The removal of the source of exposure is the most important aspect of treatment.

Dietary inorganic arsenicals (e.g., arsanilic acid) increase biliary excretion but carry with them their own set of risks.

Increasing dietary levels of sulfur-containing proteins (methionine and cysteine) is beneficial.

Vitamin E is of unproven benefit.

Prognosis

Guarded to poor. The spinal lesions are essentially permanent.

Necropsy

Focal symmetrical poliomyelomalacia of the cervical and thoracic spine with neuronal degeneration, necrosis and fragmentation and collapse of the spinal cord gray matter. Usually the ventral horns of the spinal cord are worst affected. Lesions are often most severe between vertebrae C5 and T2, the site of origin of the major nerves of the brachial plexus.

Public Health Considerations

Excessive selenium in grain used for human consumption can result in alkali disease.

Prevention

In Australia and New Zealand, the disease is most likely to be due to excessive selenium supplementation or ration formulation errors.

CHRONIC SELENIUM POISONING (ALKALI DISEASE)

Alternative Names

There are three toxicologically important chemical classes:

- Selenites (Se^{4+}). Selenites are extremely toxic and undergo reduction to elemental selenium. Damp heavy soils favor reduction of naturally occurring selenites.
- Selenates (Se^{6+}). Selenates are water soluble and toxic. Alkaline and oxidizing conditions promote the formation of selenates in soils.
- Arid, alkaline soils maintain selenium near the surface where it is available to plants; plants convert mineral Se to organoselenium compounds, particularly selenomethionine, methylselenocysteine, and selenocystathionine. This increases selenium bioavailability.

Circumstances of Poisoning

In the US, alkali disease is classically associated with the alkaline oxidizing soils of the Great Plains and consumption of obligate and facultative selenium accumulator plants.

In Australia, alkali disease has been reported from areas of the Northern Territory, northern central Queensland and Cape York. Australia has several species of obligate selenium accumulating plants in Australia: *Morinda reticulate* (mapoon; Cape York, Queensland), *Pogonolobus retuculatus* (Richmond area, Queensland), and *Neptunia amplexicaulis*. These plants require high soil selenium levels in order to grow and are thus good indicators of potentially dangerous seleniferous soils. Under Australian conditions, these plants are capable of accumulating around 4000 ppm of selenium on a dry matter basis.

Many other species of plants are facultative accumulators of selenium.

In Australia, horses are predominantly affected. However, cases of alkali disease have occurred in sheep, goats, and cattle.

Grazing animals typically avoid eating plants high in selenium because of their offensive odor and taste. The plants are more palatable because they loose their offensive odor when dried and thus large amounts of these plants incorporated into hay can be problematic.

Problems in Australia are mostly associated with drought-related grazing patterns. Chronic selenium toxicity in birds and fish has been observed in California and in Alberta. This has been associated with concentration of selenium rich soil run-off in lakes.

Selenium in the form of seleno-amino acids bioconcentrates in aquatic animals, and biomagnifies up aquatic food chains. Higher level predators (both aquatic and terrestrial) can receive toxic amounts of dietary selenium under such circumstances. Within aquatic ecosystems, sediments that are high in selenium can result in increased mortality and reproductive effects. Ecosystem-wide effects can occur very rapidly if selenium is released due to soil disturbances and mining.

Toxicokinetics

Absorption
- At high concentrations organoselenium compounds/seneo-amino acids and water-soluble selenium salts are readily absorbed.
- Speed of absorption: seleno-amino acids $>$ selenite and selenate $>$ selenides and elemental selenium.
- Selenite compounds are relatively poorly absorbed in ruminants, possibly due to reduction of selenite to insoluble, poorly absorbed, forms in the rumen.
- Primary site of absorption is the small intestine; no absorption occurs in the stomach or rumen.

Distribution
- Distributed bound to plasma proteins.

Metabolism
- Selenium is metabolized by both reduction and methylation. Glutathione is nonenzymatically oxidized as selenium is reduced and the end result is H_2Se.
- H_2Se is then either methylated for excretion or incorporated into selenoenzymes.
- Metabolism results in reactive oxygen species production and production of the selenide Se^{2-} anion.
- In marine environments, selenium forms a complex with mercury and protein, reducing the toxicity of mercury.

- A selenium—protein—cadmium complex can occur. This increases selenium tissue deposition but reduces the toxicity of both selenium and cadmium.

Deposition

- Because of its ability to replace sulfur in amino acids, Se has a high affinity for hair and epithelial structures (hooves, horns).

Excretion

- Urine is the major route of excretion in monogastric animals.
- Ruminants excrete significant amounts of Se in the feces.
- Very small amounts of Se are excreted in the bile; arsenic enhances biliary excretion.
- Methylated selenium is volatile and may be excreted by the lungs.

Toxic Mode(s) of Action

- Selenium is isostructural for sulfur in biological tissues. Thus selenium replaces S in amino acids and may affect the function of many essential proteins.
- Selenium compounds that react with thiols (i.e., glutathione) are more toxic than those that do not; glutathione depletion and lipid peroxidation are probably important mechanisms of toxicity.
- Metabolism of selenium is associated with reactive oxygen species production.
- Selenium is associated with depletion of tissue ascorbic acid that may contribute to its vascular toxicity.
- Selenium may interfere with nicotinamide and/or niacin function, particularly in pigs.
- Selenium is embryotoxic, fetotoxic, and teratogenic in birds and fish.

Clinical Signs

Affects sheep, cattle, goats, horses, and humans:

- Inactivity, anorexia, weight loss, general ill thrift, and cachexia.
- Affected animals are commonly anemic.
- Joint stiffness and lameness.
- Defects of the hair coat are often present: loss of hair of the tail/short tail hair (described as having a bob tail) and mane (roach mane), rough hair coat.
- Abnormal growth and structure of horns and hooves result in circular ridges and cracking of the hoof wall at the coronary band.
- Extremely long, deformed hooves that turn upward at the ends. Subsequent lameness is compounded by degeneration of joint cartilage and bone.

- Reduced fertility and reproductive performance occur, especially in sheep and cattle. Fertility effects may occur in the absence of overt alkali disease.
- Other lesions may include liver cirrhosis, ascites, and myocardial necrosis/scarring.
- Humans with alkali disease will commonly have damaged nails and hair.

Effects on birds

- Reduced hatchability.
- Teratogenic effects include underdeveloped feet and legs, malformed eyes, crooked beaks, and ropy feathers.

Effects on fish

- Reduced hatchability.
- Reduces smoulting success.
- Deformities present in fry and larvae.
- Increased mortality rates.

Diagnostic Aids

Clinical pathology

- Nonregenerative anemia.
- Evidence of liver disease with elevated ALT, GGT, and SDH.
- Clotting disorders, particularly decreased prothrombin activity.

  Hair and hoof selenium >5 ppm.

Treatment

Addition of copper to the diet and diets that are high in sulfur-containing amino acids may reduce the risk of alkali disease. However, these steps are rarely practical.

The addition of arsenic salts to the diet has been historically used on the basis that this will increase the biliary excretion of selenium. The technique has minimal benefit and introduces the risk of arsenic poisoning.

The removal of the source of exposure is the most effective method. If this is not possible, dietary high protein feed supplementation and/or rotation to safe pastures may reduce the risk.

Prognosis

Guarded to poor depending on the extent of disease.

Necropsy

Defects of the hair coat, particularly the mane and tail.

Hepatic cirrhosis.
Ascites.
Myocardial necrosis/scarring.

Public Health Considerations

Humans living in areas where alkali disease is common in livestock also tend to have chronic selenium poisoning.

Prevention

Given that in Australia, the problem is mostly associated with drought grazing patterns, the risk of alkali disease can be reduced by effective drought lotting and high protein feed supplementation.

Supplementation with sulfur is risky because of the potential to induce polioencephalomalacia.

Chapter 18

Industrial and Occupational Toxicants

INTRODUCTION

In human medicine, industrial and occupational toxicology is an extensive field that fills large reference books in its own right. Fortunately for veterinary toxicologists, most of this field is not relevant to veterinary medicine, which is one of the reasons that veterinary toxicology is a small field compared to human medical toxicology. The principal industrial/occupational toxicants to which domestic animals may be exposed are the petroleum hydrocarbons. In rare circumstances in which domestic animals are exposed to other industrial/occupational hazards, the available information is generally limited to human exposure and studies in laboratory rodents, and is accessible from human toxicology helplines or by online search. For these reasons, petroleum hydrocarbons are covered first in this chapter, followed by short notes on other selected industrial/occupational hazards. The subjects covered in this chapter are, therefore, in the following order:

- Petroleum hydrocarbons
- Short notes section:
  - Alcohols, ketones, esters, and ethers
  - Asbestos
  - Formaldehyde
  - Halogenated solvents

Agricultural toxicants are covered elsewhere in this book, and lead, which may be an industrial/occupational hazard, is covered in Chapter 14, Metals. Ethylene glycol is covered in the chapter covering household toxicants.

PETROLEUM HYDROCARBONS

Circumstances of Poisoning

Petroleum hydrocarbons are divided into crude (raw) oil and refined petroleum products.

Exposure to crude oil is generally limited to large domestic animals in the areas of oilfields and pipelines, and wildfowl exposed to oil slicks from marine accidents. Because Australia has only a small number of onshore oilfields and New Zealand has none, crude oil toxicosis of livestock is not the significant veterinary problem that it is in oil-producing states of North America.

Refined petroleum products are further divided into:

- Short-chain aliphatics with one to four carbons; i.e., methane, ethane, propane, butane.
- Long-chain aliphatics with five or more carbons. These include petrol (gasoline), kerosene, petroleum distillates, and a number of other petroleum-based solvents.
- Chlorinated aliphatic hydrocarbons. These include carbon tetrachloride, chloroform, trichloroethane, trichloroethylene, and tetrachloroethylene. These chemicals are commonly used as degreasing solvents and in drycleaning.
- Aromatic hydrocarbons containing one or more benzene rings. Examples are benzene, toluene, and xylene. These chemicals may be used in quick-drying paints and lacquers, and in glues. Benzene has become less readily available since it was recognized as a carcinogen.

Small domestic animals may be exposed to refined petroleum products used in the household, and in home workshops and vehicle repair. Some examples of petroleum hydrocarbon products or their synonyms commonly found in households or workshops are gasoline, diesel, kerosene, turpentine, naphtha, white spirits, Stoddard solvent, xylene, and toluene. Besides their uses as fuels, household or workshop petroleum hydrocarbon products may be used for cleaning, degreasing, paint removal, or as paint thinners. Petroleum hydrocarbons are often present in glues, lacquers, varnishes, and paints, and are detectable by odor to most people as the hydrocarbons evaporate from these products during use and drying. The use of volatile petroleum hydrocarbons, or products that release them, in confined spaces is a hazard to both the human users and any domestic animals in the confined space. Manufacturers' directions concerning use in well-ventilated areas should always be followed.

Absorption, Distribution, Metabolism, and Excretion

Petroleum hydrocarbons are highly lipophilic and unless they are of high viscosity (e.g., tar and motor oil), they are generally readily absorbed through skin and intact mucosae. Many of the refined hydrocarbons are highly volatile and are readily inhaled and absorbed through the lungs. Absorption from the gastrointestinal tract is negligible for paraffin wax and petroleum jelly, and low for refined products with high molecular weight (e.g., motor oil) but high for those with lower molecular weight (e.g., gasoline, hexane). Volatile petroleum hydrocarbons may also be partially excreted by the respiratory route, and may impart an identifying odor to the breath. Most aliphatic hydrocarbons that reach the systemic circulation undergo some hepatic metabolism, usually involving oxidation which makes the hydrocarbon more polar and therefore more readily excreted. Aromatic hydrocarbons are metabolized to phenol or to carboxylic acids, followed by conjugation. Passage through the gastrointestinal tract of petroleum hydrocarbon that is not absorbed tends to occur at a rate inverse to viscosity.

Mode(s) of Action

Pneumonia is the most common manifestation of petroleum hydrocarbon toxicosis in domestic animals. Petroleum hydrocarbons are irritant to the surfaces of the upper and lower respiratory tracts. They cause pulmonary pathology in their own right, damaging the lipid membranes of pneumocytes and altering surfactant. Viscous petroleum hydrocarbons can form a film over the larynx, facilitating the transfer of pathogens into the lower respiratory tract. The risk of aspiration pneumonia is further increased by the emetic nature of petroleum hydrocarbons. In ruminants, petroleum hydrocarbons may cause bloat and interfere with normal eructation, increasing the risk that the animal will eructate with an open glottis.

Petroleum hydrocarbons are directly irritant to skin and mucous membranes. Many act as defatting agents by dissolving the protective lipids of the skin.

At sufficient concentration, the short-chain aliphatics act as simple asphyxiants.

Volatile petroleum hydrocarbons, particularly the chlorinated aliphatic hydrocarbons, are associated with anesthetic effects. Chlorinated aliphatic hydrocarbons are also cardiotoxic, causing arrhythmias and myocardial degeneration.

Prolonged exposure to aromatic hydrocarbons in air may cause suppression of all hematopoietic cell lines in the bone marrow, leading to anemia, leukopenia, and thrombocytopenia.

Crude oil is a diverse mixture of toxicants, the ratio of which varies from oilfield to oilfield. Ruminants and horses poisoned by consumption of crude oil may also suffer from abortion and toxic effects on the liver and kidneys. Polioencephalomalacia has been reported in some crude oil poisoning cases in ruminants, and may reflect the presence of sulfur compounds or high salt content in water used in initial processing of crude oil. Ruminants may also suffer degeneration, necrosis, and sloughing of the ruminoreticular epithelium, and disrupted balance of ruminal microflora. In cases of crude oil toxicosis of livestock in the USA, ranchers are advised not to accept early offers of compensation from oil companies, but to wait for 9−12 months, because a number of animals that survive the initial risk period for aspiration pneumonia may succumb later to toxic effects on the liver and kidneys. The toxic mechanisms by which kidneys and liver are affected are not clear.

Clinical Signs

Crude oil: Bloat is a common early sign in ruminants and generally does not recur if relieved by intubation or trochar. Monogastrics are likely to vomit and ruminants may attempt to vomit. Nervous signs include ataxia, muscle tremors, confusion, central blindness, head-pressing, incoordination, and convulsions. Animals commonly develop a rapidly progressing pneumonia, and exhibit reluctance to move, low head carriage, rapid shallow respiration, and coughing. Pregnant animals may abort. There may be clinical pathology consistent with renal failure and liver damage. Animals are typically anorexic with consequent depression of blood glucose. Oil may be evident on the muzzle or in the feces. Dermal irritation may be present.

Short-chain aliphatics cause asphyxia.

Ingestion of *long-chain aliphatics* causes initial oral discomfort, salivating, head-shaking, or vomiting. These signs may be missed. The next likely clinical signs are those indicative of pneumonia. Dermal defatting and irritation may be evident. Gastroenteritis and diarrhea may develop. There may be evidence of central nervous system (CNS) depression, confusion, and narcosis, depending on the presence and proportion of volatile petroleum hydrocarbons.

As a general rule the less volatile and more viscous a refined petroleum hydrocarbon product is, the less toxic it is. Diesel fuel, home heating oil, and motor oil are relatively nontoxic, and toxicosis is likely to be limited to moderate gastroenteritis. Petroleum-derived waxes, such as paraffin wax, and petroleum jelly (Vaseline) are of very low toxicity. If a relatively viscous refined product is inhaled, it will cause less pulmonary damage than a less viscous product, because it will not spread as far. Also the more viscous products are much less likely to be absorbed through the skin or intact mucous membranes than the more fluid products.

Chlorinated aliphatic hydrocarbons are typically associated with anesthetic effects, arrythmias, and cardiotoxicity.

Aromatic hydrocarbons may cause bone marrow suppression with pancytopenia: pallor, exercise intolerance, and weakness due to anemia; increased susceptibility to infections due to leukopenia; and hemorrhagic diathesis due to thrombocytopenia. Prolonged exposure may cause central nervous damage, leading to clinical signs such as cerebellar ataxia, tremors, impaired vision, incoordination, and behavioral changes.

Diagnostic Aids

Anorexia often leads to decreased blood glucose. There may be an initial leukopenia, but this is often replaced with leucocytosis as pneumonia develops. There may be dehydration, hemoconcentration, increased serum BUN, and/or elevated liver enzymes.

Serial thoracic radiographs are useful to ascertain the extent and severity of pneumonia.

Pancytopenia may be present if toxicosis is due to aromatic hydrocarbon exposure.

Treatment

If dermal exposure occurs, act as soon as possible to prevent the animal from grooming itself, and prevent other animals from grooming the affected animal. Remove oil or liquid using warm water with a mild detergent. Hand dishwashing detergent is suitable. Ensure the mouth and nares are cleaned.

If ingestion has occurred, administration of nonabsorbed, nontoxic mineral oil may help to reduce gastrointestinal irritation and promote fecal excretion. Activated charcoal may adsorb petroleum hydrocarbons of low molecular weight such as hexane or toluene but is unlikely to be effective for viscous hydrocarbons, which will occlude the pores in activated charcoal. Gastrointestinal protectants may help to ameliorate gastrointestinal irritation.

Relieve bloat in ruminants, by intubation or by trochar and cannula. Bloat will generally not recur.

Monitor for pneumonia, and treat aggressively. The use of antibiotics has been debated, because there may be no bacterial involvement, but on the other hand bacterial infection is a common and serious complication, and there does not appear to be a compelling reason to withhold antibiotics. Corticosteroids are contraindicated. Respiratory support in the form of oxygen supplementation or even assisted ventilation may be required. However, positive pressure ventilation should be used with great caution because pneumomediastinum and pneumothorax have been frequently found on radiograph or during necropsy.

It should be borne in mind that volatile petroleum hydrocarbons are often excreted, at least in part, via the lungs and therefore if a closed system is used to provide respiratory support, it should be purged frequently to allow this excretion. Outflow from this purging, and from open systems, should be appropriately scavenged for the safety of attending personnel.

Monitor for CNS signs and treat as appropriate.

Monitor for evidence of toxic effects on kidneys and liver, which may be delayed, provide supportive care as appropriate.

Blood transfusion may be indicated in pancytopenia due to aromatic hydrocarbon exposure.

Otherwise, treatment is supportive and symptomatic. Ruminants that survive toxicosis may benefit from ruminal inoculation with ruminal fluid from healthy ruminants.

Small domestic animals that are asymptomatic 24 hours after exposure to petroleum hydrocarbons are unlikely to develop toxicosis and may be discharged, provided any contamination of the fur or feathers has been removed.

Prognosis

Prognosis for crude oil ingestion is guarded at best. Even if the animal survives the initial risk phase for aspiration pneumonia, it may subsequently succumb to renal failure or to liver failure, particularly if it is later put under the pressures of late pregnancy, parturition, and early lactation. Farmers near oilfields, pipelines, and refineries, or with livestock that have access to shorelines affected by oil slicks, are therefore well-advised to learn from North American ranchers: if compensation is offered after a spill, agree in principle to compensation but delay settling on the final compensation amount for as long as possible, because the final mortality figure may not be evident for months. The few comprehensive follow-up studies of "de-oiled" wildfowl tend to indicate that the mortality rate in the 12−15 months following release is very high, and of those that do survive, few regain sufficient health to return to breeding. This has led to debate among environmental professionals internationally about whether de-oiling and release of wildfowl caught in oil slicks is humane and/or cost-effective, notwithstanding the favorable impression the practice gives to the general public.

Follow-up studies of human beings who recovered from hydrocarbon pneumonitis or pneumonia indicate that subclinical pulmonary impairment may persist for years. This impairment may include increased susceptibility to pulmonary infections, and/or impairment of pulmonary function. This finding may be particularly relevant to athletic animals such as horses or working dogs.

Prognosis following exposure to short-chain aliphatics is generally favorable if asphyxia is not immediately fatal.

Prognosis following ingestion of long-chain aliphatics, chlorinated petroleum hydrocarbons and aromatic hydrocarbons is moderate to guarded, depending on severity of toxicosis. It should be borne in mind that benzene is carcinogenic.

Necropsy

Necropsy findings may include

- dermal, ocular, nasal, and/or oral irritation
- gastrointestinal irritation
- inflammation and sloughing of ruminoreticular epithelium
- pulmonary congestion, consolidation, abscessation. There may also be emphysema, areas of collapse, pneumomediastinum, pneumothorax, and/or pneumocoeles, and sometimes pleurisy and/or hydrothorax
- pale swollen kidneys with renal tubular necrosis
- pale or congested liver with hepatocellular hydropic degeneration and necrosis

- polioencephalomalacia with cerebral swelling, which may lead to cerebellar coning and herniation through the foramen magnum
- myocardial degeneration
- splenic congestion, but decrease in cellularity of white pulp
- in prolonged exposure to aromatic hydrocarbons, suppression of all hematopoietic cell lines in the bone marrow

The smell of volatile petroleum hydrocarbons is often evident on opening of gastrointestinal and/or respiratory tracts during the course of necropsy, and if the petroleum hydrocarbons have been ingested, agitation of gastrointestinal contents in warm water will often lead to an oily sheen developing on the surface of the water.

SHORT NOTES SECTION

Alcohols, Ketones, Esters, and Ethers

Alcohols are generally irritant to eyes, skin, and mucous membranes including the upper respiratory tract. Uses of alcohols include solvents, deicers, antifreeze, and hydraulic fluids. As a generalization, alcohols are readily absorbed and distributed widely in the body. Excretion may occur via urine or in exhaled breath. Systemic signs of toxicosis are variable but may include respiratory depression, and/or central nervous depression, and/or hypotension. The severe acidosis and central blindness associated with methanol poisoning in human beings is due to primate-specific metabolism and is not observed in nonprimate species.

Acetone is a ketone (dimethyl ketone). Other commonly encountered ketones include methyl *n*-butyl ketone, methyl ethyl ketone, methyl isobutyl ketone, isophorone, and cyclohexanone. They are typically highly volatile and are flammable. They may be encountered as solvents, degreasers, and in association with paints and lacquers. They are generally readily absorbed by inhalation and readily cause CNS depression. Other clinical signs of toxicosis may include irritation of eyes and respiratory tract.

Commonly used esters have names ending with *acetate, formate*, or *acrylate*. They are typically clear, flammable liquids and many have a pleasant odor. They are commonly used as solvents, and may be encountered in association with lacquers, plastics, paints, and resins. Some are used in perfumes. As a generalization, they are irritating to eyes, mucous membranes, and throat. They may also be irritating to the lower respiratory tract and several are known to cause CNS depression.

Ethers include ethyl ether, methyl ether, isopropyl ether, dichloroisopropyl ether, and vinyl ether. Some of these are former anesthetic agents. They are typically highly flammable or explosive. They may be encountered as solvents, for example, in resins. They cause CNS depression and some are also associated with renal and or hepatic toxicity.

The glycol ethers are commonly found as solvents in household products. They include 2-methoxyethanol, 2-ethoxyethanol, 2-methoxyethyl acetate, and 2-ethoxyethyl acetate. Clinical signs of toxicosis include CNS effects (agitation, encephalopathy, coma); hematotoxic effects including hemolysis and bone marrow suppression; metabolic acidosis; and renal tubular degeneration. Features of human poisoning have included confusion, coma, acute hemorrhagic gastritis, liver and kidney damage, cyanosis, and metabolic acidosis.

Asbestos

Asbestos is a collective term for a group of natural mineral fibers formed from hydrated magnesium silicates. Asbestos has been widely used in building in the past, before the adverse properties of asbestos were recognized, and may be found during demolition of older buildings. Asbestos fibers are subdivided into the serpentine group and the amphibole group. The only member of the serpentine group is chrysotile asbestos, also known as white asbestos. The five amphibole fibers are crocidolite (blue asbestos), amosite (brown asbestos), tremolite, actinolite, and anthophyllite. Asbestos fibers may incorporate or be contaminated by metals such as chromium, cobalt, iron, manganese, or nickel. Asbestos has properties such as heat resistance, resistance to chemicals, strength and durability that have led to very wide industrial use including manufacture of cement items and home building materials, as insulation and for fireproofing, and in building and maintenance of ships, locomotives, power plants, engine rooms, chemical plants, and brakes of motor vehicles. Chrysotile asbestos is the most important asbestos commercially, although crocidolite and amosite also have commercial applications. Asbestos is only considered to lead to adverse health effects if inhaled. The most hazardous asbestos fibers are those $<10\,\mu m$ long, because these are the most likely to reach the alveoli and persist in the lungs, while larger fibers are more likely to be removed via the mucociliary apparatus. Occasionally a long fiber may persist in the lungs if it drapes over the branching of airways. Crysotile asbestos appears to be less likely to cause adverse effects than amphibole asbestos, which may be because it is more readily degraded by pulmonary macrophages, whereas amphibole fibers are more persistent. Crocidolite asbestos is considered to be the most hazardous type of asbestos. Asbestos fibers cause an inflammatory reaction in the lungs, which may lead to asbestosis (interstitial pulmonary fibrosis), bronchogenic carcinoma, malignant mesothelioma of the pleura, or pleural effusion. Pericardial effusion and mesothelioma of the peritoneum have also been reported. Cases of mesothelioma in domestic pets have been attributed to asbestos exposure, and in some but not all cases, asbestos fibers have been found in lungs of affected dogs. Early changes in lungs of dogs chronically exposed to asbestos inhalation are very similar to those observed in human beings.

Formaldehyde

Formaldehyde is very widely used in industry. Release of formaldehyde from building materials such as particle board has been a source of concern. The acute local effects of formaldehyde such as ocular irritation, dermatitis, throat irritation, and headache are well-known. Chronic inhalation of formaldehyde by laboratory rats and mice has led to squamous cell carcinomas in the nasal cavity. Being highly reactive, formaldehyde acts at the point of contact, which in inhalation studies in rats and mice is the nasal cavity. The mechanism of carcinogenesis is considered to be chronic irritation and rapid cellular replication associated with repair. The No Observed Effect Level for carcinogenesis in rats is 2 ppm. The relevance of this carcinogenic effect to other species, particularly humans, is uncertain because of differences in the structure and function of the upper respiratory tract. Epidemiological studies in human beings chronically exposed to formaldehyde tend to indicate that human beings are not similarly susceptible to squamous cell carcinoma of the nasal cavity. The studies have also failed to demonstrate an increased risk of any other cancers. The relevance of the rodent studies to domestic animals is unknown.

Halogenated Solvents

Although the chlorinated petroleum hydrocarbons (q.v.) are halogenated solvents, they are not the only halogenated solvents. Many of these chemicals were originally developed and investigated as anesthetic agents. As a generalization they are clear, colorless liquids with a sweet odor, and they are widely used for degreasing and defatting. They are highly volatile but not flammable. The most common halogen present is chlorine, followed by fluorine. Toxicosis due to these solvents most commonly occurs by inhalation. Systemic absorption is variable depending on blood:air absorption coefficient. Once absorbed they are readily absorbed. Extent of metabolism, which largely occurs in the liver, varies between chemicals. They are excreted via the lungs and in the urine. Toxic effects include CNS depression, hepatic degeneration and necrosis, degeneration and necrosis of renal tubular epithelium, vasodilation, hypotension, and cardiac sensitization, which may lead to ventricular fibrillation. Pulmonary irritation is generally mild. CNS effects include ataxia, lethargy, incoordination, and coma. Acute toxicosis may require cardiopulmonary support, with the proviso that elimination via the respiratory route should also be supported. Hyperventilation has been used in human cases to accelerate elimination.

Chapter 19

Agricultural and Feed-Related Toxicants

INTRODUCTION

Feed in this context refers to food prepared for livestock and horses, not for domestic pets or human beings. Foods that are hazardous to domestic pets are covered in Chapter 13, Household Foods and Products. This chapter also covers issues related to water quality, and fertilizers as a source of poisoning.

This chapter does not cover overdose of element supplements. Many elements, such as iron, copper, zinc, and iodine, are essential elements but also toxic in excess. Toxicoses due to overdose of these elements are covered elsewhere in this book. Mycotoxicosis due to field or storage fungi is also covered elsewhere in this book.

New products are periodically introduced to the livestock feed market, and sometimes products are withdrawn for use in feed. It should not be assumed that this chapter provides exhaustive coverage, or that the antibiotics described here are still on the market. Chemicals used in feed must be approved in Australia by the Australian Pesticides and Veterinary Medicines Authority (APVMA), which has a searchable database on its website. In New Zealand the equivalent database is the ACVM register, which is also searchable online.

AMMONIATED FEED SYNDROME

Synonyms

"Bovine bonkers"; 4-methylimidazole poisoning.

Circumstances of Poisoning

Toxicosis is attributed to imidazoles, of which 4-methylimidazole is the best studied and appears to be the most neurotoxic. Toxicosis may occur when cattle are fed roughages that have been treated with anhydrous ammonia. Toxicosis is most likely to occur when the roughage has a high carbohydrate content and the plant material reaches a temperature of 70°C or above during

Veterinary Toxicology for Australia and New Zealand
DOI: http://dx.doi.org/10.1016/B978-0-12-420227-6.00018-9

ammoniation. Imidazoles form as a result of reaction between ammonia and reducing sugars, which is catalyzed by heat. Crops harvested when immature are the most hazardous. Toxicosis has been associated with wheat hay, Bermuda grass (*Cynodon dactylon*), sorghum, and fescue.

Toxicokinetics

There is a lack of information on the toxicokinetics of the imidazoles responsible for this toxicosis.

Relay toxicosis from affected dams to suckling calves may occur. In some cases, only suckling calves have been affected, suggesting that the toxic threshold is lower in calves.

Mode(s) of Action

There is a lack of information on the neurotoxic mechanism.

Clinical Signs

Clinical signs develop within 24–36 hours of consuming the affected feed. Cattle develop a hyperexcitability syndrome with trembling, ear-twitching, stampeding or galloping in circles, champing, hypersalivation, and convulsions. Convulsive episodes typically last approximately 30 seconds and may recur at 5–10 minutes intervals. On examination the cattle typically have dilated pupils, and clinically they appear to have impaired vision.

Diagnostic Aids

Blood urea and ammonia levels are normal.

The analytical sample of choice is the suspect feed.

Treatment

Treatment is symptomatic, with administration of barbiturates or acetylpromazine to control clinical signs. Cattle should be kept in a safe paddock if possible, although it may be impossible to safely move affected cattle.

Prognosis

Recovery is rapid once cattle are denied access to the affected feed. Deaths may occur as result of trauma incurred while affected.

Cattle do not develop tolerance to 4-methylimidazole.

Necropsy

There are no characteristic lesions. There may be evidence of trauma.

Prevention

To prevent this toxicosis, it is best to ammoniate only poor-quality roughage, avoid the use of excessive ammonia, and ammoniate during cooler seasons. Affected feed does not tend to lose toxicity while in storage, and should be discarded.

ANTIBIOTICS AND COCCIDIOSTATS OTHER THAN IONOPHORES

A number of antibiotics and coccidiostats are approved for use in feed, principally for pigs and/or poultry. These may be toxic if fed in excess to the target species, or if fed to nontarget species. The pharmacological indications and kinetics of these antibiotics will not be covered here. Table 19.1 provides brief notes on some antibiotics and coccidiostats, other than ionophores, used in livestock feed, and associated risks. Ionophores are discussed separately in the next section.

BOTULISM

Circumstances of Poisoning

Botulism of livestock appears to be rare in Australia and New Zealand, but cases in human beings, and periodic outbreaks in wildfowl, show that at least some type or types of *Clostridium botulinum* are present in both countries.

The most likely circumstances of poisoning in Australia or New Zealand are ingestions of preformed botulinum toxin by horses, cattle, or wildfowl. Adult horses and cattle may ingest preformed toxin if they are fed improperly ensiled silage, "haylage" or "bailage." Other less common sources are decaying grass, hay, or grain.

Another possible source of botulism to herbivores is contamination of hay or other feed with the dead bodies of vermin. Botulism in sheep has been recorded in Australia, in circumstances under which the sheep were protein-deficient and sought out and consumed the carcasses of rabbits and other small herbivores.

In contrast to adult horses, foals are susceptible to botulism from proliferation of *C. botulinum* in the intestinal tract; that is, rather than consuming preformed toxin, they are poisoned by toxin synthesized in their gastrointestinal tract after they consume Clostridial spores.

Wildfowl are most often affected as a result of eating rotten vegetation.

C. botulinum is a sporulating anerobic bacterium.

Toxicokinetics

Botulinum toxins are readily absorbed orally. Botulinum toxin A is the most toxic substance known. There have been documented cases of deaths occurring up to 17 days after consumption of contaminated feedstuffs.

TABLE 19.1 Risks Associated With Some Antibiotics and Coccidiostats Used in Livestock Feed

Active Ingredient	Notes on Toxicity
Apramycin	Unsafe for cats; may cause nephrotoxicity and ototoxicity
Lasalocid	See Section "Ionophores"
Lincomycin	Horses, guinea pigs, and rabbits are extremely sensitive to lincomycin and may develop severe *Clostridium difficile* diarrhea. Mortality rate from necrotizing colitis and shock is very high in horses
Maduramycin	See Section "Ionophores"
Monensin	See Section "Ionophores"
Nicarbazin	SeeSection "Ionophores"
Robenidine	Extremely toxic to aquatic organisms
Salinomycin	See Section "Ionophores"
Sulfa drugs	May cause hyperplastic goiter. May cause agranulocytosis and hypoprothrombinemia in poultry or dogs. May cause peripheral neuritis in poultry. May cause renal tubule obstruction if water supply is insufficient. Sulfaquinoxaline may cause a vitamin K-responsive coagulopathy in poultry and dogs
Tiamulin	Low toxicity by itself, but potentiates the toxicity of ionophores (q.v.) because it interferes with their metabolism and elimination
Tilmicosin	Hazardous to human beings may cause toxicity similar to lincomycin (q.v.) in horses. Used in pigs but may be cardiotoxic if overdosed
Trimethoprim	Interferes with folic acid metabolism; women in the first trimester of pregnancy should observe caution if handling this regularly
Tylosin	May cause toxicity similar to lincomycin (q.v.) in horses. May cause dermal hypersensitivity in human beings

Mode(s) of Action

Botulinum toxin cleaves neuronal proteins associated with neurotransmission of acetylcholine. The resulting toxicosis is one of progressive flaccid paralysis.

Clinical Signs

Clinical signs in adult horses include weakness, ataxia, difficulties with prehension and swallowing, recumbency, and loss of muscle tone of the tail, tongue, and jaw.

"Shaker foal syndrome" typically affects foals aged 4 weeks or less. Foals may be found dead or may develop progressive motor paralysis with stilted gait, tremors, and inability to stand for more than a few minutes. They typically also exhibit dysphagia, constipation, mydriasis, and frequent urination. Later signs are dyspnea, tachycardia, and respiratory arrest.

Clinical signs in cattle include salivation, dysphagia, and recumbency progressing from sterna to lateral. There is loss of muscle tone to the tongue, and the bladder may be full because the animal is unable to urinate.

Dermal sensitivity is unimpaired, but withdrawal reflexes of the legs are weak.

Diagnostic Aids

Samples for diagnostic testing are serum, gastrointestinal contents, and the suspect feed.

Treatment

The suspect feed should be removed immediately. Valuable animals may respond to intravenous botulinum antitoxin if it is available and treatment is instituted early in the course of the disease.

Prognosis

The prognosis is poor to hopeless, particularly if the animal becomes recumbent.

Necropsy

There are no characteristic findings in botulism of adult horses and cattle.

Foals that die of "shaker foal syndrome" may have pulmonary edema, and excessive fluid in the pericardial sac.

Prevention

Toxoids against *C. botulinum* types C and D have been used in Australia.

Appropriate care and assessment of feedstuffs is essential.

The growing popularity of haylage/bailage as feed for horses may increase the incidence of botulism cases in horses, because laypeople often lack the expertise to recognize when ensiled feed has undergone bacterial spoilage. There is a common misperception that it is normal for ensiled feed to smell unpleasant. On the contrary, feed that has been ensiled well has a pleasant sweet odor, reminiscent of breakfast cereal or even fruitcake. Ensiled feed that has an unpleasant odor like old grass-clippings or compost has been ensiled when too wet, and has undergone bacterial spoilage, but cattle and horses will accept this feed. Bacterial spoilage of this feed may include spoilage by *C. botulinum*. While *C. botulinum* is anerobic, it should be recognized that because the toxin is so potent, a lethal dose may be present even when only a very small part of the feed may be spoiled by *C. botulinum*. Therefore it is incorrect to suppose that feed is only hazardous if the silage is "slimy," although at least one New Zealand website asserts this.

Ensiled feed that has a burnt or tobacco-like odor has been ensiled when too dry and while it has a poorer feed value than well-ensiled feed, it is unlikely to pose a risk of botulism, because the toxin is heat-labile.

IONOPHORES

Circumstances of Poisoning

Ionophores are antibiotics that may be added to feed as coccidiostats or as bovine growth promotants that work by increasing propionic acid production in the rumen and thereby enhancing ruminal feed efficiency. Poisoning may occur if horses consume feed meant for poultry or cattle, or if cattle are overdosed with ionophores.

Ionophores available in Australia and/or New Zealand include monensin, lasalocid, salinomycin, nicarbazin, and maduramycin.

Toxicokinetics

Absorption of ionophores from feed is low, with most of the compound excreted unchanged in the feces. Ionophores that are absorbed are widely distributed in the body, and converted to multiple polar metabolites in the liver. Competition for metabolic pathways means that other compounds, such as tiamulin, can potentiate ionophore toxicity.

Field experience indicates that multiple sublethal exposures may be ultimately more lethal than a single acute exposure.

Mode(s) of Action

Ionophores selectively transport sodium and potassium ions between extracellular and intracellular spaces. The net results are imbalance of sodium, potassium, calcium, and hydrogen.

By interacting with the carrier mechanism that transports potassium across mitochondrial membranes, ionophores inhibit ATP hydrolysis, and decrease cellular energy production. Ionophores also cause the accumulation of calcium in mitochondria and in cytosol. Although the precise effects differ between ionophores, the key toxic event is damage to mitochondria.

Data on toxic doses in some species are presented in Table 19.2.

TABLE 19.2 Risks Associated With Some Ionophores Used in Livestock Feed

Ionophore	Species	LD$_{50}$ (mg/kg)	Field Observations
Monensin	Horse	2−3	
	Cattle	26.4	Lethality at 7.6 mg/kg/day reported
	Goat	26.4	
	Sheep	11.9	
	Pig	17−50	
	Dog	>10	Toxic at 6−7 mg/kg/day
Lasalocid	Horse	21.5	
	Cattle		Lethality at 17−28 mg/kg reported
	Pig		Toxic at 35 mg/kg. Lethal at 58 mg/kg
Salinomycin	Horse		Lethal at 190−500 mg/kg in feed
	Pig		Lethal at 166−720 mg/kg in feed
Maduramycin	Horse		Toxic at 55 mg/kg in feed
	Cattle		Toxic at 2.5−6.1 mg/kg in poultry litter
	Sheep		Toxic at 2.5−6.1 mg/kg in poultry litter
	Dog		Toxic at 12 mg/kg in feed

Clinical Signs

Onset in horses is commonly less than 24 hours, but it can be delayed for several days. Horses initially develop anorexia, diaphoresis (sweating), and polyuria. They may be febrile. By 12−36 hours after consumption, they become ataxic, and develop colic, stiffness ("tying up"), and oliguria. There is progressive posterior paresis and intermittent recumbency. Terminal signs are tachycardia, hypotension, hyperventilation, and dyspnea.

Horses that survive the acute poisoning episode may suffer ill-thrift, exercise intolerance, and arrhythmia, and may die suddenly.

Cattle develop anorexia, depression, weakness, ataxia, dyspnea, and diarrhea. Cattle may appear to recover but later collapse and die during exertion. Cattle may develop subacute toxicosis in the form of congestive heart failure.

Clinical signs in sheep are similar to those in cattle. Sheep may adopt a hunched stance, and may knuckle over when attempting to move. Sheep may take at least 3 months to recover from ionophore toxicosis.

Pigs exhibit clinical signs similar to those in sheep in cattle, and myoglobinuria has also been reported.

Dogs and cats should not be allowed to eat poultry feed or cattle feed that contains ionophores. Clinical signs reported in these species include depression, weakness, ataxia, paresis/paralysis, dyspnea, and death. These species may take months to recover from nonfatal toxicosis.

Clinical signs in poultry vary somewhat with ionophore and with species of bird, but include anorexia, depression, diarrhea, drooped head and/or wings, weight loss, dyspnea, recumbency, and death. Laying birds will show a decline in egg production, and hatchability of eggs is decreased. Chicks in the egg may fail to develop, be deformed, or be weak and unable to hatch.

Diagnostic Aids

Clinical pathology findings include:

- Increased alkaline phosphatase (bone-associated isoenzyme)
- Increased unconjugated bilirubin
- Early elevation of BUN and creatinine; may return to normal
- Moderate reduction of serum calcium for first 12−18 hours
- Marked increase in serum creatine kinase
- Elevated hematocrit
- Increased lactate dehydrogenase in first 36 hours
- Decreased serum potassium
- Increased serum AST

A range of electrocardiographic changes have been described in poisoned animals. ECG changes can vary considerably within a species, and the absence of ECG changes does not preclude myocardial damage.

Feed may be analyzed to confirm exposure. Tissue analysis is difficult and not widely available.

Treatment

Decontamination with activated charcoal may be useful if consumption is recent. Rumenotomy may be indicated in valuable livestock.

Fluids and electrolytes may be beneficial.

Prognosis

The prognosis is guarded to poor, and surviving animals are always at risk of long-term effects of cardiac damage.

Necropsy

There may be no gross lesions in acute poisoning.

Gross lesions in horses and cattle are mild hemopericardium, epicardial hemorrhages, myocardial pallor, hydrothorax, ascites, pulmonary edema, pallor of skeletal muscles. Horses may also have hepatomegaly and increased lobular pattern on the liver. Sheep may have congestion or hemorrhage of the gastrointestinal mucosa.

Histological lesions include vacuolation and degeneration of cardiac muscle fibers, and multifocal myocardial necrosis. Toxic changes may also be present in the renal tubules, the liver and skeletal muscles. In swine the damage to skeletal muscles may be more prominent than the damage to cardiac muscle.

Prevention

Feeds should be carefully managed and fed only to the species for which they were prepared. If ionophores are added as a premix, the amount should be carefully measured and thoroughly mixed.

GOSSYPOL

Circumstances of Poisoning

Gossypol is a polyphenolic compound synthesized by the cotton plant. Cotton is a significant crop in Australia, but not in New Zealand. Whole cottonseeds or cottonseed hulls remaining after extraction of cottonseed oil, may be used for stock feed.

Toxicokinetics

There is limited information on the toxicokinetics of gossypol. Ruminants are more resistant to gossypol toxicity than monogastric species, because gossypol is bound to proteins in the rumen, making it unavailable for absorption. Free gossypol is lipid-soluble and readily absorbed from the intestine. Absorbed gossypol appears to have a long half-life in the body and has been found in plasma, heart, liver, kidney, muscle, and testes, but is not excreted in milk. Gossypol is principally excreted in the feces with limited excretion of metabolites in the urine.

Mode(s) of Action

The mechanism(s) of gossypol toxicity are unclear. It is known to have cardiotoxic and hemolytic effects. Gossypol also interferes with fertility and reproduction in both sexes.

Gossypol causes gradual, progressive destruction of the myocardium, leading to congestive heart failure, and also interferes with K^+ movement across cell membranes. Gossypol was investigated as a male contraceptive in

China, and it was found that men developed hypokalemia that was not corrected by potassium supplements. Sudden deaths in gossypol poisoning may be due to hypokalemia.

The liver is damaged as a secondary consequence of congestive heart failure, and may also have impaired metabolic capability due to inhibition of glutathione-S-transferase.

Gossypol binds some amino acids, particularly lysine and methionine, leading to protein malnutrition and poor growth rate.

In male ruminants, gossypol damages the spermatogenic epithelium, inhibits enzymes in Leydig cells that are required for steroid synthesis.

Gossypol appears to have a luteolytic action in pregnancy.

Clinical Signs

Cardiotoxicity may be characterized by sudden death, or by progressive ill-thrift with dyspnea. Adult cattle may also exhibit heat intolerance, hemoglobinuria, abomasitis, and anorexia.

Decreased conception rates, increased incidence of abortions, and decreased litter sizes have been reported in sows.

Decreases in sperm count and sperm motility have been observed in cattle.

Diagnostic Aids

Gossypol may be detected in suspect feed. However in sublethal toxicosis that is not recognized for some time after the damage is done, the feed that caused the toxicosis may no longer be available.

Clinical pathology findings include elevated liver enzymes, mild anemia, erythrocyte fragility, and elevated cholecystokinin.

Treatment

There is no antidote or treatment. The affected feed should be withdrawn immediately.

Prognosis

Prognosis is guarded.

A horse that has suffered from gossypol toxicity should always be regarded as exercise-intolerant and at risk of collapsing if ridden. Recovered mares may die during parturition.

Necropsy

There may be no lesions in animals that die acutely.

In animals that survive longer, findings are those of chronic failure of both sides of the heart, with consequent lesions of lungs and liver. There may also be renal and splenic congestion, pale skeletal muscles, abomasitis, and enteritis. Testes of intact male animals will show degeneration and necrosis of the spermatogenic epithelium.

Prevention

Calves and lambs of less than 16 weeks (preruminants) should not be fed gossypol at all, and ruminants less than 6 months of age should not be fed more than 100 ppm gossypol. Adult ruminants can tolerate up to 1000 ppm gossypol. Swine should be fed less than 100 ppm, and poultry should be fed less than 200 ppm gossypol.

NONPROTEIN NITROGEN (NPN)

Synonyms

Urea poisoning, ammonia poisoning.

Circumstances of Poisoning

Sources of nonprotein nitrogen (NPN) include urea, a variety of ammonium salts, and ammoniated forages. Livestock may also be poisoned by consuming urea or other fertilizers containing ammonium or urea.

Toxicokinetics

Hydrolysis of NPN in the rumen leads to production of ammonia, NH_3. While ruminal microflora can combine ammonia with keto acids from carbohydrates to form amino acids, the microflora require weeks to adapt to increased NPN intake and lose that adaptation within a few days. Ruminants must therefore be gradually acclimatized to increased NPN. Excess ammonia in the rumen is absorbed into the systemic circulation. The liver converts ammonia from the rumen to urea, which is excreted in urine or recycled to the rumen in saliva or via the blood. However, if the capacity of the liver to detoxify ammonia to urea becomes saturated, hyperammonemia may occur.

Mode(s) of Action

Ammonia is believed to deplete α-ketoglutarate, inhibiting the citric acid cycle and production of ATP. Lactic acidosis develops.

The risk of NPN toxicity in ruminants is increased by:

- Increased ruminal alkalinity, which inhibits conversion of NH_3 to NH_4^+
- Low-energy rations with high roughage and low carbohydrate content

- Poor body condition
- Low water intake

Horses may also develop NPN toxicosis but it generally has a relatively delayed clinical course because of the greater transit time to the cecum, compared to the rumen.

Clinical Signs

Clinical signs develop when ruminal ammonia exceeds 80 mg/dL or blood ammonia exceeds 1 mg/dL.

Clinical signs typically develop with 20−60 minutes of consumption in cattle, and within 30−90 minutes in sheep.

Animals show apprehension, hypersalivation, bruxism, and polyuria. There is progression to muscle tremors, skin tremors over the face and ears, blepharospasm, stiff front legs and weakness. Ruminants may exhibit ruminal atony. When blood ammonia exceeds 7−8 mg/dL, animals become prostrate and exhibit arrhythmias, cyanosis, pronounced jugular pulse, bloat, regurgitation, terminal convulsions, and death.

Additional clinical signs observed in horses are colic and head pressing.

Progression of clinical signs is rapid and cattle often die within 2 hours, sheep within 4 hours, and horses in 3−12 hours. Ruminants may be found dead.

Diagnostic Aids

Ruminal fluid, cerebrospinal fluid, serum, whole blood, or vitreous humor may be tested for ammonia nitrogen (NH_3N). Samples should be frozen promptly and maintained frozen until analyzed. If ruminal contents are sampled, multiple samples should be collected from several locations because the ammonia content may vary within the rumen.

Diagnostic values are blood ammonia of 1−4 mg/dL, rumen ammonia >80 mg/dL, and rumen pH <7.5.

Blood for ammonia analysis is best drawn into a syringe rather than a vacuum tube, so that there is no headspace, with anticoagulant added to the syringe prior to or after blood collection.

Blood pH is low due to metabolis acidosis. Lactic acid, BUN, AST, serum potassium, and blood glucose are elevated.

Only animals that have been dead for less than 12 hours are likely to be of diagnostic value.

The feed may tested for NPN.

Treatment

Treatment is seldom successful because of the rapid progression of the toxicosis. Best results are obtained if the animal is still ambulatory.

In ruminants, the rumen should be infused with vinegar (5% acetic acid) to decrease pH. The appropriate volume of vinegar for cattle is 2−8 L, and for sheep or goats, 0.5−2 L. This infusion should be repeated every 6 hours for up to 48 hours. Cold water (<4°C) should be administered orally or by stomach tube to lower the temperature of the rumen and inhibit the activity of urease. The volume of cold water for a cow ranges from 11.5−38 L.

Rumenotomy with removal of rumen contents may be performed in valuable animals.

Bloat should be relieved and metabolic acidosis treated by IV infusion of bicarbonate or saline.

In a herd situation in which multiple animals are affected, priority should be given to treating animals that are still standing.

Prognosis

Prognosis is poor, and grave if the animal becomes recumbent.

If treatment can be given early, survivors generally recover fully in 12−24 hours.

Necropsy

Ruminal pH exceeds 8, and ruminal contents may have an odor of ammonia. Pulmonary and tracheal congestion may be present, and reflects inhalation of eructated ammonia. The abomasal mucosa may be hyperemic. Ruminants are typically bloated, and decomposition is rapid.

Prevention

NPN should not exceed one-third of the total nitrogen in the ration. Animals must be acclimatized gradually to increased NPN in the ration.

SOYBEANS, RAW

Circumstances of Poisoning

Ruminants given access to raw soybeans may develop acute toxicosis.

Mode(s) of Action

Soybeans contain high concentrations of carbohydrates and also proteins, including an active urease. Overconsumption by ruminants causes a combination of lactic acidosis and ammonia toxicosis.

Clinical Signs

Affected ruminants have ruminal engorgement, ataxia, weakness, muscle tremors, and recumbency. There may be gray, pasty diarrhea.

Treatment

Treatment is rarely successful. Rumenotomy may be effective if performed early in the course of toxicosis.

Prognosis

Prognosis is poor.

Necropsy

Raw soybeans will be present in the rumen.

Prevention

Ruminants must not be given access to raw soybeans.

SULFUR

Sulfur is discussed in detail elsewhere in this book. The following brief notes are intended to augment that information, specifically addressing sulfur in feed or water.

Circumstances of Poisoning

Excessive sulfur intake in ruminants can cause polioencephalomalacia (PEM). A variety of ruminant feeds can be high in sulfur, including but not limited to turnips, chou moellier, lucerne (alfalfa), oil-seed meals, corn by-products, sugar cane, and sugar beet. Consumption of sulfate fertilizers is a potential source of PEM. Inhalation of hydrogen sulfide gas from manure slurry may also lead to PEM in ruminants. Some water sources are high in sulfates.

PEM has been long attributed to thiamine deficiency, but in recent decades this has been questioned. There is a lack of evidence that low thiamine levels can cause PEM unless sulfur levels are high. Thiamine supplementation does appear to decrease the risk of sulfur-associated PEM. Although some plants that contain thiaminases have been incriminated in PEM, at least some of these plants are also high in sulfur.

Toxicokinetics

Regardless of whether sulfur is in an organic or inorganic form when consumed, free sulfur is liberated by ruminal bacteria, and hydrogen sulfide accumulates in the ruminal fluid and gas cap. Hydrogen sulfide is readily absorbed into the systemic circulation.

Mode(s) of Action

Hydrogen sulfide and sulfide radicals block Cytochrome C in mitochondria, leading to depletion of ATP, cellular anoxia, and death.

Clinical Signs

Animals may be found dead.

Animals with a slower clinical course exhibit central nervous signs including lethargy, twitching or drooping ears, anorexia, ataxia, fine muscle tremors over the head, bruxism, circling, head pressing, and stupor. There is cortical blindness with absence of the menace reflex but preservation of the palpebral reflex. There may be nystagmus and/or medial-dorsal strabismus of the eyeball. Terminal signs are lateral recumbency, opisthotonos, and clonic−tonic convulsions with paddling motion.

PEM as a result of sulfur toxicity is clinically and microscopically indistinguishable from PEM caused by lead poisoning, water deprivation, or water intoxication.

Diagnostic Aids

Sulfur levels are transient in ruminal contents and have often fallen to normal levels by the time the animal is clinically affected. Sulfur analysis of the diet or of the ruminal contents of unaffected herd-mates are more likely to be useful.

Treatment

The herd should immediately be removed from the suspect feed. Parenteral thiamine supplementation may be helpful. A dose of 10 mg/kg, administered three to four times per day, is suggested. The first dose should be administered by slow intravenous injection, with subsequent doses administered intramuscularly. Treatment should be continued for 3−5 days.

To relieve cerebral edema, intramuscular dexamethasone may be administered at a dose of 2 mg/kg, intramuscularly or subcutaneously.

Prognosis

Prognosis is guarded to hopeless, depending on the severity and stage of poisoning. Animals that recover may be left with permanent brain damage.

Necropsy

The brain is swollen, edematous and soft, with flattened gyri. The medulla oblongata and cerebellum are sometimes partially herniated through the foramen magnum, with cerebellar "coning." Bilateral malacia of the gray matter is often grossly visible, with focal hemorrhages and/or yellow—brown discoloration, when the brain is incised. The malacia is often fluorescent under ultraviolet light (Wood's lamp). Ultraviolet light may also reveal malacic lesions in the thalamus and/or midbrain.

Longstanding cases may feature liquefactive necrosis in the brain.

Ruminal contents may be dark gray or black. Abomasal contents may be yellow.

Prevention

Dietary sulfur concentrations should be maintained at not more than 0.40%, and preferably at less than 0.30%.

SUPERPHOSPHATE

Circumstances of Poisoning

Superphosphate poisoning is most likely if animals graze pasture that has recently been fertilized with superphosphate, particularly if the grass is short and there has been no rain to wash the superphosphate into the soil. Toxicosis may also occur if livestock have access to superphosphate that is stored prior to being spread, if superphosphate is applied while animals are grazing the pasture, or if phosphate fertilizer is added to stock feed to boost dietary phosphate or nitrogen.

Superphosphate is typically seen in late winter or spring and may be confused with pregnancy toxemia or hypocalcemia.

Mode(s) of Action

Toxicity is principally due to fluoride (q.v.), which is present in all naturally occurring phosphate deposits and therefore in all phosphate fertilizers. Calcium pyrophosphate and calcium orthophosphate may also contribute to toxicity.

The LD_{50} of superphosphate in sheep is reported to be 100—300 mg/kg.

Clinical Signs

Animals may be found dead.

Clinical signs include depression, anorexia, thirst, hypersalivation, and signs of gastrointestinal inflammation, which may include bloating, constipation, or diarrhea. Typical nervous signs are weakness, ataxia, apparent blindness, recumbency, and terminal coma.

Diagnostic Aids

Elevated fluoride in blood or urine is indicative of recent exposure.

Treatment

There is no specific, effective treatment.

Prognosis

Prognosis is poor to grave, with animals usually dying within 48 hours of onset of clinical signs.

Necropsy

Kidneys are enlarged and pale. Ruminoreticulitis and abomasitis may be present, and superphosphate granules may be visible in the ruminal contents. Microscopically, there is necrosis of the epithelial cells of the proximal convoluted tubules in the kidneys. Postmortem samples include liver, kidney, and rumen contents.

Prevention

Livestock should not be allowed to graze pasture for at least 21 days after it is topdressed, or until at least 25 mm of rain has fallen. Overgrazing, which increases the likelihood of consumption of fertilizer, should be avoided.

WATER FOR LIVESTOCK AND HORSES

Water Quality Guidelines

Water may be classified by *total dissolved solids* (*TDS*). Tolerances for TDS in water are presented in Table 19.3.

Calcium in excess of 1000 mg/L may inhibit phosphorus absorption, leading to phosphorus deficiency.

Iron in water is generally not harmful to animals.

Manganese in excess of 2000 mg/L may cause diarrhea and decreased growth.

Water for livestock should contain less than 0.5 mg/L *ammonia*.

Ideally, water should not exceed 400 ppm *nitrate* or 30 ppm *nitrite*. Nitrate is the commonest form in water, and may originate from decaying plant matter, animal waste, or fertilizers. Bacteria can convert nitrate to the

TABLE 19.3 Effects of Total Dissolved Solids (TDS) in Water on Livestock

| Livestock Class | TDS (mg/L) | | |
	No Adverse Effects	May Decrease Palatability or Cause Transient Diarrhea; Animals Will Adapt	Adverse Effects on Production and Health
Beef cattle	<4000	4000–5000	>5000
Dairy cattle	<2500	2500–4000	>4000
Sheep	<5000	5000–10,000	>10,000
Horses	<4000	4000–6000	>6000
Pigs	<4000	4000–6000	>6000
Poultry	<2000	2000–3000	>3000

more toxic nitrite, and this may happen between collection and analysis if the water is not refrigerated or acidified. Greater than 1500 mg/L nitrate in water is likely to cause methemoglobinemia sufficient to cause acute toxicity in ruminants. Nitrate levels in feed must also be considered. For further details on *nitrate poisoning*, see the section on plants containing nitrates in the chapter covering toxicity of introduced plants.

Sulfate may be in water as a result of oxidation of sulfides, or as a result of industrial pollution. Water samples for analysis should be refrigerated or formalinized. Ideally, sulfate in water should not exceed 1000 mg/L, although animals can generally adapt to up to 2000 mg/L. Sulfate in excess of 2000 mg/L is not suitable for livestock.

Coliform counts are indicative of contamination with fecal matter, and should not exceed 100 thermotolerant coliforms/100 mL.

Chapter 20

Smoke and Other Inhaled Toxicants

The first subject covered in this chapter is *smoke inhalation*, a complex multifactorial respiratory injury, followed by short notes on:

- Ammonia
- Carbon dioxide
- Carbon monoxide
- Hydrogen cyanide
- Hydrogen sulfide
- Methane
- Nitrogen dioxide
- Teflon/polytetrafluoroethylene (PTFE)

SMOKE INHALATION

Mode(s) of Action

Smoke inhalation may inflict respiratory and systemic injury by several mechanisms:

- Asphyxiation
- Carbon monoxide poisoning (q.v.), if the fire was limited for oxygen supply, which is likely to be the case in house fires
- Cyanide poisoning (q.v.), if the fire was a house fire, because many furnishings release cyanide gas during pyrolysis
- Thermal injury, which is principally an injury of the upper respiratory tract extending to, and including, the pharynx
- Upper airway injury including destruction of the epithelial layer, and edema, inflammation
- Inhalation to the lower respiratory tract of chemicals (acrolein, aldehydes, ammonia, SO_2, HCl, aromatic hydrocarbons, H_2S) and particulates that cause bronchoconstriction; denaturation of surfactant; paralysis of the mucociliary apparatus; edema, necrosis, and sloughing of airway mucosa; cast or plugs composed of fibrin, mucus, inflammatory cells, and

sloughed epithelium in the airways; alveolar edema; alveolar collapse; and impairment of alveolar macrophage function

Clinical Signs

Any animal that has been exposed to smoke and particularly one that smells of smoke should be considered to be a possible victim of smoke inhalation injury.

Clinical signs may include acute upper respiratory tract obstruction, stridor, dyspnea, dysphonia, tachypnea, wheezing, hypersalivation, lacrimation, rhonchi, coughing, and cyanosis (in the absence of CO or hydrogen cyanide (HCN) toxicosis). Note that respiratory distress may develop 12–36 hours after the initial insult, due to delayed damage to airways and alveoli, and/or secondary infection.

Diagnostic Aids

Laryngoscopy.
Tracheobronchoscopy.
Radiology for evidence of laryngeal edema, tracheal narrowing, diffuse atelectasis, pulmonary edema, or bronchopneumonia.
Blood gas analysis.

Treatment

The cornerstones of treating smoke inhalation are:

- Establish and maintain adequate gas exchange. This includes treating for CO and HCN toxicosis as required.
- Clear the trachea and bronchi of casts and plugs, as much as possible.
- Monitor for, and treat, secondary infection.

Establish and maintain a patent airway. Laryngeal edema is likely; adrenalin spray may be helpful to minimize this. The patient that is breathing spontaneously and does not have evidence of smoke inhalation injury to the pharynx and larynx may not require intubation, but should be closely monitored for the first 24 hours, and particularly the first 8 hours, because if laryngeal edema develops, intubation will become progressively more difficult. Intubation is indicated if the patient exhibits respiratory distress, stridor, hypoventilation, use of accessory respiratory muscles, edema, blistering or ulceration of the oropharynx, or burns to the face or neck.

Administer oxygen because CO poisoning is likely. Administration by mask is appropriate if the patient is conscious, but intubation and positive pressure ventilation may be required if the patient is in a stupor or coma. Persistence of metabolic acidosis when the patient has adequate resuscitation (by volume) and cardiac output suggest CO or HCN poisoning. Treat initially for CO poisoning, and treat for HCN poisoning only if the patient does not respond to oxygen. Hydroxocobalamin is recommended as the first line in HCN poisoning as part of smoke inhalation, followed by the use of sodium thiosulfate alone.

Sedation may be necessary.

If the size of the patient allows, conduct bronchoscopy to clear muco-purulent exudate, mucus plugs, and sloughing mucosa from the airways as much as possible.

Experiments in sheep have shown that administration by continuous neb-ulization of a bronchodilator such as albuterol (up to 40 mg) is beneficial. Nebulized albuterol has been used in human victims of smoke inhalation at 2.5 mg/4 hours.

Positive pressure ventilatory support should be administered with caution, because when some bronchioles are plugged by casts, it is easy to overinflate other parts of the lungs, with the risk of iatrogenic damage and even rupture of the lungs.

Corticosteroids are *contraindicated*.

Antibiotics should not be used routinely, but should be administered if clinical signs and sputum culture indicate the development of secondary bacterial pneumonia.

Fluid therapy should be guided by urinary output, because of the risk of iatrogenic pulmonary edema.

Prognosis

Prognosis depends on the severity of injury, but is significantly worse if the patient has also burns to the skin. Convalescence may be protracted and ath-letic animals should not be expected to return to full athletic capability for months, if ever. Sequelae may include asthma, pulmonary fibrosis, and chronic obstructive pulmonary disease.

Necropsy

Necropsy findings include edema of all parts of the respiratory tract, sloughed tracheobronchial mucosa, soot and casts in the airways, pneumonia, atelectasis.

AMMONIA

Circumstances of Poisoning

Ammonia accumulation is common in animal housing, largely due to the action of urease bacteria on the urea in animal urine. The use of anhydrous ammonia as a nitrogen source in fertilizer presents a source of acute ammonia poisoning, in that anhydrous ammonia can be accidentally released as an acutely toxic cloud of vapor.

Mode(s) of Action

Ammonia is acutely irritating to the eyes and to the respiratory tract.

Clinical Signs

Lacrimation, shallow breathing, nasal discharge. At 50 ppm, reduces pulmonary bacterial clearance and impairs growth rate in swine. At 400 ppm, causes immediate irritation to the throat, while at 1700 ppm, will cause laryngospasm and coughing. Ammonia may be fatal at 2500 ppm if exposure exceeds 30 minutes, and may be rapidly fatal at 5000 ppm.

Treatment

Remove animals from areas where they are exposed to ammonia.

Necropsy

No consistent lesions.

Prevention

Ammonia buildup should be prevented by attention to cleaning away animal waste, and providing adequate ventilation.

CARBON DIOXIDE

Circumstances of Poisoning

Carbon dioxide may accumulate in enclosed animal housing or from improperly vented fuel-burning heaters. Accumulation of concentrations sufficient to cause fatal poisoning is rare.

Mode(s) of Action

Carbon dioxide is a primary asphyxiant.

Clinical Signs

At 500,000 ppm, CO_2 may cause increased rate and depth of respiration. With rising concentrations, animals may exhibit agitation, ataxia, and coma. Death ensues at 400,000 ppm.

Treatment

Move affected animals to fresh air.

Prognosis

Chronic neurological damage may result from severe acute poisoning.

Necropsy

No specific lesions. Tissues may be cyanotic.

Prevention

Ensure good ventilation.

CARBON MONOXIDE

Circumstances of Poisoning

Carbon monoxide is a product of incomplete combustion. Typical sources include vehicle exhaust, portable generators, kerosene heaters, and propane-powered engines. Carbon monoxide poisoning is also common in smoke inhalation (q.v.). Carbon monoxide is colorless and odorless, and disperses readily in confined spaces.

Mode(s) of Action

Carbon monoxide combines with hemoglobin to form carboxyhemoglobin at any or all of the oxygen-binding sites of hemoglobin, and also acts to increase the stability of the bond between hemoglobin and oxygen, reducing the ability of the hemoglobin molecule to release oxygen bound to other oxygen-binding sites. The overall result is a decrease in the oxygen available to tissues. Carbon monoxide also binds to myoglobin, and with cytochrome oxidase. Binding with cytochrome oxidase causes the release of mitochondrial free radicals, which attract leukocytes. Consequences include damage to endothelial cells and the vasculature of the brain, and lipid peroxidation of brain membranes.

Clinical Signs

Clinical signs are often nonspecific and readily mistaken for other disorders. They include nausea, vomiting, ataxia, dyspnea, tachypnea, tachycardia, hypotension, and lactic acidosis. Advanced signs are those of stupor or coma, pulmonary edema, and respiratory arrest.

Textbooks often describe bright red mucous membranes, but in practice these are rarely observed. However, the animal is unlikely to exhibit cyanosis. Carboxyhemoglobin absorbs light at the same wavelength as oxyhemoglobin, so a pulse oximeter gives falsely high tissue oxygenation.

Decreased density in the central white matter, globus pallidus, caudate nucleas, and putamen may be apparent on CT scans within 12 hours.

Handheld breath analyzers for human use are available but their use has not been validated in animals.

Treatment

Oxygen, 100% should be administered by tight-fitting mask or, in the unconscious animal, by endotracheal tube.

Seizures should be treated with appropriate anticonvulsants, only after oxygen administration has been initiated.

Prognosis

Damage to the central nervous system may be permanent. A delayed neuropsychiatric syndrome is well-described in human beings.

Necropsy

There may be no findings at necropsy. However, neurodegenerative changes in cerebral white matter, myonecrosis, optic neuritis and neuroretinal edema, pulmonary edema, renal tubular degeneration.

Prevention

Engines and heaters should only be operated with excellent ventilation. Ventilation is also important for all kinds of fires.

HYDROGEN CYANIDE

Circumstances of Poisoning

HCN is released by combustion of a number of plastics, and by burning rubber. HCN is also used in a number of processes such as electroplating and metal cleaning.

In human beings, cyanide gas at 110 ppm in air is life-threatening, while 270 ppm is immediately fatal.

Mode(s) of Action

Cyanide binds to the iron of the mitochondrial oxidase system, and this inhibits the ability of cells to use oxygen in oxidative phosphorylation. The cells respond by shifting to anerobic metabolism, with decreased ATP synthesis, increased lactic acid production, leading to severe metabolic acidosis. The result is histological hypoxia, despite abundant oxygenation of the blood.

Clinical Signs

Clinical signs include tachypnea, hypotension, rapid loss of consciousness and convulsions. Pupils are dilated, although blood is typically well oxygenated giving pink or red mucous membranes. There may be tachycardia or bradycardia. Cardiac changes include ventricular arrhythmias, supraventricular arrhythmias, and atrioventricular blocks.

Although some people can smell bitter almonds on the breath of a cyanide poisoned patient, the ability to do this is genetic and some people cannot smell the odor.

Treatment

The patient should be removed from the source of the cyanide gas immediately. The patient should be treated under conditions of excellent ventilation because of risk of cyanide gas exhalation or release from fur.

The conscious patient exhibiting only agitation and hyperventilation should not be administered antidotal therapy, because all cyanide antidotes are toxic in their own right. Treat with 100% oxygen for hypoxia, and establish an IV line and initiate bicarbonate fluid therapy for acidosis. Treat symptomatically for arrhythmia and convulsions.

If the diagnosis of cyanide poisoning is certain, antidotal therapy may be administered. There are several suggested antidotal therapies for cyanide poisoning, which may or may not be available.

- Sodium nitrite is administered IV, 16 mg/kg, as a 3% solution. This induces methemoglobinemia that may be fatal if cyanide poisoning is not present. Sodium nitrite should be followed by intravenous sodium thiosulfate, 1.65 mL of a 25% solution. The sodium nitrite/sodium thiosulfate treatment may be repeated at half the initial doses after 30 minutes.
- Sodium thiosulfate may be administered alone unless cyanide poisoning is severe, and is very safe.
- Hydroxocobalamin is a precursor of vitamin B12 (cyanocobalamin). It is the preferred antidote to cyanide poisoning in human beings due to its lack of adverse side effects. The recommended regime in human beings is to reconstitute one 2.5 g ampoule with 100 mL of 0.9% saline, and administer IV over 15 minutes, followed by a second ampoule in the

same volume over the same time. This is sufficient to bind 100 mg of cyanide. The volume in which hydroxocobalamin is diluted may need to adjusted downward for small animals.

- Dicobalt-EDTA or dicobalt edetate is used in Europe and particularly in the UK, but numerous severe side effects have been reported in human beings, including seizures, vomiting, chest pain, hypotension, ventricular arrhythmias, laryngeal edema, and anaphylactic shock.
- Another agent that, like sodium nitrite, induces methemoglobinemia is 4-dimethylaminophenol, which should be followed with sodium thiosulfate.
- α-Ketoglutoglutaric acid shows promise as an antidote for cyanide, in combination with sodium thiosulfate.

Prognosis

Animals that have recovered from cyanide inhalation should be observed for at least 24 hours, but most will recover without sequelae.

Necropsy

Although textbooks often describe the smell of bitter almonds and cherry-red blood, many people are genetically unable to smell cyanide, and cherry-red blood is often not observed. There may be hemorrhage in the basal ganglia and cerebral cortex.

HYDROGEN SULFIDE

Circumstances of Poisoning

Hydrogen sulfide is a byproduct of many industrial processes, and of the breakdown of organic waste. Occupational fatalities have occurred in people entering tanks that contain liquid manure. Hydrogen sulfide is also common in geothermal areas such volcanoes, and the Rotorua area of New Zealand.

Mode(s) of Action

Hydrogen sulfide is a potent inhibitor of the cytochrome oxidase system, and thus inhibits oxidative phosphorylation, leading to cellular asphyxia.

Most information on hydrogen sulfide comes from human exposure. Concentrations of 20−50 ppm are irritating to the eyes and respiratory tract, resulting in lacrimation, cough, and nasal discharge. In humans, olfactory fatigue occurs at concentrations of approximately 150−200 ppm, so that people can no longer detect the warning smell of "rotten eggs." Inhalation of 500 ppm for 30 minutes produces clinical signs of toxicosis in human beings, and prolonged nonfatal exposure may lead to bronchitis, pulmonary edema, or bronchial pneumonia. Concentrations above 600 ppm can be fatal within 30 minutes, and 800 ppm is immediately lethal in human beings.

Clinical Signs

Clinical signs include nausea, ataxia, metabolic acidosis, tremor, convulsions, cardiac arrhythmia, fulminant pulmonary edema, coma, and death.

Treatment

The animal should be removed from the environment if it is safe to do so; however, it should be recognized that a number of human fatalities have occurred in people who went into enclosed spaces to rescue coworkers or family members who had collapsed due to hydrogen sulfide poisoning, and succumbed themselves.

The patient that is conscious and ambulatory will usually respond to oxygen but should be monitored for adverse pulmonary effects.

The patient that has collapsed should be administered 100% oxygen at high flow. In severe life-threatening toxicosis, consider administration of sodium nitrite, as for hydrogen cyanide poisoning (q.v.). Seizures should be treated with diazepam or lorazepam in the first instance, with a barbiturate as a second option. Hypotension should be treated with dopamine by IV infusion. Correct metabolic acidosis.

The patient that survives initial toxicosis should be monitored for pulmonary edema.

Prognosis

Central nervous damage has been reported in a number of human survivors of hydrogen sulfide poisoning. Effects have included impaired balance, prolonged reaction time, decrease in visual field, impaired hearing, impaired memory, mood changes, and impaired cognitive ability.

Necropsy

Necropsy findings may include pulmonary edema, pulmonary hemorrhage, petechial hemorrhages in the brain.

METHANE

Circumstances of Poisoning

Methane may be released into the environment from a variety of sources including animal waste, human sewage, geothermal activity, coal outgassing, wood pulping, landfills, and various industrial processes. Methane is part of natural gas.

Mode(s) of Action

Methane acts as a simple asphyxiant, replacing air.

Clinical Signs

Animals are often found dead. Clinical signs are those of asphyxiation.

Treatment

Animals should be moved from areas of methane exposure only if it is safe for humans to enter those areas. Supplemental oxygen will accelerate recovery. Measure blood gases and treat for metabolic acidosis if present.

Prognosis

Sequelae may include pulmonary edema, pneumonitis, and/or cerebral edema.

Necropsy

There are no specific lesions.

NITROGEN DIOXIDE

Circumstances of Poisoning

Nitrogen dioxide may form during the fermentation of ensiled feed. It is heavier than air, is yellow or yellow-brown in color, and has an odor often likened to bleach.

Mode(s) of Action

Nitrogen dioxide reacts with water of moist exposed tissues to form nitric acid, which is highly corrosive. It can pass through the upper respiratory tract with little effect and then react with water in the lungs to cause severe tissue damage. Toxicity is a function both of concentration of the gas and duration of exposure, but brief high-concentration exposures are generally more harmful than longer low-concentration exposures.

Clinical Signs

Clinical signs are those of coughing and choking. Concentrations in excess of 200 ppm may cause immediate death. Chronic low-concentration exposure may lead to chronic bronchitis or emphysema.

Treatment

Animals should be moved from a situation of exposure only if it is safe for humans to enter the area. Supplemental oxygen is beneficial, and if there is evidence of pulmonary edema, corticosteroids should be administered.

Prognosis

Prognosis is guarded. There are a number of examples of animals being moved to fresh air but dying hours to days later.

Necropsy

In acute poisoning there may be no gross lesions. Histopathology may reveal disruption of Type I alveolar cells, fibrin deposition on basement membranes, and increased numbers of alveolar macrophages. Lesions of more chronic exposure may include pulmonary congestion, pulmonary edema, and/or emphysema.

Prevention

Silage pits or stacks should only be opened in conditions of excellent ventilation.

TEFLON/POLYTETRAFLUOROETHYLENE

Circumstances of Poisoning

PTFE poisoning of birds is most often associated with overheating of Teflon-lined cookware. However, PTFE may also be found in other household appliances such as irons and ironing board covers, and from poultry equipment such as heat lamps. When heated above 280°C, PTFE breaks down to release hydrogen fluoride, carbon fluoride, carbon monoxide, and other pyrolysis products, particularly fluoropolymers of low molecular weight.

Clinical Signs

Birds, particularly pet birds, are often found dead. Birds may present with dyspnea, ataxia, or in seizures.

Exposure to pyrolysis products of PTFE can cause fever and malaise in human beings and could presumably have the same effect on domestic mammals. Human beings usually recover within hours.

Treatment

Birds should be administered supplemental oxygen, and kept warm. Treatment is otherwise symptomatic and supportive. NSAIDs may be helpful.

Prognosis

Prognosis is guarded.

Necropsy

Necropsy findings are those of severe pulmonary edema and pulmonary hemorrhage.

Prevention

Avoid the overheating of Teflon-coated appliances. Pet birds should preferably not be kept near Teflon-coated appliances.

Chapter 21

Mycotoxins and Mushrooms

MYCOTOXINS

Introduction

Mycotoxins are secondary metabolites of fungi. Fungi infecting plants or grains and producing mycotoxins may *field fungi*, which infect the plant or grain prior to harvest, or *storage fungi*, which infect the grain or plant material after it has been harvested, although some fungi proliferate both in the field and in storage. The severity of infestation varies with ambient conditions including temperature, humidity, and moisture content. In addition the seed coat of most seeds and grains is generally a barrier to fungal invasion and conditions that damage the seed coat increase the risk of fungal proliferation.

Fungi are ubiquitous but mycotoxin synthesis is variable depending on conditions, which may include climate conditions, fungal strain, and insect attack. Therefore the presence of a fungus or mold in feed does not necessarily predict the presence of mycotoxins.

Disease caused by ingestion of mycotoxins is termed *mycotoxicosis*. There are no antidotes or specific pharmaceutical treatments for mycotoxicosis. Treatment is supportive only, and prevention is therefore important. As a generalization, mycotoxins are resistant to physical or chemical destruction, although adsorbents in the feed may be helpful to reduce exposure. Commercial adsorbents are available, and activated charcoal and bentonite have also been used to adsorb mycotoxins.

Suspect feed should be transported for laboratory analysis in paper bags or fabric bags rather than plastic bags, to avoid condensation and fungal proliferation in transit. The laboratory to which the submission will be made should be contacted for details on whether to submit the sample refrigerated or frozen, or at ambient temperature after gentle oven-drying.

In this chapter, mycotoxins are covered in approximately alphabetical order in the following sections:

- Aflatoxins
- Citrinin
- *Corallocytostroma orinopreoides* toxin
- Ergot alkaloids (includes ergotism and "tall fescue poisoning")

Veterinary Toxicology for Australia and New Zealand
DOI: http://dx.doi.org/10.1016/B978-0-12-420227-6.00020-7

- Fumonisins
- Ochratoxins
- Penitrem A and roquefortine
- Phomopsins
- Slaframine (and swainsonine)
- Sporidesmin
- Stachybotryotoxins
- Tremorgenic mycotoxins associated with grasses (includes lolitrems, paspalinine, and paspalitrems)
- Trichothecenes
- Zearalenone

AFLATOXINS

Synthesizing Organism

Aspergillus flavus and *Aspergillus parasiticus*.

Distribution

Aflatoxins occur in many feed grains. Toxic levels are most often found in peanuts in Australia. Maize is also a common source of aflatoxins.

Circumstances of Poisoning

Aspergillus spp. are usually considered to be storage fungi, but aflatoxins may be synthesized under field conditions. The optimum temperature range for aflatoxin production is 25–32°C, although they may be produced at lower temperatures. Drought stress or insect attack tends to enhance production in the field, while moisture >15% supports fungal proliferation in storage.

The four major aflatoxins are aflatoxin B1, aflatoxin B2, aflatoxin G1, and aflatoxin G2.

Toxicokinetics

Aflatoxin B1 is known to be metabolized in the liver to form multiple metabolites of which one is a highly reactive epoxide which forms adducts with nucleic acids and proteins.

Aflatoxins are primarily excreted in urine. Most aflatoxin is exreted within 96 hours of cessation of exposure, but residues may persist in liver or kidney for up to 2 weeks.

Mode(s) of Action

Aflatoxins depress the synthesis of mRNA and proteins. Inhibition of protein synthesis includes, but is not limited to, inhibited synthesis of metabolic enzymes, structural proteins, clotting factors, and antibodies. The liver is the most severely affected organ.

Ruminants are generally less susceptible to aflatoxicosis than monogastric species, and adult animals are less susceptible than young animals.

Clinical Signs

Acute aflatoxicosis such as that seen in the USA is not characteristic in Australia or New Zealand, but may include depression, anorexia, and reduced production. Ruminants may exhibit transient ruminal atony or hypomotility.

Chronic aflatoxicosis is the most common presentation in Australia and New Zealand. Clinical signs include illthrift, anorexia, impaired growth, icterus, anemia, ascites, and depressed immune function.

Diagnostic Aids

Clinical pathology findings are nonspecific signs of chronic liver damage and may include mild anemia, hyperbilirubinemia, elevation of liver enzymes, decreased serum albumin and albumin:globulin ratio, and increased prothrombin time (PT).

Aflatoxin M1, a metabolite of aflatoxin B1, may be detected in milk or urine.

Examination of suspect feed with an UV lamp (e.g., Wood's lamp) may reveal intense blue-green fluorescence. This fluorescence is not the aflatoxins themselves, but kojic acid, which is often formed under similar conditions by the same fungi. Therefore this fluorescence supports but does not prove the presence of aflatoxins.

Diagnostic laboratories often offer a mycotoxin screen for aflatoxins and other common mycotoxins. There are also some commercial quick tests for use on grain.

Treatment

Gastrointestinal decontamination with hydrated sodium calcium aluminosilicate (HSCAS), which adsorbs aflatoxins with high affinity, has been shown to be useful in recent exposures of cattle and swine.

Prognosis

Prognosis is variable depending on the severity of liver damage.

Necropsy

Grossly the liver is often pale and soft. Icterus, ascites, and watery blood are other postmortem features.

Histopathological lesions are those of hydropic degeneration and necrosis of hepatocytes, with a proliferative response in hepatocytes and biliary ductules. Interlobular fibroplasia may be extensive. Regenerating hepatocytes may exhibit karyomegaly, multiple nucleoli, and atypical nuclei.

Public Health Considerations

Chronic exposure to aflatoxins is associated with increased risk of liver cancer in individuals with some hepatitis virus infections. However, grain with insect damage, damaged hulls, or high aflatoxin levels is often redirected from processing for human consumption to animal feed, so the presence of unacceptable levels of aflatoxins in animal feed does not imply that levels in human food are also excessive.

Milk from affected cattle should not be consumed.

Prevention

Harvested grains or peanuts must be appropriately stored to prevent aflatoxin formation, and sampled for the presence of aflatoxins. Mold inhibitors may be added during the mixing of processed feeds to prevent fungal proliferation, but will not destroy existing aflatoxins.

CITRININ

Synthesizing Organisms

Citrinin is synthesized by *Penicillium viridicatum* and *Penicillium citrinum*, and some species of *Aspergillus* and *Monascus*.

Distribution

Citrinin has been found in grains such as wheat, rye, and barley. Synthesis of citrinin and related compounds by an Australian isolate of *P. citrinum* has been demonstrated, but this mycotoxin does not appear to be a significant problem in Australia or New Zealand.

Citrinin has also been found in other plant products such as beans, fruits, fruit and vegetable juices, herbs, and spices, as well as in spoiled dairy products.

Circumstances of Poisoning

Penicillium proliferation most commonly occurs in storage. The optimum temperature range for citrinin production is between 12°C and 25°C. Production is most likely when the grain moisture content exceeds 16%.

Toxicokinetics

There is little information on the toxicokinetics of citrinin by the oral route, but experimental data indicate that citrinin residues may be found in edible tissues and eggs of animals that have been subject to high exposure.

Mode(s) of Action

Citrinin appears to be toxic by multiple pathways including inhibition of nucleic acid synthesis, inhibition of microtubule assembly and tubulin polymerization, alteration of mitochondrial function, inactivation of the heat shock protein 90 (HSP90) multichaperone complex, and activation of pathways that lead to apoptosis. The kidney is the most sensitive target organ. Citrinin also appears to embryotoxic and teratogenic, and may also be immunotoxic.

Clinical Signs

Acute toxicosis is rare. Chronic toxicosis causes nonspecific signs of impaired renal function including polyuria, polydipsia, dehydration, and weight loss. Affected poultry pass watery feces.

Diagnostic Aids

Clinical pathology findings are nonspecific signs of chronic renal failure including elevated BUN and creatinine. Urinalysis findings are those of hyposthenuria, cellular and granular casts, and elevations of ketones, protein, and glucose.

Treatment

Treatment is unlikely to be helpful, given that clinical signs are unlikely to become evident until the renal reserve has been irreparably destroyed.

Prognosis

Prognosis is poor.

Necropsy

Histopathology reveals degeneration and necrosis of the epithelial cells of distal tubules and collecting ducts of the kidneys. Liver necrosis may also be present.

Public Health Considerations

Citrinin is nephrotoxic to human beings and locally produced, and imported foods are subject to testing.

Animals that have suffered citrinin nephrotoxicosis should not be consumed, and nor should eggs from poultry that have suffered citrinin nephrotoxicosis.

Prevention

Sampling of harvested and stored grains or feed ingredients for citrinin, and storage of potential substrates to prevent fungal proliferation, are key.

CORALLOCYTOSTROMA ORNICOPREOIDES TOXIN

Synthesizing Organism

Corallocytostroma ornicopreoides.

Distribution

This fungus is native to Australia. Clinical cases have been reported in a relatively limited area in the Kimberley region of WA and the Victoria River district of NT.

Circumstances of Poisoning

The fungus causes galls on grasses, usually grasses of the genus *Astrebla* (Mitchell grasses). The galls are termed "corals" because of their appearance. They are typically hard, dry, white or off-white, roughly spherical and with a rough appearance. They are usually attached to the flower-heads or growing apex of the infected grass.

Toxicosis is usually seen in cattle, although it has been observed in sheep, and most often occurs following unusually high rainfall in successive wet and dry seasons, conditions that favor development of galls. Such conditions have historically occurred only once in 20 years, but may become more frequent as a result of climate change. The toxicosis occurs on "black soil" downs where *Astrebla* grass predominates. The toxicosis is consequently referred to as "black soil blindness."

Toxicokinetics

The toxin has not been identified, and the toxicokinetics are not defined.

Mode(s) of Action

Unknown.

Clinical Signs

Usually only about 5% of a herd of cattle develop overt toxicosis. Clinical signs include dehydration, apparent partial or total blindness, collapse, and death within a few hours of onset of clinical signs. Other animals in the herd may exhibit weight loss, presumably due to subclinical toxicosis. The toxin is thought to cause abortion, although it is not clear if this is a direct or indirect effect.

Diagnostic Aids

Observation of galls on grass.

Treatment

There is no specific treatment.

Prognosis

Prognosis is grave to hopeless, for those animals that develop overt toxicosis.

Necropsy

Necropsy findings include perirenal edema, pale kidneys, congestion of the ruminoreticular epithelium, and a swollen liver. There may be icterus. Histopathological findings include renal tubular necrosis, ruminoreticular inflammation, and periacinar hepatocellular necrosis. Grossly and histologically, the brain, eyes, and optics nerves are normal.

Public Health Considerations

None.

Prevention

Because the prognosis is grave to hopeless once animals are affected, prevention is key. Susceptible grass should be inspected for galls after a wet summer, and if galls are present, cattle should be denied access to the pasture until near the end of the following wet season.

ERGOT ALKALOIDS

Synthesizing Organisms

Claviceps purpurea and the fungal endophyte of tall fescue (*Festuca arundinaceae*), *Acremonium coenophialum*.

The major ergot alkaloids of *C. purpurea* are ergotamine and ergonovine, while the major alkaloid of *A. coenophialum* is the closely related alkaloid ergovaline.

Distribution

Ergot sclerotia are found on grains such as wheat, rye, barley, and oats, but may also infect ryegrasses. Tall fescue is a perennial pasture grass.

Circumstances of Poisoning

Ergot sclerotia are most likely to be found in warm, humid conditions.

Not all strains of tall fescue are infected with *A. coenophialum*, and not all strains of *A. coenophialum* produce ergovaline. Ergovaline synthesis by the endophytic fungus appears to increase with age of the host plant, and may also be increased by drought conditions or by application of nitrogen fertilizers.

Toxicokinetics

Although the pharmacokinetics of ergot alkaloids used for treatment of migraine headaches and postpartum hemorrhage have been extensively studied, there is little information on the toxicokinetics of ergot alkaloids in livestock. Clinical signs become apparent 2–6 weeks after cattle begin eating contaminated feed.

Metabolites of ergovaline in cattle are predominantly excreted in the urine, and urinary levels decline rapidly after cattle are removed from infected pasture.

Mode(s) of Action

The ergot alkaloids synthesized by *C. purpurea* act on the tunica muscularis of arterioles, causing vasoconstriction. Prolonged or high exposure may also directly harm the vascular endothelium. Blood flow to the extremities is reduced or halted, resulting in ischemic necrosis and dry gangrene. Low ambient temperature exacerbates this effect. The ergot alkaloids may also cause stimulation of the central nervous system, causing animals to be excitable, and were associated historically with mania or psychosis in human beings. Ergot alkaloids act on the myometrium in a manner similar to oxytocin, but inhibit pituitary release of prolactin in many species, resulting in inhibition of both mammogenesis during pregnancy and lactogenesis at parturition.

Ergovaline, the predominant alkaloid synthesized by *A. coenophialum*, has similar toxic properties. The inhibition of prolactin secretion causes agalactia in horses and swine and reduced lactation in cattle. Ergovaline has also a dopaminergic effect that leads to imbalances of progesterone and estrogen, which may result in early parturition for cattle and in prolonged gestation in mares. Prolactin suppression also affects the hypothalamic thermoregulatory center, causing animals to be intolerant of high ambient temperatures.

Clinical Signs

Vasconstrictive and neurological conditions caused by the ergot alkaloids of *C. purpurea* are referred to as "ergotism," while the conditions resulting from consumption of ergovaline in tall fescue are somewhat misleadingly called "tall fescue toxicosis" or "fescue foot."

The species most commonly affected by the ergot alkaloids of *C. purpurea* are cattle, pigs, sheep, and poultry.

The first sign of ischemia of the extremities in cattle is lameness, with swelling and tenderness of the fetlocks and pasterns, affecting the hindlimbs first. Within a few days a clear indented demarcation develops between the normal proximal and ischemic distal parts of the lesion. No response to stimuli can be provoked in the distal tissue, which may develop dry gangrene and slough off. Tips of ears and tail may be lost by the same mechanism. Reduced peripheral perfusion may cause pink skin of the teats or udder of cattle to appear pale, although teats do not generally become ischemic.

Abortion is not characteristic in livestock.

On the examination, body temperature heart rate and respiration rate are increased. Animals may be excitable, and there is some evidence that sheep may develop convulsions.

Necrosis of extremities is rare in pigs, which are more likely to exhibit reduced feed intake. Pregnant sows may exhibit agalactia at parturition, resulting in death of the piglets from starvation.

The ergot alkaloids of *C. purpurea* have also been associated with a heat intolerance syndrome in cattle, which resembles the "summer slump" due to ergovaline synthesized by *A. coenophialum*-infected tall fescue, described below.

Ergovaline ranges from 100 to 500 ppb in infected tall fescue, and >200 ppb is considered to be sufficient to cause toxicosis in animals grazing the pasture. Horses are the most susceptible to tall fescue toxicosis, followed by cattle and lastly by sheep.

"Fescue foot" follows a similar progression of clinical signs to ischemic necrosis caused but the ergot alkaloids of *C. purpurea*, as described above, and is likewise exacerbated by cold ambient temperatures. Affected animals also show loss of condition, rough coat and a tendency to stand with the back arched. Signs usually appear within 2−3 weeks of being turned out onto the pasture.

Cattle grazing tall fescue pasture during hot weather may develop epidemic hyperthermia, commonly known as "summer slump" or "summer syndrome." The vasoconstrictive action of ergovaline inhibits the physiological peripheral vasodilation, which is an important mechanism for temperature homeostasis in cattle. Cattle develop hyperthermia and respond with reduced feed intake, with consequent loss of weight gain and/or milk production. Affected cattle often exhibit hypersalivation and rough coat, and seek shade or ponds to stand in. Reproductive performance may also be affected. Sheep and horses may also be affected by this condition.

Feeding on endophyte-infected tall fescue pasture or hay is associated with thickened placentas, delayed parturition, birth of weak foals with dysmature lungs, and agalactia in horses. Affected foals often fail to turn into the normal presentation for birth and instead present upside-down, increasing the likelihood of dystocia. The thickened placenta may fail to rupture but present at the vulva ("red-bag") while detaching in the uterus, resulting in fetal asphyxia.

Diagnostic Aids

The ergot sclerotia of *C. purpurea* are readily visible by eye, although they may be mistaken for mouse feces. Ergot alkaloids can be extracted from suspect ground grain meals.

The presence of *A. coenophialum* in tall fescue can be confirmed by microscopic examination, although not all strains of the endophyte produce ergovaline. Extraction and identification of ergovaline may be available, but the clinical signs and history of tall fescue consumption is usually diagnostic.

Treatment

The diet should be changed immediately to prevent exposure to vasoactive alkaloid/s.

Pregnant mares that have grazed on infected tall fescue pasture may respond to domperidone, 1.1 mg/kg, PO, bid for 10−14 days.

Prognosis

Prognosis is poor if feet become ischemic.

Necropsy

Ischemic necrosis and dry gangrene of extremities are characteristic. Sheep may also show inflammation of the mouth and gastrointestinal tract.

Public Health Considerations

Recovered livestock are safe for human consumption.

Prevention

Grains or feeds containing ergot sclerotia or ergot alkaloids should not be fed. Reputable animal feed suppliers test their products for mycotoxins and can provide data to show that toxic levels of these and other common mycotoxins are not present.

Toxic tall fescue pastures should not be used during hot weather and should never be used to make hay for pregnant mares. Pregnant mares should be removed from tall fescue pasture at least 1 month before their due date, bearing in mind that the gestation period is quite variable in mares. Pregnant cows should also be removed from tall fescue pasture at least 1 month before their due date. Destruction of pastures with replacement by other pasture grasses may be indicated. Other, less desirable options are to introduce other species of grass to dilute the proportion of tall fescue in the pasture, and to frequently top the pasture to remove flower-heads. Feed additives such as glucomannans are reported to reduce gastrointestinal absorption by cattle of alkaloids from contaminated hay.

FUMONISINS

Synthesizing Organism

Fusarium verticilloides (formerly known as *Fusarium moniliforme*) and possibly also *Fusarium proliferatum*.

Distribution

Maize (*Zea mays*).

Circumstances of Poisoning

Production of fumonisins appears to be most often associated with a period of drought during the growing season of the maize, followed by cool, moist weather during pollination and kernel formation in the plant.

Toxicokinetics

There is a lack of information concerning the toxicokinetics of fumonisins in horses, one of the two species most severely affected by fumonisins. In piglets, fumonisins are readily absorbed following oral dosing, with C_{max} at approximately 2 hours. Excretion is predominantly fecal although there is some urinary excretion. Most orally administered fumonisin is excreted within 24 hours. Toxicosis generally follows prolonged dietary exposure.

Mode(s) of Action

Fumonisins inhibit the synthesis of sphingolipids by blocking the conversion of sphinganine to sphingosine.

In horses and other equids, fumonisins lead to leucoencephalomalacia, with liquefactive necrosis of the white matter of the brain. Fumonisins also cause hepatic necrosis in horses. As little as 8–10 ppm fumonisin in the diet can cause toxicosis in horses, if fed for a prolonged period.

In pigs, fumonisins at greater than 100 ppm for more than 5 days cause a rapidly progressing respiratory disease characterized by pulmonary edema and hydrothorax. Chronic exposure to lower doses of fumonisins are associated with liver necrosis and right ventricular hypertrophy.

Ruminants are comparatively tolerant of fumonisins but may exhibit anorexia if dietary levels exceed 200 ppm. Fumonisins have been incriminated in hepatopathy of farmed deer in New Zealand. Poultry are even more resistant but fumonisins at greater than 200 ppm in the diet may lead to anorexia and skeletal effects.

Clinical Signs

Clinical signs in horses include depression, drowsiness, blindness, ataxia, wandering, circling, facial and/or pharyngeal paralysis, recumbency, and coma. The clinical course is generally rapid with death ensuing within a week of onset of clinical signs, but some horses may linger for weeks. Occasional horses recover with neurological deficits. Icterus may be present as a result of liver necrosis.

Presenting signs of acute toxicosis in pigs are dyspnea, cyanosis, weakness, and exercise intolerance, with death ensuing within 4–24 hours. Sows that survive the acute toxicosis may abort, and surviving pigs or those exposed to lower concentrations of fumonisins may develop hepatopathy with icterus, anorexia, and weight loss.

Diagnostic Aids

Clinical pathology findings are those of liver degeneration and necrosis.

The most sensitive and specific test for fumonisins is the serum sphinga-nine:sphingosine ratio, but it may be difficult to find a laboratory that performs this test.

Treatment

There is no treatment for equine leucoencephalomalacia or porcine pulmonary syndrome.

Animals with only hepatic lesions may recover with appropriate supportive care.

Prognosis

The prognosis in equine leucoencephalomalacia and porcine pulmonary syndrome is poor to hopeless.

Necropsy

In horses the brain lesions are extensive malacia and liquefactive necrosis of the white matter. Microscopically, there is perivascular hemorrhage into the Virchow—Robin spaces, and macrophage infiltration in the necrotic brain tissue, but besides the macrophages there is little inflammatory response. Hepatic degeneration and necrosis is also present.

In pigs the lesions are those of severe interstitial, interlobular, and subpleural edema. Other lesions are hydrothorax, and multifocal hepatic degeneration and necrosis. Multifocal pancreatic necrosis has also been reported.

Public Health Considerations

Because of the rapid excretion of fumonisins, residues are not considered to be a public health problem.

Prevention

Grains or processed feeds should be obtained only from reputable suppliers who can provide data to show that testing for fumonisins has been conducted and that levels are within acceptable limits.

OCHRATOXINS

Synthesizing Organisms

Ochratoxins are synthesized by fungi of the genera *Aspergillus* and *Penicillium*, including *Aspergillus ochraeus*, *P. viridicatum*, and *Penicillium carbonarius*.

Distribution

Ochratoxins are most commonly found in grains such as corn, wheat, barley, and rye.

Circumstances of Poisoning

Fungal proliferation and synthesis of ochratoxins is most likely when the grain moisture content exceeds 16% and the humidity exceeds 85%. Ochratoxin production is greatest in the temperature range 12−25°C. There are at least nine different ochratoxins but Ochratoxin A is the most common and the most toxicologically significant.

Toxicokinetics

Ochratoxins are rapidly absorbed by the oral route with a C_{max} within a few hours. Ochratoxin A is converted to active metabolites by mixed function oxidases in the liver. Both biliary and renal excretion occur.

Mode(s) of Action

Active metabolites of Ochratoxin A act on the epithelial cells of the proximal renal tubules, leading to decreased renal clearance and impairment of the ability to concentrate urine.

Pigs and poultry are the species most commonly affected. Ruminants are relatively resistant to ochratoxicosis. The acute toxic range for pigs and poultry is 1−5 ppm, and concentrations in excess of 0.3 ppm may lead to chronic toxicosis if dietary exposure at this level persists for several weeks.

Clinical Signs

Acute toxicosis is rare, but may present as anorexia, diarrhea, dehydration, and depression.

Most cases diagnosed in animals are chronic toxicoses, as weight loss, depression, and polyuria, which leads to dehydration and compensatory polydipsia.

Studies in laboratory rodents have demonstrated that Ochratoxin A is immunotoxic; teratogenic, causing craniofacial abnormalities; and carcinogenic particularly to kidney and liver.

Diagnostic Aids

Clinical pathology findings are nonspecific signs of renal dysfunction including elevated BUN and creatinine. Urinalysis findings are those of hyposthenuria and increased numbers of epithelial cells and casts.

Suspect feed can be tested for the presence of ochratoxins.

Treatment

Animals should be treated for renal insufficiency with a low-protein diet and unlimited water.

Prognosis

Prognosis for full recovery is poor because by the time clinical signs develop, renal function has generally been permanently impaired.

Necropsy

Kidneys are usually enlarged, pale and with an irregular surface. On incision, the renal cortex may exhibit pale streaks indicative of fibrosis, and multiple small cysts which on microscopic examination are dilated, nonfunctional tubules. Microscopic findings are those of glomerular sclerosis, degeneration and necrosis of renal tubules, and interstitial fibrosis.

Hepatic necrosis and lymphoid depletion may occur in acute toxicosis.

Visceral gout and loss of endochondral bone may be present in poultry.

Public Health Considerations

Ochratoxin residues have been found in the meat of animals for some weeks after exposure.

Prevention

Grains or processed feeds should be obtained only from reputable suppliers who can provide data to show that testing for ochratoxins has been conducted and that levels are within acceptable limits.

PENITREM A AND ROQUEFORTINE

Synthesizing Organism

These tremorgenic mycotoxins are synthesized by a range of fungi in the genus *Penicillium*.

Distribution

Penitrems, of which the most significant is Penitrem A, and roquefortine are found on a variety of food substrates including nuts, vegetables, and dairy products, particularly if foods are allowed to grow moldy.

Circumstances of Poisoning

Although most mycotoxicoses affect livestock, these tremorgenic mycotoxins are most often associated with "garbage poisoning" in dogs that scavenge moldy food.

Toxicokinetics

Penitrem A and roquefortine are rapidly absorbed by the oral route and primarily excreted by the biliary route.

Mode(s) of Action

The mode of action of these tremorgenic mycotoxins is obscure.

Clinical Signs

Clinical signs may become evident as soon as 30 minutes after ingestion. Reported clinical signs include hypersalivation, agitation, panting, vomiting, tremors, ataxia, tachycardia, and convulsions. Affected dogs are often hypersensitive to noise and other stimuli. Dogs that recover from the acute toxicosis may have long-lasting neurological damage such as ataxia.

Diagnostic Aids

Suspect feed or vomitus may be examined for *Penicillium* spp. or for the presence of Penitrem A or roquefortine.

Treatment

Treatment is symptomatic, including control of neurological signs by diazepam, methocarbamol or barbiturates as necessary. An intravenous catheter should be placed and maintained by slow intravenous fluid administration so that the dog can be monitored and treated as required for hyperthermia, dehydration, metabolic acidosis, or rhabdomyolysis.

Prognosis

Prognosis is usually favorable, although convalescence may be prolonged and some dogs have long-standing neurological deficits after recovery.

Necropsy

There are no specific necropsy findings. Stomach contents or bile may be collected for mycotoxin analysis.

Public Health Considerations

Tremorgenic mycotoxins have caused toxicosis in human beings consuming moldy food.

Prevention

Food waste, particularly if it appears moldy, should be discarded in such a way that dogs cannot scavenge it.

PHOMOPSINS

Synthesizing Organism

Phomopsis leptostromiformis, a fungus that causes stem blight in white and yellow sweet lupins (*Lupinus* spp.).

Distribution

The mycotoxicosis, somewhat misleadingly known as Lupinosis, is most common in Australia but has been reported occasionally in New Zealand. *P. leptostromiformis* grows on both living and decaying sweet lupin. Production of toxic levels of phomopsins often occur after rain.

Circumstances of Poisoning

Poisoning is most common in sheep but has also been reported in cattle, pigs, and sheep, and may result from using sweet lupins as a forage crop or from feeding the sweet lupin plants to animals after the seeds have been harvested for human consumption.

Toxicokinetics

There is a lack of information on the toxicokinetics of phomopsins.

Mode(s) of Action

Phomopsins are hepatotoxic.

Clinical Signs

Clinical signs include anorexia, depression, icterus, ketosis, and hepatogenous photosensitivity.

Diagnostic Aids

Clinical pathology findings are those of toxic liver injury including elevated liver enzymes and hyperbilirubinemia.

Treatment

Animals should be removed from the affected feed. Animals exhibiting photosensitivity must be provided with deep shade. Treatment is supportive and should include palatable, easily digested food.

Prognosis

Prognosis varies based on the severity of liver injury.

Necropsy

In acute toxicosis the liver is typically enlarged, pale and orange or yellow. In chronic toxicosis the liver may be small, bronze-colored, and firm on cutting due to fibrosis. Copious transudate may be present in the abdominal and thoracic cavities and the pericardial sac.

Public Health Considerations

Phomopsins in the human food supply are attracting increasing attention from regulatory agencies around the world, because phomopsins have been shown to be potent hepatotoxins in all species in which they have been tested.

Prevention

Oral zinc supplementation, at not less than 0.5 g/day, may protect sheep from liver injury. Cultivars of sweet lupin that are resistant to *P. leptostromiformis* are available and their use should be encouraged.

SLAFRAMINE AND SWAINSONINE

Synthesizing Organism

Rhizoctonia leguminicola.

Note that swainsonine is also produced by some higher plants, including Darling pea (*Swainsona canescens*) in Australia and locoweeds (*Astragalus* spp.) in North America. For more information on swainsonine toxicity, refer to the section on Darling pea.

Distribution

R. leguminicola infects clovers (*Trifolium* spp.) and other legumes including soybean (*Glycine max*), lucerne (alfalfa; *Medicago sativa*), and blue lupin (*Lupinus angustifolius*), causing "black patch."

Circumstances of Poisoning

"Black patch" lesions are most like to occur on legumes in summer during periods of high rainfall and high humidity.

Toxicokinetics

Slaframine is rapidly absorbed and is converted to an active metabolite by microsomal flavoprotein oxidase in the liver. There is a lack of information on excretion of slaframine.

Swainsonine: See section on Darling pea (*S. canescens*).

Mode(s) of Action

Slaframine, also known as "slobber factor," acts as a parasympathomimetic on endocrine and exocrine glands, particularly the salivary glands and pancreas. Salivary secretion can be increased up to 50%, and secretion of pancreatic fluid and enzymes are also increased. Slaframine does not directly affect cardiovascular function in most species, with the exception of the dog and the guinea pig.

Slaframine toxicosis has been reported in cattle, sheep, horses, goats, pigs, cats, dogs, guinea pigs, and poultry.

Swainsonine: See section on Darling pea (*S. canescens*).

Clinical Signs

Effects of slaframine become evident within hours in cattle and may be evident in 15 minutes in small herbivores such as guinea pigs. Animals exhibit pronounced hypersalivation, which may last for hours or days. Animals may also exhibit anorexia, ruminal tympany, diarrhea, frequent urination, and lacrimation. Dairy cows may have decreased milk production. Sheep, pigs, and guinea pigs have been reported to develop dyspnea and cyanosis, with open-mouth breathing.

Decreased cardiac and respiratory rates, and decreased left ventricular and aortic pressure and consequent decreased cardiac output have been observed in dogs. Guinea pigs may also develop bradycardia, as well as hypothermia.

Abortion has been reported in cattle and experimentally induced in guinea pigs.

The extent to which swainsonine and other, as yet unidentified, toxins produced by *R. leguminicola* may contribute to the clinical features of poisoning is uncertain.

Diagnostic Aids

Slaframine may be detected in suspect feeds.
Swainsonine: See section on Darling pea (*S. canescens*).

Treatment

The contaminated feed should be removed. Atropine may be helpful but in many cases, once clinical signs are evident the toxicosis is refractory to atropine. Water should be provided *ad libitum*, and fluid therapy instituted if the animal is clinically dehydrated. Respiratory distress or hypothermia should be treated symptomatically. There is a lack of information on effective treatment of cardiovascular changes in dogs.

Prognosis

Prognosis is good. Most animals recover uneventfully and deaths are rare.

Necropsy

There is a lack of information on necropsy findings in slaframine toxicosis, because deaths are rare.
Neurological lesions associated with swainsonine have not been reported in slaframine toxicosis, but this may reflect the fact that deaths are rare and brains of affected animals have not be collected, rather than an absence of lesons.

Public Health Considerations

None.

Prevention

The feeding of pasture or hay containing slaframine or swainsonine should be avoided. There is a lack of information on how to detoxify feeds containing either of these mycotoxins.

SPORIDESMIN

Synthesizing Organism

Sporidesmins are found in the spores of the saprophytic fungus *Pithomyces chartarum.*

Distribution

P. chartarum grows on dead plant material such as pasture litter, and is found worldwide, although strains vary in their ability to synthesize sporidesmins. In New Zealand, 86% of *P. chartarum* isolates produce sporidesmins, compared to 67% in Australia. More than 90% of sporidesmin produced is Sporidesmin A.

Circumstances of Poisoning

Clinical cases occur in ruminants grazing improved pastures and are usually associated with perennial ryegrass (*Lolium perenne*) in New Zealand. Toxicosis is most likely to occur when there is close grazing of pastures so that leaf litter is consumed. *P. chartarum* is most likely to sporulate when minimum night temperatures exceed 14°C, day temperatures exceed 20°C, and humidity is near 100%. These conditions are most likely in late summer or early autumn after at least 4 mm of rain.

Toxicokinetics

There is a lack of information on the toxicokinetics of sporidesmins, although they are known to be excreted in urine. Repeated moderate doses tend to cause greater overall liver pathology than single large doses. Clinical signs are typically delayed for 3 days in high exposures, and 10−14 days in moderate exposures.

Mode(s) of Action

Sporidesmins are acutely toxic to the biliary canilicular membranes of the liver, causing reduction in bile flow. Animals develop obstructive cholangitis with impairment of the excretion of phylloerythrin, a photodynamic porphyrin pigment produced by microbial breakdown of chlorophyll. As a result, blood levels of phylloerythrin become elevated. In areas where the blood is exposed to sunlight through unpigmented skin, photosensitization develops. Sporidesmins promote apoptosis, and may also cause direct capillary injury. In sheep and goats in particular, urinary excretion of sporidesmins is associated with hemorrhagic ulcerations in the urinary bladder.

Ruminants and laboratory animals are susceptible to sporidesmin toxicosis. Sheep and fallow deer are the most susceptible ruminant species on a μg/kg basis, followed by cows, red deer, and goats in ascending order of resistance. Merino sheep are less susceptible than breeds of English origin. Among English breeds, Wiltshire sheep appear to be relatively resistant to sporidesmins when compared to wool-producing breeds. Pigs may suffer mild cholangitis without clinical signs, while horses are highly resistant to sporidesmins.

Clinical Signs

Clinical signs in sheep are those of dermal photosensitization, particularly of ears, eyelids, face, and lips. Affected areas are edematous and erythematous, and may exude serum. The lesions are pruritic and self-trauma by scratching or rubbing is superimposed on the initial lesions. Secondary bacterial infection and/or cutaneous myiasis (flystrike) is common. On the examination, sheep exhibit icteric mucous membranes and urine deeply colored by bilirubin and in some cases also by whole blood or heme. Sheep may exhibit urinary incontinence. When only some sheep in a flock may exhibit clinical signs, it is probable that others in the flock are subclinically affected and will exhibit decreased growth, feed conversion, wool production, and reproductive performance. Some fibrosis of hepatic triads and bile ductule proliferation, indicative of subclinical sporidesmin toxicosis, is ubiquitous in sheep in the North Island of New Zealand, with only unweaned lambs having normal hepatic triads.

Lesions in goats are similar to those in sheep but usually less severe.

In dairy cattle the first sign of toxicosis is a sudden decrease in milk production, followed by development of dermal lesions of photosensitivity, usually 14−24 days after sporidesmin ingestion. Lesions are confined to lightly pigmented or pink skin, particularly that with little or no hair cover such as ears, lips, udder, teats, and coronets. Initial lesions of erythema and edema progress to exudation, ulceration, and eschar formation. Cattle develop icterus and bilirubinuria. Some cattle develop erythrocyte fragility with intravascular hemolysis, hemoglobinuria, and anemia.

Dark-skinned cattle with few or no white markings may suffer severe liver injury. These cattle may only show signs of decreased milk production, growth, and reproductive performance, but have impaired hepatic reserve.

Fallow deer develop clinical signs after 7−14 days and exhibit violent shaking of head and ears, severe pruritis, restlessness, icterus, and frequent urination with bilirubinuria. The tongue is often ulcerated as a result of photosensitization while licking pruritic sites. Mortality may be as high as 50% in affected herds.

Diagnostic Aids

Clinical pathology findings are those of elevated GGT, free and conjugated bilirubin, cholesterol, AST, and GDH. Serum albumin is decreased but globulins are increased. PT is increased. Occasional cattle develop an acute hemolytic anemia. In subchronic and chronic cases, all ruminants may develop a normocytic, normochromic anemia. Urinalysis findings are those of bilirubinuria, and may also include hemoglobinuria or hematuria. Secondary bacterial cystitis may be present.

Treatment

Treatment is supportive. Deep shade should be provided and affected animals only put out to graze at night, because severe lesions may result from only a few minutes' exposure to sunlight. Secondary bacterial infections or myiasis should be treated as required.

Prognosis

Prognosis is poor for fallow deer. Most sheep and cattle eventually recover fully, with residual hepatic fibrosis, although breeding animals may succumb the next spring because loss of hepatic reserve leaves them unable to cope with the increased metabolic demands of late pregnancy and early lactation.

Necropsy

On necropsy the tissues are icteric. In acute toxicosis the liver is pale and swollen, although later it develops a greenish color. The gall bladder is typically distended and the mucosal surface may be severely ulcerated. Extrahepatic bile ducts are distended.

Livers of convalescent or recovered animals have bile ductule proliferation and periportal fibrosis, and may be grossly misshapen.

Ulceration of the mucosal surface of the bladder, cystitis, and pyelonephritis may be present.

Sheep may have adrenal cortical hyperplasia.

Fallow deer may have severe pulmonary edema and interstitial emphysema, ulceration of the tongue, and gastric or intestinal ulcerations, which may have perforated with consequent peritonitis. Liver and urinary tract lesions are similar to those in sheep. Pulmonary lesions have also been reported in goats.

Public Health Considerations

None.

Prevention

In New Zealand, high spore counts may be considered to be predictive of risk because most strains of *P. chartarum* are toxigenic. District advisories on spore counts are available by radio and internet. On-farm monitoring of spore counts is recommended because there may be multiple microclimates within the property. Commercial services exist to conduct spore counts on samples collected by farmers, or the farmer may purchase a microscope and hemocytometer slide to perform the counting. Information on sample collection and submission is readily available on the internet.

When spore counts are high, a daily dose of a zinc salt, equivalent to 25 mg/kg zinc, should be administered. Intraruminal devices that provide a slow-release depot of zinc are commercially available. Administration of zinc sulfate through drinking water is effective in dairy cows because of their high water intake but less reliable in other livestock. Cows should be habituated to the taste in advance of anticipated rises in spore counts, to avoid a transient decline in water intake. Other options are drenching with zinc oxide, or application of zinc oxide to pasture or to a supplement with which the animals are familiar.

Pasture may be sprayed with benzimidazole fungicides to inhibit the proliferation of *P. chartarum*, although this approach may not be suitable for hill country because it requires that the land is accessible to a vehicle with a spray boom. Sprayed pasture may remain safe for up to 6 weeks but must be sprayed again if, within 3 days of spraying, more than 25 mm of rain falls in a 24-hour period. Pasture that already has a high spore count may be made safe by fungicide spraying provided it is withheld from grazing for at least 5 days.

Ruminants should not be forced to graze pasture closely when spore counts are high, because this increases the risk of ingesting leaf litter. Hay or crops may be provided as alternative feed. Pasture with a high spore count can be made into hay because the sporidesmin level declines rapidly under normal conditions of haymaking and storage.

Rams bred for resistance to sporidesmin toxicosis should be used as replacement sires in severely affected areas.

STACHYBOTRYOTOXINS

Synthesizing Organism

Stachybotrys species, of which the best known is *Stachybotrys atra*.

Distribution

Stachybotrys species grow on cellulose-rich materials including grains, paper (including wallpaper), wood, and straw, under circumstances of high moisture. Heavy growth in buildings is colloquially known as "black mold" and incriminated in "sick building syndrome."

Circumstances of Poisoning

Toxicoses in animals have been associated with the feeding of moldy straw or the use of moldy straw as bedding.

Toxicokinetics

There is a lack of information on the toxicokinetics of the stachybotryotoxins.

Mode(s) of Action

Stachybotryotoxins include satratoxins F, G, and H, verrucarin J and roridin E, and trichoverrols A and B. The satratoxins, verrucarin J, and roridin E are macrocyclic trichothecenes, which are irritant to skin and mucous membranes, and disrupt protein synthesis. Cells with the highest rate of mitosis, including gastrointestinal mucosal cells (enterocytes), lymphoid tissues, and bone marrow, are the most susceptible to this effect.

Clinical Signs

Clinical signs in the horse include erythema and edema of the nose, lips, oral cavity, and tongue, progressing to malodorous necrotic lesions in the mouth. Regional lymph nodes may be hypertrophied and develop necrotic areas. Horses may develop gastroenteritis and diarrhea.

Lambs fed contaminated wheat straw have developed anorexia, hypersalivation, inflammation of lips and nose, and depression. Some animals may develop dyspnea, nasal discharge, diarrhea, and/or pyrexia. Similar clinical signs have been reported in cattle. Immunosuppression may lead to death from secondary infections.

Contact dermatitis is the first sign of toxicosis in pigs, and may occur on the lips and nose, on the udder of sows and around the mouth in piglets. The dermatitis progresses from serous to necrotizing. Pigs are typically depressed. *Stachybotrys* toxicosis has been suspected of causing abortion in pregnant sows.

Clinical signs in poultry include depression, anorexia, necrotic lesions of the oral cavity and tongue, and contact dermatitis on the legs.

Diagnostic Aids

Initial hematology findings are those of acute leukocytosis, followed by thrombocytopenia and leukopenia with relative eosinophilia.

Suspect bedding or feed may be tested for the presence of stachybotryotoxins.

Treatment

Treatment is symptomatic. It should be borne in mind that animals are likely to be immunosuppressed and may need broad-spectrum antibiotic cover to prevent secondary infection, even with pathogens against which the animals have previously been vaccinated. Vaccines given during toxicosis are unlikely to stimulate a protective antibody response.

Prognosis

Prognosis varies with severity of poisoning, but is guarded if leukopenia is present.

Necropsy

Postmortem findings in horses include oral, esophageal and gastric ulcerations, gastrointestinal inflammation and hemorrhage, hemorrhages in muscle, and lymphoid necrosis. Extensive hemorrhages have been reported in dogs in the subcutis, pleura, and diaphragm. Sheep develop multiple ecchymoses, as well as oral, forestomach, and gastroenteric inflammation. Tonsils, Peyer's patches, and other gut-associated lymphoid tissue may have necrotic areas. Histologically, areas of B-lymphocyte predominance in lymph nodes and spleen are most severely affected.

Liver, kidney, and ruminal or gastric content should be collected and frozen for possible later analysis for stachybotryotoxins.

Public Health Considerations

In human beings, stachybotryotoxins are associated with contact dermatitis, upper respiratory tract irritation, fever, malaise, headache, and fatigue. It has been suggested that at least some cases of sudden infant death syndrome may be caused by stachybotryotoxin exposure.

Prevention

Straw for bedding or feed should be stored dry (<20%) moisture and should not be used if it has areas of black mold. Animal housing should be kept as dry as possible and monitored for "black mold."

TREMORGENIC MYCOTOXINS ASSOCIATED WITH GRASSES (LOLITREMS, PASPALININE, AND PASPALITREMS)

Synthesizing Organism

Lolitrems are synthesized by *Neotyphodium lolii*, an endophytic fungus of perennial ryegrass, *L. perenne*.

Paspalinine and paspalitrems A and B are synthesized by *Claviceps paspali*, which infects paspalum grass (Dallis grass; *Paspalum* spp.).

Distribution

Both tremorgenic mycotoxins are found in pastures in Australia and New Zealand.

Circumstances of Poisoning

The levels of lolitrems and related compounds increase in ryegrass in late spring and persist into autumn. The highest levels of endophyte and mycotoxins are found in the lower leaves and the stems of ryegrass plants, and therefore staggers is most likely when pastures are heavily grazed.

The sclerotia containing the mycotoxins of *C. paspali* mature in autumn.

Toxicokinetics

There is little specific information on the toxicokinetics of lolitrems, but signs develop gradually over a few days and may persist for up to 7 days after animals are removed from pasture.

Similarly, there is very little information on the toxicokinetics of the mycotoxins of *C. paspali*, but in experimental cases, clinical signs take more than 48 hours to appear after exposure commences, and clinical signs may persist for several days after animals are removed from the pasture.

Mode(s) of Action

Lolitrem B, paspalitrems A and C, and paspalinine have been shown to inhibit the function of high-conductance calcium-activated potassium channels, and to reduce concentration or function of inhibitory amino acids including GABA and glycine.

Clinical Signs

"Ryegrass staggers" is most often reported in cattle but may also occur in sheep, deer, llamas, and horses. "Paspalum staggers" has been reported in cattle, sheep, and horses.

Signs are mild or absent when animals are at rest but become more severe when animals are moved or otherwise agitated. Signs include fine tremors of the head and neck, stiffness, ataxia, hypermetria, and opisthotonus, and may progress to seizures. However, clinical signs generally subside rapidly if animals are left undisturbed. Occasionally animals may become aggressive.

Diagnostic Aids

The presence of the endophyte in perennial ryegrass may be confirmed by microscopic examination, while the sclerotia of *C. paspali* are visible on seedheads of infected *Paspalum* species.

Some laboratories may offer a mouse bioassay to confirm the presence of tremorgenic mycotoxins.

Treatment

There is no specific treatment. Animals should be removed from the suspect pasture and kept in a quiet safe place.

Prognosis

Prognosis is generally excellent, although recovery may take several days. Mortality is rare and usually associated with accidents such as falling off banks or cliffs, or drowning in water.

Necropsy

There are no specific signs or samples at necropsy.

Public Health Considerations

These mycotoxins do not accumulate in fat or muscle, so meat from affected animals is safe to eat.

Handling of affected horses should be the minimum required to move them from affected pasture, and riding should be avoided, until they are fully recovered.

Prevention

Prevention of ryegrass staggers is complicated by the widespread reliance on perennial ryegrass pastures, particularly in New Zealand, and by the fact that the endophyte confers on the grass resistance to insect attack, so that infected pastures tend to grow better than pastures that are endophyte-free. Heavy grazing of infected perennial ryegrass pastures in late summer or early autumn should be avoided if possible, in order to minimize consumption of stems and lower leaves. Cultivars of perennial ryegrass infected with a strain of endophyte that does not produce lolitrem B or ergovaline are available in New Zealand.

Infected paspalum pastures should either be avoided when the sclerotia are present, or, if the terrain allows mowing, topped to remove infected seedheads.

TRICHOTHECENES (OTHER THAN STACHYBOTRYOTOXINS)

Synthesizing Organism

Principally fungi of the genus *Fusarium*.

Distribution

The trichothecenes deoxynivenol (DON), diacetoxyscirpenol (DAS), and T-2 toxin are most likely to be in cereal crops such as corn, wheat, and barley.

Circumstances of Poisoning

Contamination of grains with these mycotoxins is most likely to occur in the field prior to harvest, under conditions of high rainfall, high humidity, and delayed harvesting.

Toxicokinetics

Trichothecenes are readily absorbed by the oral route. Hydroxylated metabolites are excreted by both biliary and renal routes, within a few days in ingestion.

Mode(s) of Action

DON causes mild to moderate gastroenteric lesions in pigs, and is also a centrally acting emetic. DAS and more particularly T-2, like the trichothecenes produced by *Stachybotrys* species (q.v.), are radiomimetic substances that affect rapidly dividing cells of the bone marrow, lymphoid tissues, and intestinal mucosa, and cause lesions similar to those of ionizing radiation. Mechanisms of this effect include inhibition of protein synthesis and inhibition of nucleic acid synthesis.

Clinical Signs

All these trichothecenes are associated with gastroenteritis and diarrhea.

Dietary levels of DON ≥ 1 ppm cause a dose-related reduction in feed consumption in pigs, with feed refusal at ≥ 20 ppm. DON also causes decreased feed intake and vomiting in dogs, but is well tolerated by ruminants and horses.

DAS and T-2 toxin at levels ≥ 2 ppm cause decreased food comsumption in pigs, and at 4 ppm or more, oral irritation, dermal irritation, and immunosuppression may develop. At 16 ppm, both mycotoxins are likely to cause emesis and complete feed refusal in pigs.

Dermal lesions in pigs are often manifested as crusting lesions on the snout, buccal commissures, behind the ears and around the prepuce. Poultry may also develop oral ulcers and exhibit feed refusal.

Diagnostic Aids

Immunosuppression in pigs may be evident as leukopenia. Anemia and thrombocytopenia may also be present. There is limited evidence that T-2 toxin may be associated with increased activated partial thromboplastin time and PT.

Mycotoxin screens, including rapid tests, are available for these mycotoxins.

Treatment

The feed refusal helps to limit toxicosis. Contaminated feed should be removed and replaced. Dermatitis and, if it occurs, diarrhea should be treated as required. Stress, and exposure to pathogens, particularly novel pathogens should be avoided, due to possible immunosuppressed state, and vaccinations should be delayed until normal leukocyte counts are present.

Prognosis

Prognosis is generally good in moderate toxicosis, provided that contaminated feed is removed, appropriate supportive care is provided, and opportunistic infection is avoided or treated.

Necropsy

Lesions reported for DAS and T-2 toxicosis include oral ulceration, gastrointestinal ulceration, enteritis, ulceration of tonsils and Peyer's patches, and lymphoid depletion. Broiler chickens ingesting high doses of T-2 toxin may grow small, misshapen feathers.

Public Health Considerations

Because trichothecenes are rapidly excreted, residues in animal products do not pose a public health hazard.

Prevention

Grains or processed feeds should be obtained only from reputable suppliers who can provide data to show that testing for trichothecene mycotoxins has been conducted and that levels are within acceptable limits.

ZEARALENONE

Synthesizing Organisms

Fusarium species, particularly *Fusarium graminarium* and *F. moniliforme*.

Distribution

Substrates include maize, wheat, and barley. Zearalenone has been detected in grains grown in warmer parts of Australia such as Queensland, but at low levels, and zearalenone toxicosis does not appear to be a significant problem.

Circumstances of Poisoning

Fungal proliferation and mycotoxin synthesis are most likely in humid conditions. The practice of rapidly drying grain in Australia is likely to be a significant protective factor against zearalenone toxicosis. Zearalenone synthesis in North America is often associated with considerable fluctuation in ambient temperature during maturation and harvesting of the grain substrates, whereas in Australia, temperatures during maturation and harvesting tend to be more stable.

Toxicokinetics

Zearalenone is rapidly absorbed following ingestion. It is metabolized to zearalenols and excreted by both the biliary and renal routes. Enterohepatic cycling delays excretion. Small amounts of zearalenone may be secreted in milk.

Mode(s) of Action

Zearalenone acts as a potent nonsteroidal estrogen, binding to receptors for estradiol-17β.

Clinical Signs

Clinical signs are those of excessive estrogen administration, and are most often observed in pigs. Gilts may show estrous behavior, vulval swelling that may lead to prolapse, and mammary development. Signs in mature breeding sows may be of nymphomania, or anestrus and pseudopregnancy, depending on the stage of the estrus cycle when exposure commences. Barrows may develop preputial and nipple enlargement. Mature boars are resistant to toxicosis, but young boars and young bulls may suffer testicular atrophy. Mammary enlargement in heifers, and vaginitis in mature cows, have been reported. Ewes may exhibit reduced ovulation rates and increased duration of estrus. Pregnant ewes may abort.

Diagnostic Aids

Zearalenone may be detected in suspect feed, bearing in mind that clinical signs, particularly pseudopregnancy, may persist for some time after exposure ceases.

Treatment

Exposure to dietary zearalenone must be halted, and prolapse or vaginitis treated. Anestrous sows may respond to prostaglandin $F_2\alpha$ injections.

Prognosis

Most animals will recover in 1–4 weeks after cessation of exposure, but sows may remain in pseudopregnancy for up to 10 weeks and young boars and young bulls may be permanently infertile or subfertile.

Necropsy

Necropsy and histopathology findings in pigs include ovarian atrophy, follicular atresia, squamous metaplasia in cervix and vagina, uterine edema and hypertrophy, and cystic, degenerative endometrial glands. Lesions in mammary gland include ductal hyperplasia and epithelial proliferation.

Public Health Considerations

Although zearalenone has been found in human foods, it is principally found in grain-derived foods rather than as residues from animal products.

Prevention

Rapid drying of harvested grain, and storage under dry conditions, is an important preventative measure. Grain containing 1 ppm or more of zearalenone is unsuitable for feeding to gilts, while grain containing 3 ppm or more is unsuitable for sows. Corresponding thresholds of toxicological concern are 10 ppm for maiden heifers, 15 ppm for pregnant sows, 20 ppm for young boards and 25 ppm for mature cows.

MUSHROOMS

Introduction

In both Australia and New Zealand, there are numerous species of mushroom for which the edibility or toxicity is unknown. Toxicosis due to ingestion of mushrooms nevertheless appears to be extremely rare in domestic animals.

Only the most significant species in Australia and New Zealand are discussed here. They include:

- *Agaricus xanthodermus* and *Agaricus pilatianus*
- *Amanita phalloides* and *Amanita pantherina*
- *Amanita muscaria*
- *Aseroë rubra*
- *Chlorophyllum molybdites*
- *Phallus* species
- *Psilocybe* species (and other psilocybin-containing mushrooms).

AGARICUS XANTHODERMUS AND *AGARICUS PILATIANUS*

Alternative Names

These mushrooms share the common name "Yellow Stainer."

Distribution

Both species commonly grow wild in lawns and gardens, often in clusters or fairy rings.

Appearance

The caps of these mushrooms typically range from 50 to 200 mm in diameter. The cap is white. The gills are white but make become brown with age. *Agaricus xanthoderma* stains bright yellow, fading to brown, when bruised, but only young specimens of *A. pilatianus* exhibit this characteristic. The yellow staining is most distinctive at the base of the stalk. Young mushrooms may have a somewhat square cap.

Both species have a characteristic unpleasant odor, which becomes even more apparent when they are cooked. The odor is variously described as resembling phenol, disinfectant, iodine, kerosene, or ink. It is likely that this odor serves to warn domestic animals not to eat the mushrooms.

Circumstances of Poisoning

Yellow Stainer mushrooms have caused human cases of poisoning because of their resemblance to the field or meadow mushroom *Agaricus campestris* and the cultivated mushroom *Agaricus bisporus*. Most cases of poisoning have occurred in preschool children.

Absorption, Distribution, Metabolism, and Excretion

Clinical signs usually develop within 30–120 minutes in human beings, indicating rapid absorption.

Mode(s) of Action

The substance or substances responsible for toxicosis are not clearly defined, although phenol and related compounds have been isolated from *A. xanthodermus* in sufficient concentrations to cause toxicosis.

Clinical Signs

Symptoms and clinical signs in human beings include headache, nausea, abdominal cramps, vomiting, and diarrhea. Dizziness, diaphoresis (sweating), and drowsiness have also been reported. In most adults, clinical signs resolve within a few hours, but in some cases recovery has been delayed 48 hours. Fluid loss may be life-threatening in small children.

Curiously, some human beings can eat Yellow Stainer mushrooms with impunity.

Diagnostic Aids

There are no specific diagnostic aids.

Treatment

Treatment is symptomatic.

Prognosis

Prognosis is favorable in adult human beings, but may be guarded in small children. The prognosis in domestic animals is unknown.

Necropsy

There are no specific lesions. Nonspecific lesions of gastroenteritis, intestinal congestion, or hemorrhage, and dehydration would be expected.

Public Health Considerations

Poisoning with Yellow Stainer mushrooms is common in human beings, particularly in Australia, but does not appear to be a problem in animals.

Prevention

People should be warned to always smell mushrooms they collect, and to check for yellow staining. Mushrooms with an offensive odor should not be eaten. It should be noted that the edible Horse Mushroom, *Agaricus arvensis*, also exhibits yellow staining but has a pleasant odor resembling anise or licorice. *A. arvensis* is prized in North America, Britain, Europe, and Western Asia, and immigrants from any of those areas may collect Yellow Stainer mushrooms in error, misled by the yellow staining, if they have a poor sense of smell.

AMANITA PHALLOIDES

Alternative Names

Death Cap, Death Angel.

Distribution

A. phalloides is typically found in groups, most commonly under deciduous or less commonly coniferous trees. They are often found under oak trees. They are believed to have originated in Europe but are now found worldwide.

Appearance

A. phalloides initially appears to be a white ball at the soil surface. As the mushroom grows, this ball forms a characteristic cup, the volva, at the base of the stalk, but this may be inapparent because it may be located underground. The cap is usually white but may be pale yellow or greenish, and does not have striations at the margins. The gills are white, and are initially covered by a veil that breaks to form a skirt-like annulus near the top of the stalk. Younger specimens may have an odor said to resemble that of rose petals, but older mushrooms may have an offensive odor. The cap may reach up to 16 cm in diameter. From above, on cursory examination, *A. phalloides* may be mistaken for the field or meadow mushroom *A. campestris*.

Asian immigrants to Australia or New Zealand have been poisoned because they mistook *A. phalloides* to the very similar, and edible, Asian species *Volvariella volvacea*, which is also known as the Paddy Straw Mushroom or simply as the Straw Mushroom.

Note: There are a number of other *Amanita* species, which share the common name Destroying Angel, that contain the same toxins as *A. phalloides* and which also have the volva, the annulus, and the characteristic white gills, although they differ from *A. phalloides* in that the color of the cap is not as variable. It is safest to assume that mushrooms with white gills should never be consumed.

Amatoxin toxicosis has also occasionally resulted from consumption of mushrooms in other genera, notably *Lepiota* and *Galerina*.

Circumstances of Poisoning

A. *phalloides* is by far the leading cause of fatal mushroom poisoning worldwide, due to their passing resemblance to A. *campestris* and their extremely toxic nature. A. *phalloides* are reported to be palatable. Amatoxins are water-soluble, extremely thermostable, and resistant to acids and enzymes, and are not destroyed by cooking, boiling, soaking, or drying.

One mushroom is likely to contain enough amatoxins to kill an average adult human being.

A. *phalloides* mistaken for edible species and added to dishes such as casseroles could pose a risk to domestic pets as well as humans. Experimentally, dogs have been shown to be susceptible to poisoning with amatoxins.

Absorption, Distribution, Metabolism, and Excretion

The toxic principles in A. *phalloides* are amatoxins and phallotoxins, but phallotoxins are not absorbed by the gastrointestinal route, so toxicity following ingestion of mushrooms is due to amatoxins.

Amatoxins are rapidly absorbed, and severely hepatotoxic concentrations in the liver may be reached within an hour of ingestion. Amatoxins are detectable in human plasma for 24–48 hours after ingestion of A. *phalloides*, although plasma levels are not well correlated to severity of toxicosis. Amatoxins are excreted into the bile but undergo extensive enterohepatic cycling, resulting in prolonged exposure of liver cells. Effective clearance from the body is principally by the urinary route.

Mode(s) of Action

Amatoxins bind with a subunit of DNA-dependent RNA polymerase II, the enzyme responsible for the transcription of DNA to mRNA. As a result, formation of mRNA is inhibited and protein synthesis disrupted. The lack of essential proteins leads to cellular necrosis. Cells with a high rate of protein synthesis are the first to be affected by this mechanism, with the result that gastrointestinal effects are the first observed. Liver necrosis is delayed due to the slow degradation of the preexisting reservoir of mRNA in the liver. In later stages of toxicosis, necrosis of the proximal renal tubules may also occur, due to the direct effects of amatoxins, the secondary effects of hepatic failure, or both.

The length of time that amatoxins are present in the cell at a concentration sufficient to inhibit transcription is critical, and enterohepatic cycling extends this time for hepatocytes, with the result that fulminant hepatic failure is the most serious consequence of A. *phalloides* consumption.

Clinical Signs

In human beings, gastrointestinal signs including abdominal pain, nausea, vomiting, and severe watery diarrhea develop 6−24 hours after ingestion of *A. phalloides*. These clinical signs resolve 24−48 hours after ingestion, giving a false impression that the patient is recovering, but hepatic necrosis is progressing. The patient then deteriorates with acute liver failure, severe coagulopathy, hypoglycemia, acidosis, and hepatic encephalopathy. Acute renal failure with oliguria or anuria may also develop.

Diagnostic Aids

Clinical pathology findings are those of rapidly progressing hepatic failure, including steep rises in serum transaminases and rapidly developing coagulopathy. Elevation of bilirubin occurs in severe cases, and findings indicative of renal failure occur in the most severe cases.

Treatment

Treatment includes supportive measures including fluid and electrolyte replacement.

In human cases, intravenous therapy with silibinin has made a significant difference to mortality rates from *A. phalloides* poisoning. The recommended protocol in human beings is a single loading dose of 5 mg silibinin/kg, followed by 20 mg silibinin/kg via continuous infusion over 24 hours. If treatment is delayed while silibinin is obtained, aggressive hydration therapy to avert oliguric renal failure should be performed.

N-Acetyl cysteine (NAC) may also be helpful in conjunction with silibinin. NAC is usually administered intravenously in 5% dextrose, although 0.9% saline may be also used. The suggested dosage in human beings is 150 mg/kg over 15 min intravenously, followed by 50 mg/kg over 4 hours intravenously, followed by 100 mg/kg over 16 hours intravenously.

Hemoperfusion and plasmaphoresis have not been shown to useful in human cases of *A. phalloides* poisoning. The use of a Molecular Adsorbent Recirculating System appears to be useful.

Advances in treatment have significantly reduced the mortality rate from *A. phalloides* consumption in human beings, but this mushroom remains a significant cause of liver transplants and of death.

Prognosis

Mild toxicosis, characterized by gastrointestinal effects but minimal to mild evidence of hepatic dysfunction, has a hopeful prognosis. The prognosis is very poor to grave if there is evidence of severe hepatic dysfunction, with or without bilirubinemia, and grave to hopeless if renal dysfunction also develops. Liver transplant is often required in human patients if there is severe hepatic dysfunction, even in the absence of renal dysfunction.

Necropsy

Lesions are those of severe hepatocyte degeneration and necrosis, and necrosis of proximal renal tubules. Petechiae and ecchymoses are likely to be present, and icterus may also be present.

Public Health Considerations

Mushroom hunters should never collect or consume mushrooms with white gills, and should also be aware of the characteristic annulus and volva. The field mushroom, *A. campestris*, has gills that are never lighter than a medium pink-beige, but which progress to a deep seal-brown as the mushroom matures and ages. It may have an annulus, but does not have a volva. The Paddy Straw Mushroom, *V. volvacea*, has a volva but does not have an annulus, and the gills are pale pinkish-brown. *V. volvacea* does not grow in Australia or New Zealand.

Prevention

Mushrooms or toadstools growing in dog pens should be removed, particularly if the dog is a puppy and at risk of playing with strange objects out of boredom. Grazing animals do not appear to be attracted to mushrooms or toadstools.

AMANITA MUSCARIA AND *AMANITA PANTHERINA*

Alternative Names

A. muscaria: Fly agaric, Fly amanita.
  A. pantherina: Panthercap.

Distribution

These mushrooms are introduced species in both Australia and New Zealand. *A. muscaria* is commonly found under pine trees, but may be spreading into native forest in Australia.

Appearance

A. muscaria is the distinctive mushroom often illustrated in childrens' books, with a red or orange-red cap with white or pale warty spots, a white stem with a white skirt-like annulus, and a volva that forms two or three scaly rings around the base of the stem. Gills are white. The cap may be up to 25 cm in diameter and the stem may be up to 22 cm. It often grows in groups.

A. pantherina is similar to *A. muscaria* but has a tan or brown cap rather than a red or orange one, although it also has the pale spots on the cap, which in both species are remnants of a universal veil. The annulus, volva, and white gills are as for *A. muscaria*.

Note: The native Australian species *Amanita xanthocephala* is a similar color to *A. muscaria*, but is smaller and has no annulus. It is typically found in eucalyptus forests.

Circumstances of Poisoning

These mushrooms do not appear to be attractive to domestic livestock or pets, but appeal to some people because of the presence of psychoactive chemicals, primarily muscimol and ibotenic acid, in both species. As for other recreational drugs, there is a possibility that dried material may be deliberately fed to domestic pets, or that puppies in particular may chew on dried material when teething.

Immature *A. muscaria* has been mistaken for puffballs and collected and cooked in error.

There are some traditional preparation and cooking procedures that make *A. muscaria* safe for human consumption, but toxicosis may occur if these are not followed correctly.

Absorption, Distribution, Metabolism, and Excretion

The rapid onset of clinical signs indicates that absorption of muscimol and ibotenic acid is rapid. Both ibotenic acid and muscimol readily cross the blood—brain barrier. Ibotenic acid is metabolized to muscimol by decarboxylation, and this metabolism occurs in the brain. Consequently it is thought that most of the toxic effects are due to muscimol. Excretion is via the renal route. Muscimol has been detected in urine within 1 hour of ingestion.

Mode(s) of Action

Muscimol binds to GABA receptors, inhibiting the uptake of GABA by neurons and glia. Ibotenic acid acts on inhibitory glutamate receptors.

Clinical Signs

Reported clinical signs of *A. muscaria* or *A. pantherina* ingestion in human beings are variable but may include incoordination, light-headedness, mood elevation progressing to euphoria, spatial distortion, heightened visual and auditory sensitivity, mydriasis, anxiety, agitation, depression, and alternating periods of lethargy and agitation. Seizures and coma may occur in severe intoxication, but respiration is usually not depressed unless the patient requires heavy sedation due to agitation. Recovering patients report residual headache for several days.

Note: Although it was long thought that the toxic principle in *A. muscaria* was muscarine, in fact there is generally very little muscarine in this mushroom and muscarinic clinical signs, such as hypotension and hypersalivation are not part of the typical toxidrome.

Diagnostic Aids

Dried mushroom material may be analyzed for muscimol and ibotenic acid, which are stable at room temperature for at least 3 months.

Treatment

Treatment is supportive. Due to the rapid absorption, decontamination is very unlikely to be useful. Agitation or seizures are generally responsive to diazepam or other benzodiazepines. Intubation is not indicated unless there are seizures. Most patients require only observation and confinement to a safe, quiet environment with monitoring.

The use of atropine or physostigmine is not recommended.

Prognosis

Prognosis is excellent provided that the patient is protected from traumatic misadventure, and provided any seizure activity or severe agitation is controlled to prevent exhaustion and acidosis.

Necropsy

There are no typical necropsy findings.

Public Health Considerations

A. muscaria or *A. pantherina* may be tried as recreational drugs although they are not particularly popular, because the effects are highly unpredictable and it may result in mood depression rather than elevation. Also, use may be followed by prolonged headaches, episodes of somnolence, and amnesia.

Prevention

These species and all mushrooms and toadstools, other than *A. campestris*, should be removed from dog pens or runs to prevent dogs or puppies from gnawing on them out of boredom.

ASEROË RUBRA

Alternative Names

Red starfish fungus.

Distribution

This species is common and widespread in QLD, NSW, VIC, SA, and TAS. It grows in leaf litter and may grow in bark chip mulches.

Appearance

This distinctive species has a white or pinkish hollow stem, at the top of which 4–10 pink or red forked "arms" radiate out from a dark olive-brown disk. The fungus has a foul odor like sewage or rotting flesh, which is attractive to flies.

Circumstances of Poisoning

Dogs have been poisoned, presumably because they were attracted by the foul odor.

Absorption, Distribution, Metabolism, and Excretion

No information.

Mode(s) of Action

No information.

Clinical Signs

Clinical signs are those of severe gastrointestinal irritation, which may include hematemesis and dysentery. Loss of consciousness has been reported in one dog.

Diagnostic Aids

Identification of the fungus can be confirmed by a professional mycologist.

Treatment

Treatment is symptomatic and supportive, but should be aggressive because fatalities have been recorded in dogs.

Prognosis

Guarded; may be favorable with aggressive therapy.

Necropsy

Lesions are those of severe gastrointestinal irritation and inflammation.

Public Health Considerations

These fungi are unlikely to pose a risk to human beings because of their repulsive smell.

Prevention

Dog owners with bark mulches in their gardens should be warned to watch for these fungi and to remove them promptly.

CHLOROPHYLLUM MOLYBDITES

Alternative Names

Green-gilled parasol, false parasol.

Distribution

This mushroom is native to Australia but also found in other countries, particularly in the tropics. It is one of the most common causes of mushroom poisoning in North America. There is only one record of this mushroom being found in New Zealand, and this record may be an error.

Appearance

The cap is 10–30 cm in diameter, white to cream in color with concentric rings of brown scales and often with a small central peak of darker color. The cap tends to mature from conical to flat. The gills are white at first but then mature to green. The stem is usually sepia with a prominent annulus. When cut or bruised, the flesh darkens to a pink or red shade.

Circumstances of Poisoning

Dogs have been poisoned. Human beings have been poisoned after mistaking this mushroom for an edible species.

Absorption, Distribution, Metabolism, and Excretion

Onset of toxicosis in human beings may be within 30 minutes of ingestion, and is usually within 2 hours, indicating rapid absorption.

Mode(s) of Action

The toxin is a gastrointestinal irritant. It not fully characterized but has a molecular weight >400 kDa, is water-soluble and is moderately heat-labile, losing all activity if heated to 70°C for 30 minutes. The toxin is present in all parts of the mushroom, with highest concentrations in the cap. The concentration of toxin appears to be variable based on factors such as climatic conditions and age of mushroom. Tolerance of the toxin also appears to be variable between individual people.

Clinical Signs

Clinical signs are those of nausea and vomiting, followed by diarrhea. Human victims of poisoning have reported chills, abdominal pain, and cold sweats. In human beings, toxicosis can last up to 7 days, but usually resolves within 24 hours.

Diagnostic Aids

The mushroom can be identified by a professional mycologist if photographs of the fresh mushroom, dried mushrooms, and a spore print are submitted.

Treatment

Treatment is symptomatic and supportive. In dogs, diarrhea resulting from eating this mushroom is often severe, leading to hypovolemic shock and electrolyte imbalances.

Prognosis

Favorable with prompt, aggressive treatment.

Necropsy

No specific necropsy findings.

Public Health Considerations

This mushroom also poses a risk to human beings, especially small children.

Prevention

Do not allow dogs access to this mushroom.

PHALLUS SPECIES

Alternative Names

Stinkhorns.

Distribution

There are thought to be seven species of *Phallus* in Australia. They have been found in QLD, NSW, VIC, TAS, and SA. *Phallus* species do not appear to occur in New Zealand.

Appearance

Phallus species are so-named because their shape bears some resemblance to that of an erect penis. They vary in color depending on species. They typically have an offensive odor like that of sewage or rotting flesh. This odor is attractive to flies.

Circumstances of Poisoning

Because of their odor, like that of sewage or rotting flesh, stinkhorns are attractive to dogs.

Absorption, Distribution, Metabolism, and Excretion

Onset of clinical signs in some dogs within 2 hours of consumption indicates rapid absorption of the toxin/s.

Mode(s) of Action

Unknown.

Clinical Signs

Clinical signs have included vomiting, dysentery, ataxia, miosis, hypersalivation, cardiopulmonary dysfunction, collapse, and sudden death.

Diagnostic Aids

Liver enzymes may be elevated in serum. Clotting times may be prolonged.
   Fungal identification can be confirmed by a professional mycologist.

Treatment

Treatment is symptomatic and supportive, but should be aggressive.

Prognosis

Prognosis varies depending on dose and on whether treatment is prompt and aggressive.

Necropsy

Necropsy findings may include pulmonary congestion; severe gastroenteritis, which may be hemorrhagic; and hepatic degeneration/necrosis.

These fungi are unlikely to pose a risk to human beings because of their repulsive smell.

Prevention

Dog owners should be warned that dogs should not be allowed to consume these fungi.

PSILOCYBE SPECIES AND RELATED HALLUCINOGENIC SPECIES

Alternative Names

Magic mushrooms, shrooms.

Distribution

These species grow in pasture or on rotting wood, dung, or compost. The most common species in Australia are *Psilocybe cubensis*, *Psilocybe subcubensis*, *Psilocybe subaeruginosa*, *Copelandia cyanescens*, and *Gymnopilus junonius*, while the most common species in New Zealand are *Psilocybe semilanceata* and *C. cyanescens*.

Appearance

Psilocybe species are "little brown mushrooms" (LBMs) that closely resemble a number of other species such as *Galerina* spp. Although *Panaeolina foenisecii* has been reported to contain serotonin and related compounds, and is often mistakenly reported to contain psilocybin, it is not psychoactive or toxic, although it is not particularly palatable. *Galerina* species, on the other hand, often contain highly hepatotoxic amatoxins and may therefore cause toxicosis similar to that of *A. phalloides*. For this reason, it is recommended that LBMs should never be consumed.

G. junonius is a large golden-brown mushroom typically found on rotting wood. Caps may be up to 15 cm in diameter. Gills range from cream to brown. Stems are up to 10 cm tall and up to 25 mm thick, golden or tan with silky brown "hairs." Common names for the mushroom are spectacular rust-gill, big laughing gym, and laughing mushroom. It is found in NSW, VIC, TAS, SA, and WA.

The appearance of hallucinogenic mushrooms varies between species. Many but not all species of psilocybin-containing mushrooms bruise blue when handled or damaged, and blue discoloration may also be present at the base of the stem.

Circumstances of Poisoning

Psilocybe and related genera of mushrooms are consumed fresh or dried, or as an infusion in tea, for their hallucinogenic properties, and domestic pets in the households of magic mushroom users may be deliberately or accidentally exposed.

Absorption, Distribution, Metabolism, and Excretion

Absorption is very rapid, with the result that clinical effects may be manifested in as little as 10 minutes. Psilocybin (4-phosphoryloxy-*N,N*-dimethyltryptamine) is dephosphorylated in the liver to psilocin (4-hydroxy-*N,N*-dimethyltryptamine), largely on first pass, so the principal active compound is psilocin. Psilocin is further metabolized to a variety of circulating metabolites, or is glucoronidated for renal excretion. Most of an ingested dose is excreted, principally in urine, within 8 hours.

Mode(s) of Action

Psilocin has a high affinity for the 5-HT2A serotonin receptor in the brain, and mimics the effects of serotonin.

Clinical Signs

The effects of psilocybin ingestion begin 15 minutes to 2 hours after eating and typically last for 6 hours.

The active compound, psilocin, is a hallucinogen with lysergic acid diethylamide-like effects. The effects are highly variable, but human users also report euphoria, visual or auditory perceptual disorders. A "bad trip" may occur, with feelings of anxiety or panic. Other effects of psilocin may include muscle weakness, ataxia, paresthesias, hyperreflexia, mydriasis, dry mouth, nausea, vomiting, loss of urinary control, and drowsiness. Blood pressure and heart rate may be increased. Some users report swings in body temperature and temperature perception, with successive episodes of sweating and shivering.

There may be a posttrip headache. There have been occasional reports of protracted psychosis in some individuals, although it is speculated that these individuals had latent mental illness.

Diagnostic Aids

In human beings, metabolites in urine may be detectable in urine for up to 7 days. If psilocybin ingestion is suspected in an animal, law enforcement authorities may be able to provide information on urine testing.

Treatment

Psilocybin and psilocin are of low toxicity, and are among the least toxic of all recreational psychoactive drugs. The principal risks of ingestion are physical injury due to accidents or self-trauma while hallucinating, and the risk that the mushrooms are not a psilocybin-containing species, but a highly hepatotoxic *Galerina* species.

The patient should be kept in a safe, quiet place with moderate ambient temperature, and monitored.

Prognosis

Prognosis is excellent provided that the patient is kept safe.

Psilocybin is not addictive, but repeated use may result in tolerance, so that the user is refractory to the effects.

Necropsy

Death is highly unlikely unless the patient has an accident while hallucinating. The postmortem sample of choice to confirm exposure is urine, aspirated from the bladder.

Public Health Considerations

Possession, sale, transport, or cultivation of psilocybin mushrooms is illegal in both Australia and New Zealand.

Prevention

Domestic pets and livestock do not appear to be inclined to eat psilocybin mushrooms.

Chapter 22

Venomous and Poisonous Vertebrates

Part 1: Venomous and Poisonous Terrestrial Vertebrates in Australia

The venomous and poisonous terrestrial vertebrates in Australia include the following:

> Cane toads, *Rhinella marinus* (formerly *Bufo marinus*)
> Platypus
> Snakes—endemic *Elapidae* of Australia.

CANE TOAD *RHINELLA MARINUS*

Alternative Names

The former Linnaean name was *Bufo marinus*.

Distribution

The cane toad was introduced to Queensland and is now well established across northern Australia including Northern Territory, northern New South Wales, and northern Western Australia. There have been occasional findings of cane toads in Victoria, South Australia, and Tasmania, although it is thought that some of these were stowaways in shipments of furniture belonging to people moving interstate. The range of the cane toad is expanding.

Appearance

The cane toad is a large toad, up to 24 cm in length, but averaging 10−15 cm. Females are significantly larger than males. They have a dry warty skin and are generally a brown/yellow color, although color varies, including gray, red/brown, and olive/brown. The ventral surface is lighter in

Veterinary Toxicology for Australia and New Zealand
DOI: http://dx.doi.org/10.1016/B978-0-12-420227-6.00021-9

color; cream or pale gray, with or without darker splotches. They have pronounced ridges above their eyes, which have golden irises and horizontal pupils. There is a prominent parotid gland caudal to each eye in adults. The toes of the front limbs are free from webbing, although the toes of the hind limbs are partially webbed. Juvenile cane toads have darker, smoother skin than mature adults. Tadpoles are black.

Circumstances of Poisoning

The cane toad is poisonous rather than venomous, i.e., it does not inject venom but excretes it from glands under the skin. Severe poisoning is most likely to occur when domestic animals, most commonly dogs and less commonly cats, mouth the cane toad. The toad defends itself by contracting periglandular muscles in the skin to secrete a thick cream/white, irritating secretion. The secretion comes from the parotid glands caudal to the eyes, and from smaller glands that are distributed throughout the skin. The secretion contains bufogenins, bufotoxins, catecholamines, dopamine, and serotonin.

The toxic secretion of cane toads can contaminate water supplies or animal feed.

Toxicokinetics

The irritant effects of the secretion on the oral mucosa are immediate. The other toxic components of the secretion are readily absorbed across mucous membranes into the systemic circulation. They can also be absorbed through conjunctiva, through contact with open wounds, and from the gastric mucosa. Onset of systemic signs occurs within a few minutes and death may occur in approximately 15 minutes if exposure is sufficient.

Bufogenins are excreted via the urine by first-order kinetics.

Mode(s) of Action

Bufotoxins and bufogenins are cardioactive, having digitalis-like effects, and they also have vasopressor effects. They bind to Na−K ATPase, inhibiting the enzyme, leading to increased extracellular concentration of potassium and increased intracellular sodium.

Clinical Signs

Initial signs are hypersalivation, pawing at the mouth, head-shaking, vocalization, retching, and vomiting. Mucous membranes are often brick-red. Within a few minutes the animal becomes disorientated, may appear blind, and becomes ataxic. Some dogs may exhibit opisthotonus. Severe toxicosis progresses to seizures and coma.

Diagnostic Aids

Auscultation may reveal tachycardia or bradycardia, arrhythmia, ventricular tachycardia progressing to ventricular fibrillation, and terminally, heart failure.

Clinical pathology findings include increased PCV, glucose and BUN, hyperkalemia, and hypercalcemia. There may be a reduced WBC count.

Treatment

Immediate first aid is copious flushing of the animal's mouth with running water, unless the animal is having seizures or is unconscious.

Diazepam, 0.5 mg/kg IV, should be administered to control seizures.

Cardiac function should be monitored, preferably by ECG.

Atropine should not be administered as a treatment for hypersalivation, but is appropriate for cases of marked bradycardia.

Tachycardia may respond to beta-blockers such as propranolol (up to 2 mg/kg, repeated every 20 minutes if necessary). Ventricular arrhythmia may be treated with lidocaine or procainamide HCl.

Severe hyperkalemia should be treated with an infusion of insulin, glucose, and sodium bicarbonate.

Calcium is *contraindicated*.

Digoxin-specific Fab (Digibind) has been used in human beings.

Prognosis

Mortality in untreated cases ranges from 20% to 100%.

Prognosis in treated cases varies depending on the amount of secretion absorbed, and timeliness and aggressiveness of treatment.

Necropsy

There are no characteristic lesions and analysis for the toxins is not practical. Pulmonary congestion may be present. If the dog ate a toad rather than merely mouthing one, there may be identifiable remnants in the stomach.

Public Health Considerations

Cane toads also pose a risk to human beings, especially small children, who may not wash their hands between investigating a toad and eating, and people with cuts on their hands.

Prevention

Pet owners in areas in which cane toads are established should be warned of the dangers that cane toads pose, and educated about the need for immediate first aid by flushing the mouth with copious running water.

PLATYPUS

Alternative Names

Duck-billed platypus.
The Linnaean name of the platypus is *Ornithorhynchus anatinus*.

Distribution

The natural range is along eastern Australia from Queensland from Victoria, with a slight extension into South Australia, and also Tasmania, King Island, and the Furneaux group. The platypus has also been successfully introduced to Kangaroo Island. The platypus is semiaquatic and is always found in proximity to lakes and streams.

Appearance

The platypus is a monotreme of distinctive appearance, with a dense brown fur, a snout that superficially resembles the bill of a duck, and a broad flat tail. The feet, particularly the fore feet, are webbed. Adult males are generally approximately 50 cm in length while females are approximately 43 cm in length.

Only males deliver venom, via mobile spurs on the hindlegs. The venom is synthesized in crural glands and delivered to the spur through ducts. The spurs of the female are rudimentary and generally fall off in the first year, and the crural glands of the female are not functional.

Circumstances of Poisoning

Reports of platypus envenomation of dogs are anecdotal.

Toxicokinetics

There is a lack of information on the toxicokinetics of platypus venom, but human victims of envenomation report immediate severe pain.

Mode(s) of Action

Platypus venom is a mix of proteins, principally defensin-like proteins.
There is little information on the mechanism by which these proteins exert their toxic effects.

Clinical Signs

Human beings envenomated by platypuses report immediate excruciating pain that may be incapacitating. Edema develops rapidly around the wound and spreads. Some people have reported a long-lasting hyperalgesia follow-ing platypus envenomation.

Diagnostic Aids

None.

Treatment

On the basis of human accounts of envenomation, analgesia would be appropriate.

Prognosis

Reports of fatal envenomation of dogs are anecdotal only.

Necropsy

No information.

Public Health Considerations

People unfamiliar with Australian fauna should be warned not to try to catch or handle platypuses.

Prevention

Platypuses are a protected species and should not be interfered with.

SNAKES

General

Although the distribution of individual species varies, all parts of Australia have dangerous venomous snakes. Most although not all species are shy and avoid confrontation, and all snakes should be left alone and allowed to escape if possible. Snakebite is rare in the winter months in the more temperate parts of Australia, but snakes are active all year in the warmer northern areas.

Almost all venomous terrestrial Australian snakes are members of the Elapidae family (the exception being the Brown Tree Snake, *Boiga irregularis*, which is not of veterinary importance). The action of their venoms is predominantly neurotoxic. Some species also produce venom that causes hemorrhaging. Other toxic effects of venom may include hemolysis, nephrotoxicity, myotoxicity, and cardiotoxicity. Local necrosis at the site of the bite is not generally a significant problem.

For color illustrations of the dangerous venomous snakes of Australia, and detailed descriptions of their appearance and distribution, the reader is referred to the following paper, which is in the public domain and available online:

Shea, GM (1999). The distribution and identification of dangerously venomous Australian terrestrial snakes. *Australian Veterinary Journal* Vol. 77, No. 12, December 1999. http://onlinelibrary.wiley.com/doi/10.1111/j.1751-0813.1999. tb12947.x/epdf.

Another source of color photographs of dangerous venomous snakes is the *CSL Antivenom Handbook*, which is in the public domain and can be read online or downloaded as a pdf file.

The venomous snakes of greatest importance in Australian veterinary practice are the Brown Snake (*Pseudonaja* spp.), the Tiger Snake (*Notechis* spp.), and the Red-Bellied Black Snake (*Pseudechis porphyriacus*). Brown Snakes are found throughout continental Australia but the other two species are distributed along the Eastern seaboard. Of the three, only the Tiger Snake is found in Tasmania. Cats and dogs are the domestic animals most often bitten by venomous snakes. Other species that suffer venomous snake-bites less commonly are horses and cattle. Most cases are attributed to the domestic animal deliberately investigating or, in the case of dogs and cats, trying to catch the snake, but herbivores may be bitten by snakes hiding under hay placed on the ground. Cases of snake envenomation are most common in rural areas, but also occur in urban areas.

In cases in which the snake is not identified, there is a Snake Venom Identification Kit available from CSL Ltd, Parkville, Victoria, although it is expensive. A swab from the bite site is considered to be the sample of choice for this kit, although other body fluids can be used. A study in cats has shown that plasma is a useful sample for this kit only for the first 8 hours, but urine is useful for 24 hours. A very high level of venom in the sample may result in a false-negative reaction. Identification of the venom, either directly, by identi-fication of the snake, or by familiarity with the moderate differences in clinical presentation, is desirable because monovalent antivenom is cheaper than polyvalent, and less likely to be associated with adverse side effects.

CSL Ltd is also the source for antivenoms. The quantity of antivenom required is correlated with the amount of venom in the bite/s, not with the size of the bitten animal, and therefore horses, for example, do not necessar-ily need more antivenom than small animals. Antivenom should be adminis-tered according to clinical response. The *CSL Antivenom Handbook* is in the public domain and can read online or downloaded as a pdf file. It includes photographs of the snakes for which the antivenoms are effective.

Weakness, tremors, hypersalivation, ataxia, and mydriasis are characteris-tic clinical findings in small animals envenomated by snakes. Neurological signs may progress to paralysis particularly if the bite was from a Tiger Snake or Brown Snake. Discoloration of the urine with hemoglobin or myoglobin may be evident. Emesis may occur.

Therapeutic measures for envenomated small animals include administration of antivenom, establishment, and maintenance of intravenous fluid therapy, and respiratory support as required. Prompt administration of antivenom is associated with a significantly improved prognosis. Blood transfusion may be required.

Clinical pathology parameters that should be monitored are PCV and clotting function. BUN and creatinine monitoring may also be useful. Evidence of renal failure worsens prognosis.

Some veterinarians use premedications such as antihistamines, corticosteroids, or adrenalin prior to the administration of antivenom. These premedications are also commonly used in human envenomations but their importance in animal envenomations does not appear to have been the subject of controlled trials. Adrenalin should not be administered IV because it has been suggested that it may be associated with cerebral hemorrhage if coagulopathy is present.

Survival of small animals treated with antivenom is $\geq 75\%$. Cats show a higher survival rate, with or without treatment, than dogs, even though the time from envenomation to presentation tends to be longer for cats, and there is experimental evidence that cats have a higher innate tolerance to the venom of Australian snakes. However, data may be confounded in part by the presentation of cats that have been bitten by small nonvenomous snakes of brown color, mistaken for venomous *Pseudonaja* spp. by the owner. Survival without antivenom treatment is reported to be 66% for cats and 31% for dogs.

Megaesophagus, which slowly but spontaneously resolved, has been reported in a small number of dogs following Tiger Snake envenomation.

There are few published reports of the management of venomous snakebite in horses or cattle. The muzzle seems to be the most common location of bites. Horses may sweat profusely due to pain. Reported clinical signs associated with confirmed Tiger Snake bite in a horse included muscle fasciculation, tachycardia and tachypnea, reluctance to move, myoglobinuria, neutrophilia with left shift, and elevations in CK and AST.

Genus- and Species-Specific Notes and Comments

- *Acanthophis* spp.—Death Adders

    Death Adders are found in all Australian states and territories except Victoria and Tasmania. They are short, thick-bodied snakes with triangular heads. A small number of envenomations of dogs have been reported. As for human envenomations, the clinical effects are neurotoxic, without evidence of coagulopathy or myotoxicity. There is a specific CSL Death Adder Antivenom.

- *Austrelaps* spp.—Copperheads

  It is important to note that these snakes are not closely related to the North American snake *Agkistrodon contortix* that shares the same common name but is a pit viper of the family Crotalidae. These shy snakes are found near water in southeastern Australia and in Tasmania. They do not always have copper-colored heads. The appropriate antivenom is CSL Tiger Snake Antivenom.

- *Hemiaspis daemeli*—Gray Snake

  There is one reported case of fatal envenomation of an adult dog. CSL Polyvalent Antivenom should be administered in the event of envenomation by this snake.

- *Hoplocephalus* spp.—Broad-headed Snakes

  Envenomation of domestic animals has not been reported, but it is thought that the venom in a bite would be sufficient to kill a small domestic animal. CSL Tiger Snake antivenom should be used.

- *Notechis* spp.—Tiger Snakes

  The principle neurotoxin is notexin, which depletes acetylcholine and is also a myotoxin. There is also a procoagulant in the venom and extensive thrombus formation has been reported postmortem in a dog and a cat. However, the clinical presentation, due to the depletion of circulating prothrombin, is a coagulopathy.

  Envenomation has been comparatively well described. The first phase is the preparalytic phase featuring hypersalivation, tremor, vomiting, defecation, and tachypnea.

  This is followed by the paralytic phase that includes skeletal muscle paralysis, coagulopathy, and oliguria. Myoglobinuria and/or hemoglobinuria may be present. Later effects include mydriasis with reduced pupillary reflex, rigidity, and renal failure. If renal failure develops, the prognosis is poor.

  CSL Tiger Snake antivenom should be used.

- *Oxyuranus* spp.—Taipans

  A recent report of envenomation of a dog by a Coastal Taipan is in the public domain:

  Judge PR (2015). Coastal taipan (*Oxyuranus scutellatus*) envenomation of a dog. *Australian Veterinary Journal* 2015;93:412−416. doi: 10.1111/avj.12375.

  Briefly, the dog presented with evidence of neurotoxicity, hemolysis, coagulopathy, and myotoxicity. The appropriate antivenom was identified using Snake Venom Identification Kit, which returned a positive result to Taipan venom. The dog required mechanical ventilation for 4 days, enteral nutrition via nasogastric tube, and intensive fluid therapy.

  CSL Taipan Antivenom should be used.

- *Pseudoechis* spp.—Black Snakes

  The most significant species to the veterinary field is *P. porphyriacus*, the Red-Bellied Black Snake. Venom is both hemolytic and neurotoxic, and the clinical presentation may include intravascular hemolysis, rhabdomyolysis, and anuric renal failure.

- *Pseudonaja* spp.—Brown Snakes

  It should be noted that a number of snake genera and species in Australia are brown, including some nontoxic species, the King Brown that is actually of the genus *Pseudoechis* (Black Snakes) and the Taipan *Oxyuranus scutellatus*. Therefore, if a client reports that an animal was bitten by a snake of brown color, it does not necessarily follow that the snake was a member of the genus *Pseudonaja*.

  Characteristics of Brown Snake envenomation in domestic pets are coagulopathy, hypotension, and ascending paralysis with respiratory muscle failure, while human cases of *Pseudonaja* envenomation do not usually feature significant neurotoxicity. Cardiac output is reduced. The heart rate typically increases initially and then decreases. Hematology findings include thrombocytopenia and decreased fibrinogen, and prothrombin time and activated partial thromboplastin time are increased. The venom promotes coagulation, which depletes fibrinogen (venom-induced consumptive coagulopathy).

  CSL Brown Snake Antivenom should be used.

- *Rhinoplocephalus nigrescens*—Small-eyed Snake

  The venom of this snake caused myolysis when experimentally injected into dogs. They may be mistaken for Red-Bellied Black Snakes, but the appropriate antivenom is CSL Tiger Snake antivenom.

- *Suta suta*—Curl Snake

  There is a report of a cat fatally envenomated by this species. CSL Polyvalent Antivenom should be used.

- *Tropidechis carinatus*—Rough-scaled Snake

  This species is also known as the Clarence River Snake. This snake bites readily. It may be mistaken for the Tiger Snake, but fortuitously, CSL Tiger Snake antivenom is the appropriate antivenom.

Part 2: Venomous Aquatic Vertebrates

INTRODUCTION

This chapter is largely devoted to aquatic vertebrates that synthesize their own toxin or venom. Some fish employ a toxin synthesized by an invertebrate, such as ciguatoxin or tetrodotoxin. For detailed information on toxicoses associated with those toxins, see Chapter 23, Venomous and Poisonous Invertebrates.

Fish that employ *tetrodotoxin* are those in the order Tetraodontiformes, and include fish with common names such as puffer fish, porcupinefish, blowfish, balloonfish, boxfish, or globefish. These marine fish are not infrequently found washed ashore. Because of the extremely harmful nature of the toxin, and the manner in which the fish acts as a delayed release mechanism for the bacterial toxin, *inducing emesis is indicated* if a dog consumes a puffer fish or blowfish that it finds dead on a beach.

Ciguatoxin is not generally a problem in fish caught in New Zealand waters. Most cases of ciguatera poisoning are associated with fish caught in northern Australian waters, such as those caught off the coast of Queensland. Ciguatoxic fish include:

Epinephelus species	Rock cods
Gymnothorax species	Moray eels
Lethrinus species	Emperors
Lutjanus species	Includes paddletail, red bass, tropical snappers
Plectropomus species	Coral trout
Scomberomorus commersoni	Spanish Mackerel
Sphyraena species	Barracudas
Symphorus nematophorus	Chinamanfish

The aquatic vertebrates of possible veterinary significance in Australia and/ or New Zealand, that produce their own toxin or venom, include the following:

- Fish
  - Eeltail catfish, *Tandanus tandanus*
  - Old Wife, *Enoplosus armatus*
  - Rabbitfishes, *Siganus* species and Scat (family Scatophagidae)
  - Stonefish, Scorpionfish, Bullrout, Lionfish, and relatives (Scorpaenidae family)
- Sea Snakes
- Stingrays (Dasyatididae, Gymnuridae, Myliobatidae, and Urolophidae families)

EELTAIL CATFISH, *TANDANUS TANDANUS*

Alternative Names

Tandan, jewfish, freshwater catfish, catfish, cobbler fish.

Distribution

This is a freshwater species, native to the Murray-Darling river system. They are more common in relatively still water, such as slow moving streams, lakes, and ponds with fringing vegetation, than in running water.

This fish is sometimes kept in home aquariums, although they require a large tank.

There are also some marine catfish, such as the striped catfish *Plotosus lineatus* that are similar in shape and are also referred to by the common name eeltail catfish.

Appearance

Usually about 50 cm long, but can grow larger. The skin is smooth, with olive-green, brown, or gray coloration dorsally and a pale underside. There are four pairs of barbels around the mouth. The tail tapers and resembles that of an eel.

Circumstances of Poisoning

The eeltail catfish has sharp, serrated, venomous spines on the dorsal and pectoral fins. Anglers are occasionally stung and pet dogs accompanying anglers could also be potentially stung. Eeltail catfish have a reputation as "escape artists" from home aquariums, and a domestic pet could potentially be stung by an escaped fish.

Toxicokinetics

Little information. Pain is immediate and may persist for several hours.

Mode(s) of Action

No information.

Clinical Signs

Acute pain.

Diagnostic Aids

Radiography or ultrasound may be helpful to determine if spines remain in the wound.

Treatment

Treat for pain. Infiltrate the wound with local anesthetic.

Prognosis

Unknown for domestic animals.

Necropsy

Unknown for domestic animals

Public Health Considerations

Anglers and other people wading in water in which this species is found, should be advised that immersing the sting site in hot water, up to 45°C, for up to 20 minutes is the appropriate first aid measure.

Prevention

Avoid allowing dogs to wade in water where the fish is found, or to investigate fish that have been caught.

OLD WIFE, *ENOPLOSUS ARMATUS*

Distribution

This species is unique to the southern Australian coast, and is particularly common in inshore reefs and around the pylons of piers and jetties.

Appearance

This fish resembles tropical angelfish in shape, and has attractive vertical black and silver-white. It has two dorsal fins, of which the caudal one is long.

Circumstances of Poisoning

This fish has long spines on the tall dorsal fins. There is no obvious groove or venom gland associated with the spines, but people have reported receiving painful stings. Instances of people being stung are primarily those of marine aquarists collecting or keeping this species. Domestic pets could be stung if, for example, a fish was dropped while being moved between tanks.

Toxicokinetics

No information. Pain is immediate.

Mode(s) of Action

No information.

Clinical Signs

Pain and swelling.

Diagnostic Aids

None. Radiography may be useful to ensure that no spine is left in the wound.

Treatment

Treat for pain. Infiltrate the wound with local anesthetic.

Prognosis

Unknown for domestic animals.

Necropsy

Unknown for domestic animals.

RABBITFISHES, *SIGANUS* SPECIES AND SCAT (FAMILY SCATOPHAGIDAE)

Alternative names

Rabbitfish may also be known as spinefoots or foxfaces.

Distribution

Estuaries, lagoons, reefs, and coastal waters. They are tolerant of variable salinity.

Both the genus *Siganus* and the family Scatophagidae include attractive species that are popular for aquariums.

Appearance

Various.

Circumstances of Poisoning

These species are often encountered by anglers. Stings usually occur when these fish are being removed from nets, spears, and hooks.

Fish kept in aquariums may sting if they are handled carelessly or become alarmed, and could pose a hazard to household pets if, for example, a fish was dropped or an aquarium broke.

When alarmed or handled carelessly, the fish erect their dorsal and anal fin spines, which can easily puncture the skin and deliver venom.

Toxicokinetics

No information. Pain is immediate.

Mode(s) of Action

No information.

Clinical Signs

Human victims of stings report severe pain, marked to severe swelling, and sometimes delirium. Some victims report numbness.

Diagnostic Aids

None. Radiography may be useful to ensure that no spine is left in the wound.

Treatment

Treat for pain. Infiltrate the wound with local anesthetic.

Prognosis

Unknown for domestic animals.

Necropsy

Unknown for domestic animals.

Public Health Considerations

Immersing the sting site in hot water, up to 45°C, for up to 20 minutes is the appropriate first aid measure.

FISH OF THE ORDER SCORPAENIFORMES

This Order includes, but is not limited to, Stonefish (Synanceiidae family), Scorpionfish and Lionfish (Scorpaenidae family), and Sailback Scorpionfish, Waspfish, Soldierfish, and Bullrout (Tetrarogidae family).

The most venomous fish are stonfish belonging to the Synanceiidae family, genus *Synanceia*, and significant envenomation may also result from stings from fish in the Scorpaenidae family and Tetrarogidae family. There are numerous members of these families in Australian waters. There are also numerous members of the Scorpaenidae family in New Zealand coastal waters, although stinging incidents appear to be very rare in New Zealand. Most cases that have occurred in New Zealand waters appear to be due to *Scorpaena cardinalis*.

Stonefish have caused fatalities in human beings and in dogs.

Comprehensive information on the members of the Order Scorpaeniformes can be found at http://fishesofaustralia.net.au/home/order/44.

If the links on the left side of the webpage are followed through to the species level, color photographs of the individual species are shown, as well as a map showing their distribution in Australian waters.

Distribution

All members of these families are carnivores. Some are ambush predators with very effective camouflage (e.g., stonefish and bullrout), while others have dramatic coloration that warns of their venomous nature, e.g., lionfish. Most are marine, but some, e.g., estuarine stonefish and bullrout, are found in fresh or brackish water.

Despite their venom, many species of lionfish and scorpionfish are popular aquarium fish, because of their unusual and attractive appearance. Bullrout and stonefish are also sometimes kept in home aquariums.

Appearance

Appearance varies greatly with species. However, general characteristics include ridges and/or spines on the head, a dorsal fin with 11−17 long, well-separated spines, and well-developed pectoral fins are with 11−25 rays. Venom glands are found at the bases of the dorsal, pelvic, and anal pelvic fins. Stonefish, the most dangerous members of the order, have 13 dorsal spines.

Circumstances of Poisoning

Envenomation most often occurs when people are wading and tread on one of these fish, although it may occur as a result of keeping of these fish in aquariums.

Stonefish include the reef stonefish (*Synanceia verrucosa*) and the estuarine stonefish (*Synanceia horrida*). Their common names indicate their preferred locations. Estuarine stonefish are somewhat tolerant of fresh water and may be found in brackish canals.

Toxicokinetics

Pain is immediate, severe and radiating, and lasts approximately 12 hours in untreated human cases.

Mode(s) of Action

Stonefish venom is a complex mixture and differs between the two species in the genus *Synanceia*. Toxic elements in stonefish venom include the following:

- hyaluronidase that promotes spreading of the venom;
- cardiovascular toxins, including cardioleputin, that are mediated by muscarinic receptors and adrenoreceptors, and which cause bradycardia;
- neuromuscular toxins that cause massive release of acetylcholine and lead to depolarizing neuromuscular blockade;
- trachynilysin, which forms nonselective membrane pores that contribute to the neuromuscular blockage;
- stonustoxin, which produces depolarizing paralysis of the diaphragm, and is also a potent hemolytic and edema-forming toxin, and an inducer of hypotension, counteracting the activity of noradrenalin;
- neoverrucotoxin that has similar activity to stonustoxin;
- verrucotoxin that blocks calcium channels and affects myocardial K + (ATP) channels, inducing hypotension. It also has hemolytic action.

There is less information on the venoms of other fish in the Order. Some venom characteristics are as follows:

Pterois volitans venom acts on muscarinic cholinergic receptors and adrenoceptors. Stonefish antivenom neutralizes many of the in vitro effects of *P. volitans* venom. Experimentally, *P. volitans* venom has caused profound hypotension and myocardial injury when injected intravenously into rabbits.

Venom of *Scorpaena* species has been shown in experimental animals to induce hypotension, tachycardia, and polypnea, and to exhibit hemorrhagic, hemolytic, cytolytic, and proteolytic activities.

Bullrout (*Notesthes robusta*) venom contains a proteinaceous nocitoxin, which stimulates polymodal nociceptors. Bullrout venom has also mild proteolytic and hemolytic activity.

Soldierfish (*Gymnapistes marmoratus*) venom exhibits esterase, acid phosphatase, alkaline phosphatase, and phosphodiesterase activity, contains serotonin or a similar substance that acts on serotonin receptors, appears to stimulate the release of acetylcholine to act at muscarinic receptors, and also appears to stimulate the release of prostaglandins. Soldierfish venom also appears to stimulate the release of nitric oxide from endothelial cells to produce relaxation of vascular smooth muscle.

Clinical Signs

Clinical signs in dogs stung by stonefish, according to anecdotal reports, include severe pain, rapid collapse, severe hypotension, bradycardia, and death. There are no reports of dogs surviving stonefish envenomation.

Stonefish envenomation in humans is excruciatingly painful, and there is severe edema and tissue discoloration. Clinical signs may include dizziness, nausea, vomiting, diarrhea, abdominal cramps, arrhythmias, tremor, weakness, paralysis, collapse, hypotension, bradycardia, pulmonary edema, seizures, and death.

Diagnostic Aids

Radiography or ultrasound may be appropriate to ensure that there is no spine retained in the wound.

Treatment

Infiltrate the wound with local anesthetic, or use a regional block. Human experience with the effectiveness of systemic pain relief, e.g., pethidine, is variable.

There is an antivenom for stonefish venom that is effective in human beings and is administered according to the number of wounds from stonefish spines. Unfortunately the antivenom is expensive and not likely to be held at veterinary practices. There are no published case reports of successful use of stonefish antivenom in dogs, although there are anecdotal reports of domestic dogs being stung by stonefish in Australia.

Stonefish antivenom is effective against lionfish venom in vitro, but clinically does not appear to be effective against bullrout envenomation.

Otherwise, treatment is symptomatic and supportive.

In all cases the wound should be thoroughly cleaned and explored to ensure there are no spines remaining in the wound. Do not suture wounds. Provide antibiotic cover because of the likelihood of tissue necrosis and secondary infection.

Prognosis

Prognosis is grave in the case of stonefish envenomation of dogs. There is a lack of information on the prognosis in domestic animals of envenomation by other members of the Order.

Necropsy

Pulmonary edema may be present.

Public Health Considerations

For all these fish the immediate first aid measure is to immerse the stung body part in hot water, up to 45°C, for 20 minutes. However, victims of stonefish envenomation should not delay seeking medical attention.

SEA SNAKES

Distribution

The yellow-bellied sea snake, *Pelamis platurus* has the greatest range and has washed up on beaches of New South Wales and the North Island of New Zealand.

Sea snakes found in Australian, but not New Zealand, waters include the following:

Genus or Species	Common Name/s	Distribution
Acalyptophis peronii	Spiny-headed Sea Snake, Peron's Sea Snake, Horned Sea Snake	NT, QLD, WA
Aipysurus spp.	Olive Sea Snakes	NT, QLD, WA
Astrotia stokesii	Stoke's Sea Snake or Large-headed Sea Snake	Northern and eastern waters
Emydocephalus spp.	Turtlehead Sea Snakes	NT, QLD, WA
Enhydrina spp.	Beaked Sea Snakes	NT, QLD
Ephalophis greyae	Grey's Mudsnake, North-Western Mangrove Sea Snake	Northwestern waters
Hydrelaps darwiniensis	Port Darwin Mud Snake, Port Darwin Sea Snake, Black-Singed Sea Snake, Black-Ringed Mangrove Snake	Northern waters
Hydrophis spp.		Northern and northwestern waters
Lapemis curtus	Shaw's Sea Snake or Short Sea Snake	Indo-Australian waters
Laticauda spp.	Sea Kraits	Indo-Australian waters
Parahydrophis	Northern Mangrove Sea Snake	Northern waters

Sea snakes are tolerant of fresh water, can be found in estuaries and occasionally swim up rivers.

Appearance

Appearance varies with species. In contract to terrestrial snakes, sea snakes typically have a laterally compressed body with a paddle-like tail. The ventral aspect of the snake is smooth, making them helpless if washed ashore.

Sea snakes typically have short venom fangs. Although sea snakes produce venom, and some produce highly potent venom, most species are not aggressive. Furthermore the great majority (60%−80%) of bites are "dry" or "blank"; that is, no venom is injected.

Circumstances of Poisoning

Sea snakes are not generally of veterinary concern but if a sea snake was stranded on a beach, it could possibly bite a dog if threatened by one, or bite a large animal that trod on the snake.

Toxicokinetics

There is little information, but clinical signs usually become evident within 4 hours in human beings.

Mode(s) of Action

All the sea snakes of Australian and New Zealand waters are Elapidae and their venoms are similar to those of Australian terrestrial snakes (q.v.). having neurotoxic (paralytic) and myotoxic effects.

Clinical Signs

As for terrestrial Elapidae of Australia.

Treatment

CSL manufacture a sea snake antivenom, but there is no information on the use of this antivenom in domestic animals. It is prepared from the venoms of the Beaked Sea Snake, *Enhydrina schistosa* and the Australian tiger snake, *Notechis scutatus*, and there is clinical evidence that it is effective against venoms of many sea snakes. The usefulness of this polyvalent antivenom suggests that if it is not readily available, tiger snake antivenom could be a beneficial alternative for use by veterinarians in the more southern parts of Australia. No antivenom is likely to be available to New Zealand practitioners.

Otherwise, treatment is symptomatic.

Prognosis

The venom of many sea snake species is extremely potent, so in the unlikely event of envenomation, prognosis must be guarded.

Necropsy

No information for domestic animals.

Public Health Considerations

People encountering sea snakes stranded on beaches are advised to use a long stick or similar implement to push the snake back into the sea.

Prevention

Do not allow dogs to bother stranded sea snakes.

STINGRAYS (*DASYATIDIDAE, GYMNURIDAE, MYLIOBATIDAE,* AND *UROLOPHIDAE* FAMILIES)

Alternative Names

Ray, stingaree.

Distribution

There are many species of stingray in Australian waters, and they often rest motionless, and partially buried in bottom sediment, in shallow water. Stingrays are also common in the waters around the North Island and top of the South Island of New Zealand, but have been sighted as far south as Foveaux Strait.

Appearance

Varies with species.

Circumstances of Poisoning

Rays are generally docile, but if they are stepped on, if their spinal column is touched, or sometimes if they perceive a threat from above, they will lash their tail which has one or two sharp, serrated spines at the tip. Spines are grooved to allow venom to travel to the tip. The venom gland or glands are at the base of the tail. Dogs and horses taken to the beach and wading in shallows may be at risk of stepping on rays, just as people are.

Toxicokinetics

No information. Pain is immediate and persists for up to 48 hours in human beings.

Mode(s) of Action

Ray venom contains serotonin, 5-nucleotidase, and phosphodiesterase. Serotonin causes severe pain when injected, and the enzymes cause tissue necrosis.

Clinical Signs

Severe pain and laceration, followed by local tissue necrosis. Systemic effects observed in human victims of stingray stings include nausea, vomiting, diarrhea, hypotension, muscle cramps, cardiac arrhythmia, delirium, tremors, and seizures. Stingray stings are reported to bleed profusely.

Diagnostic Aids

Ultrasound is recommended because the stinging spine has numerous small, backward-directed barbs that may break off in the wound, and which may not be radio-opaque. Sometimes the spine itself may break off and remain in the wound.

Treatment

Immersion of the wound in hot water (45°C) provides significant pain relief. Infiltration of the wound with local anesthetic, or regional nerve block, is also highly effective. Also treat for foreign bodies (barbs), and laceration, and antibiotic cover is recommended because there is a high potential for infection. Suturing of wounds is not recommended because of the high risks of tissue necrosis, of infection, and of retained foreign bodies. The edges of the wound should be approximated and the wound allowed to heal by second intention.

Prognosis

Human victims report that pain persists for 48 hours.

Public Health Considerations

People are advised to wear sturdy footwear with ankle protection when wading in shallows.

Chapter 23

Venomous and Poisonous Invertebrates

Part 1: Aquatic Invertebrates

The toxigenic or venomous aquatic organisms and/or toxicoses described in this chapter are as follows:

- Cyanobacteria (sometimes incorrectly referred to as "blue-green algae")
- Ciguatera poisoning
- Conotoxins
- Dinoflagellate and diatom toxins responsible for "*shellfish poisonings*"
- Tetrodotoxin. This includes toxicoses from *sea slugs* and *blue-ringed octopi*, as well as a range of vertebrates that employ this bacterial toxin
- Cnidaria. This includes *bluebottles*, the *Portuguese Man-of-War*, and large and small *box jellies*
- Fire coral
- Sponges
- Sea urchins

CYANOBACTERIAL TOXINS (CYANOTOXINS; "BLUE-GREEN ALGAL" TOXINS)

Note: Although some cyanobacteria produce saxitoxin, it is also produced by dinoflagellates and toxicity is most commonly associated with consumption of shellfish. It is therefore discussed in detail under "Dinoflagellate toxins."

Synthesizing Organisms

Cyanobacteria of toxicological significance to animals in Australia include *Anabaena circinalis* (saxitoxins); *Aphanizomenon ovalisporum*, *Cylindrospermopsis raciborskii*, and *Lyngbya wollei* (cylindrospermopsin and deoxy-cylindrospermopsin); *Microcystis aeruginosa* (microcystin);

Veterinary Toxicology for Australia and New Zealand
DOI: http://dx.doi.org/10.1016/B978-0-12-420227-6.00022-0

Nodularia spumigena (nodularin); *Phormidium* spp. (anatoxin-a and related compounds) and *Limnothrix* (unidentified toxins).

Cyanobacteria of toxicological significance to animals in New Zealand include *N. spumigena* nodularin); *Microcystis* spp. (microcystin); Anabaena spp., *Oscillatoria* spp., *Aphanizomenon issatschenkoi*, and *Phormidium autumnale* (anatoxin-a and related compounds).

With regard to cylindrospermopsin, toxigenic strains of *C. raciborskii* and *A. issatschenkoi* have been detected in New Zealand but have not been associated with toxicoses. Likewise, in addition to *Microcystis* spp., a number of other genera of cyanobacteria in New Zealand are known or suspected producers of microcystin. These genera include *Anabaena*, *Planktothrix*, and *Nostoc*. Saxitoxin has been detected at low levels in New Zealand fresh waters, although the synthesizing organism is uncertain.

Dermal toxicity reported in human beings swimming in water containing blue-green algae is likely to be caused either by aplysiatoxins synthesized by *Lyngbya, Schizothrix* or *Oscillatoria* spp., or lyngbyatoxin-a synthesized by *Lyngbya* spp. Although animals are relatively resistant to dermal toxicity, dogs should not be allowed to swim in water where dermal toxicosis from cyanobacteria has been reported, because lyngbyatoxin-a is also a gastrointestinal toxicant, and because of the possible presence of the other toxins produced by *Oscillatoria* and *Lyngbya*.

The use of the term "blue-green algae" to describe the cyanobacteria is obsolete and biologically incorrect.

Distribution

With the exception of *Nodularia*, which is found in estuarine or marine waters, the cyanobacteria are found in fresh water.

Circumstances of Poisoning

Animals are poisoned when their drinking water is contaminated with cyanobacteria. Acute deaths of dogs from anatoxin-a poisoning has resulted from dogs consuming mats of *Phormidium* or *Oscillatoria*. Dogs may also be poisoned by water ingested while swimming.

Toxin production by cyanobacteria is generally greatest at temperatures between 18°C and 25°C, and declines substantially at temperatures below 10°C or above 30°C. Eutrophication of water by nitrogen-rich runoff increases the likelihood of blue-green algal proliferation.

Toxicokinetics

There little specific information on the toxicokinetics of the cyanobacterial toxins, although clinical experience shows that all are rapidly absorbed.

Microcystin is taken up by hepatocytes by carrier-mediated transport, and sublethal doses are retained in the liver for days after a single dose, at least in mice.

Modes of Action

Cylindrospermopsin, microcystin, and nodularin are primarily hepatotoxic whereas anatoxin-a is neurotoxic. There is limited information on the toxicity of *Limnothrix*, but extracts have caused necrosis of liver and other organs in mice.

The toxic mechanism of microcystin and nodularin is irreversible inhibition of protein phosphatases 1 and 2A, key regulatory enzymes that catalyze dephosphorylation of serine/threonine residues in various phosphoproteins including both structural proteins and enzymes. The toxic mechanism of cylindrospermopsin appears to be less well determined, but it is cytotoxic to liver and kidney.

Cylindrospermopsin and nodularin are both carcinogenic, while microcystin is a tumor promoter.

Anatoxin-a is a potent prostsynaptic depolarizing neuromuscular blocking agent.

Anatoxin-a(S), a potent anticholinesterase, has not been detected in Australia or New Zealand.

Clinical Signs

Clinical signs of poisoning with microcystin or nodularin begin within 1−4 hours of ingestion and include depression, diarrhea that may be hemorrhagic, weakness, pale mucous membranes, and shock. Animals that can vomit, such as dogs, are likely to do so. Death may occur in 1−24 hours. In severe outbreaks, large numbers of livestock may be found dead in the vicinity of the contaminated water source.

Cattle poisoned by drinking toxic levels ($\sim 50\,\mu g/kg/day$) of cylindrospermopsin generally succumb to liver failure within 10 days.

Ruminants that do not die acutely from ingestion of hepatotoxic cyanotoxins may develop hepatogenous photosensitization.

Onset of anatoxin-a toxicosis is typically abrupt and may begin within 30 minutes of ingestion. Clinical signs are muscle rigidity, tremors or seizures, paralysis, respiratory failure, and death within 30 minutes of the onset of clinical signs.

Diagnostic Aids

Water may be tested for cyanobacteria or their toxins. If analysis is likely to be delayed, a water sample can be fixed by addition of formalin to make 10% formalin (4% formaldehyde) solution, or by use of Lugol's iodine. The recommendations of the analyzing laboratory should be sought and followed. Samples are best collected in glass containers and should be stored in the dark.

Water may be frozen if toxin detection by mouse bioassay is planned. However, for ethical reasons, a request for a mouse bioassay may be refused unless there is substantial risk to human health.

Treatment

Cholestyramine, 172 mg/kg/day orally, has been credited with contributing to recovery from microcystin poisoning in a dog and, based on studies in laboratory rats, may also be helpful in other species. Cholestyramine is believed to work by binding microcystin in the intestines and therefore treatment should be initiated as early in the toxicosis as possible. There are no controlled trials in domestic animals that prove that cholestyramine is beneficial.

Besides the use of cholestyramine, all treatment is symptomatic and supportive.

Prognosis

Prognosis in acute toxicosis is poor to hopeless. Chronic poisoning with the hepatotoxic cyanotoxins may leave an animal permanently debilitated by liver damage.

Necropsy

Lesions of the hepatotoxic cyanobacterial toxins are those of acute gastroenteritis, swollen congested liver, and edematous gall-bladder. Histopathological lesions range from centrilobular necrosis to complete disintegration of the cord-like arrangement of hepatocytes.

There are no characteristic findings of neurotoxic cyanobacterial toxicosis.

Public Health Considerations

All the cyanobacterial toxins are also extremely hazardous to human health.

Prevention

The use of bacteriocides and/or filtration systems may be practical in some bodies of water, particularly in cooler areas when the season for cyanobacterial proliferation is short, and local government authorities may be able to provide locally relevant information on this. Eutrophication of water supplies by nitrogen-rich runoff should be prevented as far as possible. If prevention of cyanobacterial proliferation cannot be instituted, prevention of exposure is the only option.

CIGUATERA POISONING

Synthesizing Organism

Gambierdiscus toxicus, a dinoflagellate, is considered to be the predominant but not necessarily the only organism that synthesizes the toxins responsible for ciguatera poisoning.

Distribution

The dinoflagellates, which synthesize poisons including ciguatoxin, maitotoxin, scaritoxin, and palytoxin, grow on macroalgae adhering to corals and are ingested by herbivorous fish that eat the macroalgae. These are in turn ingested by carnivorous fish. The toxin content is progressively magnified moving up the food chain.

Circumstances of Poisoning

Ciguatera poisoning is common in tropical waters and is a significant problem in northern parts of Australia. In Australia, human poisoning has been associated with ingestion of fish such as Barracuda (*Sphyraena jello*), Chinaman fish (*Symphorus nematophorus*), Cobia (*Rachycentron canadus*), Coral cod (*Cephalopholis miniata*), Coral trout (*Plectropomus* spp.), Flowery cod (*Epinephelus fuscoguttatus*), Groper (*Epinephelus lanceolatus*), Paddle tail (*Lutjanus gibbus*), Queenfish (*Scomberoides commersonnianus*), Red bass (*Lutjanus bohar*), Red emperor (*Lutjanus sebae*), Spanish mackerel (*Scomberomorus commerson*), Spotted mackerel (*Scomberomorus munroi*), Sweetlip emperor (*Lethrinus miniatus*), and Trevally (*Caranx* spp.)

The toxins responsible for ciguatera poisoning cannot be detected by taste of the fish, and are not destroyed by cooking.

Cats are reported to be extremely susceptible to ciguatera poisoning and have been used as a bioassay species. There appears to be no basis for the legend that a cat will not eat fish that contains ciguatera toxins.

Toxicokinetics

Toxicokinetics vary depending on the toxin involved, but as generalizations, the toxins that cause ciguatera poisoning are very rapidly absorbed by the oral route and are also absorbed by the dermal route, for example, by filleting fish. They are widely distributed in the body, including crossing the placenta, and only slowly excreted, being sequestered in adipose tissue and possibly also bound to proteins. Excretion is at least partly by the renal route. These findings are consistent with clinical experience in humans that shows that symptoms of poisoning develop within 1−8 hours of ingestion and the neurologic manifestations in particular may persist for weeks, months, or even years.

Mode(s) of Action

Ciguatoxin and scaritoxin sodium lower the threshold for opening voltage-gated sodium channels in synapses of the nervous system, while maitotoxin increases the calcium ion influx through excitable membranes. Palytoxin binds to $Na + K + $-ATPase, a sodium pump found in all vertebrate cell membranes, and while bound, may change the sodium channel back and forth from open to closed, although the open conformation is more common. While it is open, there is free diffusion of sodium and potassium ions through the channel.

Clinical Signs

Reported clinical signs in cats include emesis, hypersalivation, lachrymation, ataxia, ascending paralysis, arrhythmia, dyspnea, and terminal cyanosis.

Ciguatera poisoning has also been occasionally reported in dogs, with clinical signs including emesis, diarrhea, head shaking, nystagmus ataxia, and paralysis.

Clinical signs in human beings include gastrointestinal, neurologic, and cardiovascular signs. Gastrointestinal signs include vomiting, diarrhea, and abdominal pain and cramps.

Neurologic signs include paresthesias, dental pain, dysuria, visual blurring, weakness, pruritis, depression, headache, myalgia, and arthralgia. Reversal of temperature perception is very characteristic of this poisoning but does not always occur.

Cardiovascular signs in human beings include arrhythmia, bradycardia, hypotension, and cardiac block.

Miscarriages have been reported in human beings, and human infants have been poisoned through breastmilk.

Treatment

There is no specific treatment. Treatment should be supportive, with monitoring of vital signs.

Prognosis

Variable depending on dose.

Necropsy

There are no specific findings on necropsy. Urine, kidney, liver, and adipose tissue may be collected as fresh tissue and frozen if immediate analysis is not available.

Public Health Considerations

Ciguatera poisoning is one of the most common food poisonings in the world. Marine anglers should be warned that domestic pets are also susceptible to ciguatera poisoning.

Prevention

Do not feed carnivorous fish to cats and dogs, particularly if outbreaks of ciguatera poisoning have been reported in the area.

CONOTOXINS

Synthesizing Organism

Marine molluscs of the genus *Conus* (cone shells; cone snails), which includes more than 600 species. There are at least 70 species in Australian waters.

Distribution

Most cone shells are found in warm tropical waters with a few species adapted to temperate waters. Cone shells occur in the waters off both Australia and New Zealand but are more likely to be encountered in Australian waters. They are largely nocturnal but may be found in rock pools or burrowed in sand during the day.

Circumstances of Poisoning

Cone shells stab with a small chitin tooth of the radula, when picked up or disturbed. They are carnivorous and predatory, and use chemosensors on the siphon to detect potential prey. The cone shell fires the venom-loaded radula tooth into prey like a harpoon, by means of muscular contraction, and then retracts the radula to draw the prey in. Cone shells have multiple such "harpoons" and can "fire" in any direction. The attack is extremely rapid, occurring in milliseconds.

Accidental cone shell envenomation in domestic animals has not been reported in the peer-reviewed literature, but the most likely candidate would be a curious dog.

Toxicokinetics

It is difficult to generalize about conotoxins because there are some 200 different conotoxins so far identified and it is estimated that there may be more than 50,000 in total. Each *Conus* species synthesizes 100−200 different conotoxins. However, in the clinical sense, effects of envenomation by

conotoxins are generally felt within minutes. In survivors of severe envenomation, clinical signs may persist for weeks.

Mode(s) of Action

The modes of action of conotoxins, which are small peptides are diverse,
as a generalization they are inhibitors of ion channels, involved in the transmission of neuromuscular signals in animals, including calcium channels,
sodium channels, and potassium channels.

Clinical Signs

Clinical signs reported by human victims of envenomation by cone shells
include immediate sharp burning or stinging sensation, local numbness or
paresthesia, oral or generalized paresthesia, nausea, blurred vision, weakness,
dysphagia, areflexia, paralysis and apnea.

Diagnostic Aids

There are no specific diagnostic aids.

Treatment

There is no specific antivenom. Monitor and support vital functions. Airway
maintenance and protection is vital, bearing in mind that the pharynx may be
paralysed. Respiratory support may be required.

Prognosis

Likely to be guarded to poor in a significant envenomation.

Necropsy

No significant findings.

Public Health Considerations

People should be aware that they should never collect live *Conus* species, or
handle them for any reason, even to move them out of the way of an inquisitive
pet. The *Conus* radula can penetrate wetsuits, so even gloves are not
protective.

Public awareness of the dangers of *Conus* species is generally high in
Australia, but people in New Zealand tend to be surprised to learn that
Conus species occur in New Zealand waters.

Prevention

Dog owners need to be vigilant when taking dogs to the beach or in the vicinity of rock pools.

DINOFLAGELLATE AND DIATOM TOXINS ("SHELLFISH POISONINGS")

Synthesizing Organism

Paralytic Shellfish Poisoning

Dinoflagellates in Australian waters that can synthesize the toxins to cause paralytic shellfish poisoning (PSP) include members of the genera *Alexandrium* (*Gonyaulax*), *Gymnodinium*, and *Pyrodinium*. A number of toxigenic species of *Alexandrium* are found in New Zealand waters.

Neurotoxic Shellfish Poisoning

Neurotoxic shellfish poisoning (NSP) in New Zealand has been caused by brevetoxin synthesis by an organism similar to *Gymnodinium breve* (*Ptychodiscus brevis*), which is the organism responsible for NSP in the Gulf of Mexico. Similar organisms have been found in Australian waters. Compounds similar to brevetoxin can also be synthesized by some other marine algae found in Australian waters.

Diarrhetic Shellfish Poisoning

Potentially toxic diarrhetic shellfish poisoning (DSP) dinoflagellates in Australian waters include species of the genera *Dinophysis* and *Prorocentrum*. The toxicity of these species is variable, and sometimes dense blooms occur with no toxin synthesis. DSP is relatively rare in New Zealand.

Amnestic Shellfish Poisoning

The toxin responsible for amnestic shellfish poisoning, domoic acid, is synthesized by diatoms of the genus *Pseudo-nitzschia*.

Distribution

PSP and DSP have been reported in both Australia and New Zealand, and NSP has been reported in New Zealand.

Circumstances of Poisoning

Poisoning follows consumption of shellfish that have concentrated the toxins through filter feeding. Proliferation of the synthesizing organisms is most common in the summer months when sea water is warm.

Shellfish poisoning has been reported in cats and dogs, although cases in which dogs refused to eat contaminated shellfish have also been reported. Cats have sometimes been used as a bioassay species to determine whether shellfish are safe for human consumption.

The toxins are not destroyed by cooking.

Mode(s) of Action

Paralytic Shellfish Poisoning

PSP toxins, of which the best known and most potent is saxitoxin, block the sodium channels of excitable membranes, inhibiting action potentials and nerve transmission impulses. In vertebrates the peripheral nervous system is particularly affected.

Neurotoxic Shellfish Poisoning

Brevetoxins and their derivatives exert their toxic effect by specific binding to site-5 of voltage-sensitive sodium channels.

Diarrhetic Shellfish Poisoning

The toxins that cause DSP include okadaic acid, dinophysis toxins, pectenotoxins, yessotoxins, and spiramino acid. The diarrhetic effect may be linked to the ability of some of these toxins to act as potent inhibitors of protein phosphatases.

Amnestic Shellfish Poisoning

The causative compound, domoic acid, is an excitatory amino acid which acts as a glutamate antagonist on the kainate receptors of the central nervous system.

Clinical Signs

Paralytic Shellfish Poisoning

In human beings, typical symptoms of poisoning include parasthesias of the extremities, progressing to muscular incoordination, respiratory distress, and muscular paralysis leading to death by asphyxiation in extreme cases. Onset of symptoms may occur only 30 minutes after ingestion, and fatalities, if they occur, generally occur within 12 hours.

Neurotoxic Shellfish Poisoning

The time to onset of symptoms of NSP in human beings is usually around 3 hours, but may range from 15 minutes to 18 hours. Reported symptoms include parasthesias, reversal of perception of hot and cold, myalgia, vertigo, clumsiness, abdominal pain, vomiting, diarrhea, headache, tremor, dysphagia, slow pulse, and dilated pupils. Symptoms and clinical signs last from 1 to 72 hours. Treatment is supportive. Respiratory difficulty is rare. Brevetoxins can also lead to cough, wheezing, and ocular irritation, if the toxin is aerosolized by wave action during red tides. NSP has not been associated with human fatalities.

Diarrhetic Shellfish Poisoning

Clinical signs include severe vomiting, nausea, and diarrhea. No human fatalities have been reported and recovery is generally complete within 3 days.

Amnestic Shellfish Poisoning

Clinical onset ranges from 15 minutes to 38 hours but the average is 5 hours.

Gastroenteric clinical signs including nausea, vomiting, abdominal cramps, and diarrhea occur first, followed by neurological symptoms. In human beings, neurological symptoms include dizziness, headache, seizures, disorientation, short-term memory loss, respiratory difficulty, and coma. The mortality in human cases is approximately 2%, with immunosuppressed and elderly patients most at risk. Ten percent of victims suffer long-term memory problems and/or muscular and sensory problems.

Diagnostic Aids

Suspect shellfish can be tested for toxins.

Treatment

Treatment in all forms of shellfish poisoning is symptomatic. Assisted ventilation may be required in PSP.

Prognosis

Prognosis depends on the toxin(s) ingested and the severity of poisoning.

Necropsy

There are no distinctive findings on necropsy in any of the "shellfish poisonings."

Public Health Considerations

All of these toxins pose a risk to human health.

Prevention

Pet owners should be warned that domestic pets are also susceptible to shell-fish poisonings.

TETRODOTOXIN

Synthesizing Organism

Tetrodotoxin is synthesized by symbiotic bacteria including *Pseudoalteromonas tetraodonis* and certain species of the genera *Pseudomonas* and *Vibrio*, as well as some other species.

Organisms That Employ Tetrodotoxin

Organisms in Australian waters that use tetrodotoxin include the blue-ringed octopus (*Hapalochlaena* spp.) and the sea slug (*Pleurobranchaea maculata*) as well as blowfish, pufferfish, and toadfish (family Tetraodontidae, which includes the genera *Arothron, Canthigaster, Chelonodon, Contusus, Feroxodon, Lagocephalus, Marilyna, Omegophora, Polyspina, Reicheltia, Sphoeroides, Tetractenos, Tetraodon, Torquigener, Tylerius*). In New Zealand, tetrodotoxin poisoning is most commonly a result of dogs eating sea slugs that have washed up on beaches, but some species of pufferfish are found in New Zealand waters and also pose a hazard to dogs if washed ashore.

Distribution

Puffer fish and related fish species that employ tetrodotoxin are found in waters all around Australia and both main islands of New Zealand. The blue-ringed octopus is found on shallow reefs, in coral rock pools and in tidal pools to a depth of approximately 20 m. Sea slugs are found around New Zealand and southeastern Australia.

Circumstances of Poisoning

Most veterinary cases of poisoning in Australia and New Zealand have occurred as a result of dogs consuming sea slugs or puffer fish that have washed ashore.

The blue-ringed octopus may bite if disturbed. Tetrodotoxin is the major venom in the bite, although histamine, tryptamine, octopamine, taurine, acetylcholine, and dopamine are also present. The bite is often painless.

Toxicokinetics

There is little specific information on the toxicokinetics of tetrodotoxin. Clinical signs often develop within 30 minutes of ingestion, and usually within 3 hours, indicating rapid absorption. One human fatality occurred at 17 minutes after ingestion. Rare cases of delayed toxicosis are likely due to late release of the toxin from the ingested material.

If the patient survives for 24 hours, chances of survival are good, so it appears that C_{max} is reached within 24 hours. Excretion appears to be primarily via urine.

Absorption from the bite of a blue-ringed octopus is much more rapid than from ingestion of a species employing tetrodotoxin, and may cause death within minutes.

Mode(s) of Action

Tetrodotoxin blocks fast voltage-gated sodium channels, affecting action potential generation and impulse conduction.

Clinical Signs

Clinical signs of tetrodotoxin poisoning in dogs include emesis, tremors, incoordination, hyperesthesia, muscle fasciculation, seizures, nystagmus, and diarrhea.

Diagnostic Aids

Tetrodotoxin acts as an emetic in dogs and it is common for the dog to regurgitate recognizable fish or sea slugs.

Treatment

Ingestion of a fish or invertebrate that contains tetrodotoxin is one of the rare situations in which inducing emesis as soon as possible, although it should be recognized that the rapid absorption of tetrodotoxin means that this measure, or gastric lavage as an alternative decontamination measure, may be futile.

Diazepam or phenobarbital should be administered to control tremors and muscle fasciculation. Severe cases will require general anesthesia and artificial ventilation. Intravenous fluid therapy should be initiated, and the patient's urine output, blood gas balance and cardiac functions monitored.

4-Aminopyridine has been shown experimentally to act as a tetrodotoxin antagonist and there is anecdotal evidence supporting its use, but controlled clinical trials have not been conducted.

Prognosis

Dogs that survive for 24 hours have a good prognosis.

Necropsy

There are no specific findings on necropsy. Urine and fresh liver are the analytical samples of choice.

Public Health Considerations

Tetrodotoxin is also deadly to human beings, and public awareness of the dangers of the species that employ it is critical.

Prevention

To prevent tetrodotoxin poisoning, dogs should not be permitted to wander unattended on beaches, and owners need to be vigilant to ensure that dogs do not eat organisms that employ tetrodotoxin. In areas where blue-ringed octopi are found, dogs should not be allowed to play in rock pools.

CNIDARIA

Synthesizing Organisms

The medically important sea jellies of Australian waters are:

- *Physalia* (bluebottles and Portuguese Man-of-War).
- *Chironex fleckeri* (major box jellyfish).
- *Carukia barnesi* and other box jellyfish causing Irukandji syndrome.

Physalia utriculus (bluebottle) and *Physalia physalis* (Portuguese Man-of-War) are also found in New Zealand waters, but the box jellies listed above are not.

A number of other species of sea jelly can cause painful stings, but care in excess of basic first-aid as not required. All sea jellies, in the water or beached, alive or apparently dead, should be regarded as capable of envenomation.

Distribution

C. fleckeri is restricted to tropical waters along the northern coast of Australia, and is also found in the seas off Papua New Guinea, the Philippines, and Vietnam.

In Australia, Irukandji syndrome is most often reported north of Cairns. Irukandji syndrome has also been reported from a number of other countries in the tropical Pacific and in the Caribbean.

Circumstances of Poisoning

Human envenomations are most likely to occur while the victim is swimming.

The fur of domestic animals provides protection against envenomation while swimming or wading in shallow water, but the potential for dogs to be stung on poorly haired areas such as the nose, abdomen, or scrotum should not be overlooked.

Dogs should be discouraged from investigating beached sea jellies.

Most human cases of Irukandji syndrome occur between October and May inclusive.

Toxicokinetics

There is a lack of information on the toxicokinetics of the venoms of any of these cnidarians.

In human beings, *Physalia* stings and *C. fleckeri* stings are associated with immediate pain. The pain from a *C. fleckeri* envenomation may last up to 8 hours, and pruritis at the site of the sting may persist for up to 2 weeks. In contrast the sting in Irukandji syndrome is often not felt, but severe systemic symptoms develop from 30 to 120 minutes later and generally subside within 12 hours.

Mode(s) of Action

The modes of action of the venoms of the dangerous cnidarians are not fully elucidated, although there is some information. *P. physalis* venom increases the permeability of plasma membranes in vitro, and induces calcium and sodium influx into cells. It also causes histamine release from mast cells. *C. fleckeri* venom is directly toxic to cardiac myocytes, while Irukandji syndrome features release of cytokines and nitric oxide. In severe envenomation, human beings may develop toxic cardiomyopathy and pulmonary edema. Intracerebral hemorrhage, attributed to uncontrolled hypertension, has been reported in some human victims.

Clinical Signs

Physalia species: Most human envenomations lead only to localized pain and pruritis. On human skin the stings can be seen as a weal with a "string of beads" appearance. In rare cases, human victims have developed systemic symptoms that may include nausea, vomiting, headache, chills, drowsiness, dyspnea, cardiovascular collapse, and death.

C. fleckeri: Human victims report immediate severe pain, and on human skin the stings cause linear welts, characteristically a crosshatched pattern.

The tentacles are often still adherent on human skin when the patient is presented for treatment, but the likelihood adherence of the tentacles to various types of animal fur is unknown. Cardiac effects in severe envenomation include tachycardia, impaired contraction, and arrhythmia. There may be hypertension or hypotension. Death may occur within a few minutes. A delayed hypersensitivity reaction, in the form of pruritic dermatitis, is common in human patients.

Irukandji syndrome: The envenomation may not be noticed and skin lesions are not typically observed. In humans, systemic symptoms develop from 30 to 120 minutes after envenomation, and include apprehension, agitation, vomiting, hypertension, tachycardia, and severe pain in the back, limbs, or abdomen.

Diagnostic Aids

Physalia species and *C. fleckeri* may be observed, but the sea jellies responsible for Irukandji syndrome are small and easily overlooked, and are not excluded from swimming areas by stinger nets.

Nematocysts may be recovered from the skin or fur. Recovery of *C. fleckeri* nematocysts from human skin can be performed with "sticky tape," but skin scrapings are required to recover nematocysts of the small species that cause Irukandji syndrome.

Treatment

All possible cases of cnidarian envenomation must be handled with great care to avoid envenomation of handlers, as undischarged nematocysts may be present on the skin or in the fur.

Physalia species: Flush the affected area with sea water to remove any adherent tentacles. Do NOT use vinegar, which causes additional discharge of *Physalia* nematocysts. Fresh water may also cause a discharge of nematocysts to a lesser extent, but may be used in an emergency if salt water is not available. The envenomated area should be immersed in hot water at 45°C for at least 20 minutes. Analgesia may be indicated, and the patient should be monitored for pruritis and prevented from inflicting self-trauma. Hypersensitivity reactions are rare complications. There is no antivenom available for *Physalia* stings.

C. fleckeri: As soon as possible, remove any tentacles and apply vinegar liberally. Vinegar inactivates undischarged nematocysts. Monitor vital functions, particularly cardiac function and provide emergency cardiorespiratory support as necessary. Intravenous magnesium, 10 mmol, may be beneficial, but is controversial.

There is an antivenom available for *C. fleckeri* envenomation, although its use is controversial and its effectiveness in human beings is debated. The number of ampoules that would be appropriate for a domestic animal is unknown. The appropriate dose for a human being is 3−6 ampoules, diluted in 100 mL saline and administered IV.

Irukandji syndrome: Apply vinegar liberally to all visible sting sites to inactivate undischarged nematocysts. Fentanyl or morphine analgesia is recommended in human envenomations, but pethidine is not, because of possible complications including histamine release, tachycardia and myocardial depression. Monitor for hypertension and/or pulmonary edema and treat as required. Glyceryl trinitrate is the recommended therapy for hypertension in human victims of Irukandji syndrome.

Envenomations by other sea jellies: Wash the sting site with sea water or saline, and remove any tentacles. Hot water immersion or ice packs may be helpful. Do NOT use vinegar.

Note: Because vinegar is only recommended for envenomation by *C. fleckeri* or the small cnidarians that cause Irukandji syndrome, it is currently not indicated for any cnidarian envenomations occurring in New Zealand waters.

Prognosis

Prognosis varies based on the severity of envenomation, but is likely to be favorable in most cases.

Necropsy

With the exception of pulmonary edema in Irukandji syndrome, there are no distinctive internal lesions.

Public Health Considerations

The same precautions against exposure, and first-aid measures (such as hot water for Physalia envenomations, vinegar for *C. fleckeri* envenomation) apply to human beings.

Prevention

Owners in coastal areas should be warned that they should not allow dogs or other animals to investigate beached cnidarians, or allow dogs to wade or swim in the sea when cnidarians are numerous.

FIRE CORAL

Synthesizing Organism

Venomous corals of Australia, fire corals, belong to the genus *Millipora*.

Distribution

Fire corals are found in tropical waters. They are generally located in areas of high water movement. However, they are also popular as aquarium species.

Circumstances of Poisoning

Veterinary poisoning would be unlikely unless a dog was to mouth a fire coral that a diver had brought ashore, or that an aquarium owner had allowed the dog access to. The coral is unable to sting people through the thick skin of the fingers or palm of the hand, so it would unlikely to be able to envenomate a domestic animal unless mouthed.

Toxicokinetics

There is little information. Human victims of envenomation report that pain occurs immediately.

Mode(s) of Action

The toxin is a water-soluble, heat-sensitive protein.

Clinical Signs

Clinical signs in human beings include pain, swelling, and blisters. Extensive stinging may induce nausea and vomiting. There may be local lymphadenitis.

A Type IV hypersensitivity reaction, with prolonged swelling and pruritis, has been reported by some human victims.

Corals often harbor numerous bacteria, so secondary infection is a common complication.

Diagnostic Aids

None.

Treatment

Soak the affected are with hot sea water. Fresh water is reported to increase the pain in human victims. Application of vinegar may be helpful. Any visible parts of the coral should be removed with tweezers. Analgesia may be indicated.

Prognosis

Prognosis is excellent.

Necropsy

Not applicable.

Public Health Considerations

Divers and owners of reef aquariums should be aware of the risks of fire coral.

Prevention

Do not allow domestic species access to fire coral that has been brought ashore or that is kept as an aquarium species.

SPONGES

Synthesizing Organism

Sponges, phylum *Porifera*. Most sponges are harmless.

Distribution

Venomous sponges occur around the coastline of Australia and Tasmania.

Circumstances of Poisoning

The most likely situation of exposure would be if a dog investigated a sponge that had been washed ashore, using its nose or mouth.

Toxicokinetics

There is little information. Envenomation by a sponge causes delayed rather than immediate clinical signs.

Mode(s) of Action

Venom is delivered via spicules made of silicon.

Clinical Signs

Clinical signs are those of erythema, swelling and pain at the contact site. The pain may last for days.

Diagnostic Aids

None.

Treatment

Treatment is symptomatic. Self-trauma should be prevented. If the dog's mouth is affected, very soft or liquid food may be required until the swelling subsides.

Prognosis

Prognosis is excellent.

Necropsy

Not applicable.

Public Health Considerations

People should be aware that not all sponges are harmless.

Prevention

Dogs should not be allowed to investigate sponges that have washed ashore, or pick them up in their mouths.

SEA URCHINS

Synthesizing Organism

Sea urchins, which belong to the class *Echinoidea*.

Distribution

Sea urchins are found in marine habitats throughout the world.

Circumstances of Poisoning

Sea urchin envenomation of a domestic animal would be most likely to occur if the animal was wading in shallow water and therefore dogs and horses would be the most likely victims. Sea urchins are not aggressive but have spines and pedicellariae, which are short pincer-like structures that they use for defense. Both spines and pedicellariae may contain venom, depending on the species of sea urchin. However, most sea urchin injuries in Australian and New Zealand waters do not involve significant envenomation but are primarily traumatic injuries due to the spines.

Toxicokinetics

There is little information on toxicokinetics of sea urchin venoms of the species found in Australian and New Zealand waters.

Mode(s) of Action

There is little information on the modes of action of sea urchin venoms of the species found in Australian and New Zealand waters.

Clinical Signs

Human victims of sea urchin envenomation report that the stings are intensely painful. Severe envenomation has been associated with muscle spasms, faintness, and dyspnea.

Diagnostic Aids

Radiographs should be taken to check for broken sea urchin spines left in the puncture wound.

Treatment

Immerse the wound in water, as hot as the victim can comfortably bear, for at least 30 minutes. Sea urchin venoms are proteinaceous and heat-labile. Remove spines, by surgery if necessary. Note that spines tend to dye pink or light-colored skin, giving the impression that the spine is still present when it is no longer there. Monitor vital functions, and provide respiratory support as required. Also provide antibiotic cover, and tetanus prophylaxis if the victim is a horse that has been ridden into the sea.

Prognosis

Good.

Necropsy

No specific findings.

Public Health Considerations

Sea urchin injury, with or without envenomation, may occur in people who wade or dive in areas where sea urchins are plentiful.

Prevention

Avoid exposure.

Part 2: Venomous and Poisonous Terrestrial Invertebrates in Australia

The venomous and poisonous terrestrial invertebrates of veterinary significance in Australia include the following:

Australian paralysis tick, *Ixodes holocyclus*
Australian tarantulas or whistling spiders (*Selenotholus, Selenotypus, Coremiocnemis, Phlogius* spp.)
Ants
Caterpillars
Sawflies (*Lophyrotoma interrupta*)
Redback spiders, *Latrodectus hasselti*
Tasmanian paralysis tick, *Ixodes cornuatus*

Note: Venomous effects of *bees, wasps, and bumblebees* are covered in the following section on Venomous Terrestrial Invertebrates in New Zealand, and in the interests of brevity are not repeated in this section.

At the end of this section, brief remarks are also presented on:

Funnel-web spiders (*Atrax, Hadronyche, Illawarra* spp.)
Fiddleback/hobo spiders (*Loxosceles* spp.)
Scorpions, centipedes, and millipedes

AUSTRALIAN PARALYSIS TICK, *IXODES HOLOCYCLUS*

Alternative Names

Paralysis tick, dog tick, scrub tick.

Distribution

This species of tick is generally found in a 20-km wide strip that follows the eastern coast of Australia, although in some moist places, such as the Bunya Mountains and the Lower Blue Mountains its range may extend more than 100 km inland. The distribution of the tick is limited by its susceptibility to desiccation in areas where temperature is high and humidity is low. As a result, these ticks are most abundant in areas with persistent high humidity and little direct sunlight, such as rainforests. The major host *of I. holocyclus* is the bandicoot, but they are also found on echidnas, possums, kangaroos and a variety of other native animals. Because exposure to *I. holocyclus* is continuous or near-continuous in native fauna, native fauna tend to have a high immunity to the toxic effects.

Appearance

There are numerous tick species in Australia. Features by which adult *I. holocyclus* may be distinguished from other species are:

- Of the four pairs of legs, the most cranial and the most caudal pairs are distinctly darker than the middle two pairs of legs.
- Complete encirclement of the anus by the anal groove, which is pear-shaped.

Larvae of the tick have six legs and the body (excluding legs) is approximately 0.5 mm in length and 0.4 mm wide. Nymphs and adults have eight legs. The body of the nymph is approximately 1.2 mm in length and 0.85 mm wide. Unengorged adults are 3.8 mm in length and 2.6 mm wide, whereas fully engorged adult females are 13.2 mm long and 10.2 mm wide.

The adult female has very long mouthparts with which to feed. She also has a dorsal *scutum*, or shield, that covers only the cranial part of the body, whereas that of the male covers the entire dorsum. The adult male has short mouthparts and poses no direct risk to human beings or animals. However, the presence of a male does indicate the likely presence of a female or females.

A professional identification service is available at the Department of Medical Entomology Level 3, ICPMR, Westmead Hospital, Westmead, NSW 2145.

Circumstances of Poisoning

I. holocyclus are most active in Spring and early Summer. To find a host, *I. holocyclus* climb up to 50 cm in vegetation and wave their forelegs slowly, a behavior known as "questing." Both sexes quest but of adult ticks, only the female feeds off the host. The adult male quests to find females in order to mate, and males may also feed off females.

Domestic animals are at risk of picking up *I. holocyclus* when moving through vegetation. All domestic mammals, as well as domestic poultry may be parasitized by *I. holocyclus*, although the most common victims are dogs, cats, and human beings. The tick saliva has a local anesthetic effect so that animals are not stimulated to find the tick, and in addition, some areas such as the back of the head are inaccessible to self-grooming.

The ticks can be carried on items such as clothing or camping equipment and then parasitize indoor pets.

I. holocyclus larvae and nymphs need to feed off hosts in order to mature, secrete a small amount of holocyclotoxin and are capable of exerting toxic effects if present in sufficient numbers. However, most cases of serious toxicosis are associated with the adult female tick.

Toxicokinetics

Clinical signs are typically delayed, and usually not observed in small animals until the tick has been feeding for 3–5 days, but this is because the adult female does not start injecting holocyclotoxin until Day 3 of feeding, rather than any significant delay in holocyclotoxin taking effect once injected. On the contrary, it appears that once secretion commences, holocyclotoxin enters the systemic circulation rapidly and may induce clinical signs within hours. Toxin injection peaks on days 4–6. In some cases, by the time the animal is presented for veterinary care, the tick has already detached itself and it is necessary to search for a crater in the center of a raised, inflamed area rather than a tick.

Once a tick has started injecting toxin, the removal of the tick does not prevent some further absorption of toxin from the attachment site. Nevertheless, removal of ticks is a necessary part of treatment.

The delay in clinical signs following attachment of *I. holocyclus* is greater in calves, ranging from 6 to 13 days in controlled trials.

A single adult female *I. holocyclus* secretes enough holocyclotoxin to kill a large dog or a sheep.

Mode(s) of Action

The neurotoxin injected by *I. holocyclus* is holocyclotoxin, which acts by inhibiting release of acetylcholine at the neuromuscular junction. Holocyclotoxin, a proline-rich glycoprotein, is produced in the salivary glands of the tick.

Death from tick paralysis is commonly due to a combination of primary hypoventilation due to paralysis of the respiratory muscles, and myocardial depression leading to pulmonary congestion and congestive heart failure. However, the rapidly ascending neuromuscular paralysis can also cause other life-threatening complications such as aspiration pneumonia.

Clinical Signs

Early signs include change in vocalization (e.g., softer bark), weakness in the hindlegs, mydriasis, anorexia, and vomiting. This progresses to rapidly ascending paralysis, progressively worsening dyspnea, moist cough, difficulty swallowing, cyanosis, coma and death. Clinical signs progress rapidly over 24–48 hours.

Thermoregulation is typically impaired so body temperature may be above or below normal.

Some dogs present as cases of acute congestive heart failure, while some cats present as acutely asthmatic. Tick paralysis should also be considered in cases of sudden development of megaesophagus.

Affected cats often exhibit significant anxiety that may lead to sudden death. Clinical signs in large animals are similar to those observed in dogs. Tick paralysis is a significant cause of morbidity and mortality in young ruminants and foals. Adult livestock and horses often develop some immunity.

Diagnostic Aids

Identification of any ticks found.
Laryngeal palpation may reveal a thrill due to respiratory difficulty.
Extensive radioopacity of the lungs is indicative of a poor prognosis.

Treatment

Provide emergency supportive therapy, such as oxygen, as required by the presentation.

Removal of any tick or ticks still attached is a priority. *I. holocyclus* are often but not always found cranial to the forelegs on domestic pets. Sites of attachment may include lips, inside the mouth or nares, external ear canals, around the eyes, between the toes, and around the anus. *I. holocyclus* can be removed with forceps, a commercial tick remover, or by twisting the body of the tick. If the mouthparts of the tick remain attached they will not continue to inject toxin, but may cause a local foreign body reaction. Clinical signs often worsen in the 24 hours after all *I. holocyclus* are removed, because of toxin being absorbed from the attachment site, but removal of ticks is nevertheless essential.

Administer APVMA-approved tick antiserum (tick antivenom), minimum dose 0.5−1.0 mL/kg, or according to manufacturer's recommendations. There are a number of APVMA-approved suppliers of tick antiserum in eastern Australia. Slow IV administration (over 20 minutes) is recommended in dogs to minimize adverse reactions. Intraperitoneal administration is safest in cats and can also be done in dogs. Antiserum is only able to neutralize circulating toxin, and is therefore most effective early in toxicosis. In advanced cases, most holocyclotoxin is already tissue-bound.

Tick antiserum can also be administered to large animals, e.g., foals and calves, but treatment is often prohibitively expensive for all but the most valuable animals.

Monitor tissue oxygenation and support respiration and oxygenation as required. Oxygen may be administered by tracheostomy. If the animal shows evidence of exhaustion due to respiratory effort, consider administering oxygen as part of general anesthesia under pentobarbitone. Reassess every 6−8 hours.

Animals should be maintained in a dark, quiet environment. Sedation may be helpful in the agitated or noncompliant patient, although the benefits of calming the patient must be balanced against effects on body temperature and blood pressure. Body temperature should be monitored and extremes of hyperthermia or hypothermia prevented; however, mild hypothermia can be tolerated because it reduces oxygen requirement.

The animal should be positioned in sternal recumbency with the head low if possible, otherwise in left lateral recumbency, to minimize aspiration. Vomiting should be prevented with an anti-emetic, e.g., metoclopramide. Vomiting animals should be maintained in a position that minimizes risk of aspiration, and suction of esophageal contents may be required. A low dose of atropine may be used to minimize fluid secretion, but this must be balanced against the effects of atropine on the heart and on body temperature. Monitor for complications such as aspiration pneumonia and treat as necessary.

Broad-spectrum antibiotic cover is a recommended protective measure in all cases of tick paralysis. Application of an acaricide may be advisable particularly for long-haired pets.

The blink reflex is reduced or absent, so the eyes should be monitored. Artificial tears may be required. The urinary bladder should also be monitored and emptied as necessary.

Postdischarge care is important and includes keeping the animal cool and calm, because of the potential for delayed cardiotoxic effects, and also monitoring water intake and urine output.

Prognosis

Prognosis depends very much on the severity of clinical signs and accordingly, how early in the course of toxicosis the animal is presented for treatment. Nonfatal cases frequently require hospitalization for several days.

The prognosis is grave if the animal is presented when it can no longer stand or worse, cannot right itself from lateral to sternal recumbency. Such animals also typically have moderate to severe compromise of respiratory function.

Necropsy

Lesions are nonspecific.

Public Health Considerations

The Australian paralysis tick also poses a hazard to human beings, with toxicosis most commonly observed in preschoolers. Untreated tick paralysis can be fatal in human beings. Symptoms include unsteadiness, progressively increasing weakness of the limbs and ascending symmetrical paralysis, slurred speech, multiple rashes, headache, mydriasis, double vision, fever, swollen lymph nodes, partial facial paralysis. Deep-tendon and gag reflexes are diminished. Dyspnea, bradycardia, decreased oxygen saturation, and asystole may develop. Myocarditis has occurred in children. Some people develop a hypersensitivity reaction to *I. holocyclus*.

Prevention

The use of topical, long-acting acaricides should be strongly recommended to owners living in or near areas where *I. holocyclus* is found. However, owners should be warned that none of the various sprays, collars, rinses, or spot-on products are 100% effective, and therefore regular (at least weekly) examinations are necessary. Owners should be educated on how to remove ticks if found. Application of kerosene, turpentine, or other substances should be discouraged because these substances are irritant and potentially toxic in their own right, and may cause the tick to inject more toxin before it dies.

Owners should be educated to recognize subtle early signs of toxicosis such as change in voice, frequent sitting, or difficulty negotiating stairs. The importance of presenting the animal for veterinary attention as early as possible should be stressed. Owners who do not live in areas where *I. holocyclus* is endemic should be warned to examine their animals for at least 7 days after taking their animals into such an area, and also warned that *I. holocyclus* can be brought home on camping equipment or clothing.

AUSTRALIAN TARANTULAS (*SELENOTHOLUS, SELENOTYPUS, COREMIOCNEMIS, PHLOGIUS* SPP.)

Alternative Names

Whistling spider, barking spider, bird-eating spider.

Distribution

Tarantulas are widely distributed throughout continental Australia, but most of the limited number of documented cases of dog fatalities have been from northern Queensland.

Appearance

Adult spiders have a body approximately 6 cm long, with leg-span of 16 cm. They are hairy, particularly on the legs, and vary in color from fawn to deep brown. They have large fangs.

Circumstances of Poisoning

Dogs appear to be particularly sensitive to the venom of these spiders. Dogs may encounter these spiders outdoors, on when the spiders are kept as pets. Female spiders typically live in burrows, while males live under rocks or logs.

Toxicokinetics

Absorption of venom is rapid, and dogs often die within 30–120 minutes of a bite. Human beings who suffer systemic effects following a bite generally recover in 6–8 hours, suggesting that metabolism and excretion are also rapid.

Mode(s) of Action

Tarantula venom contains a complex mixture of peptides with different mechanisms of action, but neurotoxic action has been demonstrated experimentally.

Clinical Signs

Experimentally and in the limited number of reports in the literature, the clinical signs are apnea and cardiac arrhythmia.

Treatment

There is no specific antivenom. Treatment is symptomatic.

Prognosis

Based on the limited number of documented cases, prognosis in dogs appears to be grave to hopeless.

Necropsy

No specific findings.

Public Health Considerations

Australian tarantula bites are painful to human beings. Some people have developed systemic signs of nausea, vomiting, and fever.

Prevention

Dogs should be prevented from provoking these spiders.

ANTS

There are approximately 90 species of venomous ants of the genus *Myrmecia* in Australia. The bulldog ant *Myrmecia pyriformis* and the jack jumper *Myrmecia pilosula* (actually a complex of several closely related species) in particular have caused a number of human fatalities.

Myrmecia ants are characteristically large, aggressive ants. Some grow up to 40 mm long. They have characteristic large eyes and long mandibles. They have good vision, and can track and even follow intruders from a distance of 1 m. Some species will jump toward intruders. Depending on species, *Myrmecia* ants may be black, red, or a combination of black and either red or orange. They characteristically grip their victim with their mandibles and curl their body to inflict multiple stings.

Compounds found in *Myrmecia* venom include histamine, dopamine, noradrenalin, mellitin, apamin, mast cell degranulating peptide, secapin, tertiapin, protease inhibitor, procamine A and B, phospholipase A and B, hyaluronidases, acid phosphomonoesterase, and α-D-glucosidase.

In human beings, these ants can inflict very painful stings, and can induce an anaphylactic reaction in approximately 1%–3% of the population. *Myrmecia* stings are responsible for approximately 90% of hospital admissions for anaphylaxis. In the absence of an anaphylactic reaction, stings in humans can be treated by application of ice packs.

Cases of acute renal failure have been documented in dogs that were tethered over *Myrmecia* ant nests and unable to escape the consequent mass attacks and multiple stings. In a dog that died as a result of multiple *Myrmecia* stings, lesions included hemorrhage and necrosis of the small intestine and myocardium, bilateral nephrosis with tubular necrosis, and patchy hemorrhage of the lung alveoli, pancreas, and adrenal cortices.

The Green-head Ant *Rhytidoponera metallica* can sting if disturbed, and the sting has caused anaphylaxis in some human beings. The yellow crazy ant *Anoplolepis gracilipes* and the Green Tree Ant *Oecophylla smaragdina* can spray formic acid which causes dermal and ocular irritation. A number of other native ants can inflict a painful bite that is not venomous.

There have also been a small number of introductions of fire ants, of the genus *Solenopsis*, into Queensland and New South Wales. These ants inflict a painful sting and can cause anaphylactic reactions in humans.

CATERPILLARS

Processionary caterpillars, the caterpillars of *Ochrogaster lunifer*, have been incriminated in mid- to late-term abortions in mares. Experimental dosing with the caterpillars or shed exoskeletons of caterpillars caused abortions in mares, with few impending signs. On postmortem examination, setal fragments were found in multiple organs including the liver, gastrointestinal tract, and reproductive tract, and were associated with lesions of amnionitis, serositis, ulceration, and inflammation. It is not clear whether the caterpillars are toxic in their own right, or whether the setae act as vectors for introduction of bacteria.

In addition, a number of caterpillars of Australian *Lepidoptera* have hairs or spines that can cause urticarial reactions, and may cause oral and gastric irritation if caterpillars are consumed.

SAWFLIES (*LOPHYROTOMA INTERRUPTA*)

Alternative Names

Sawfly larval poisoning (SLP).

Distribution

In Australia, SLP occurs in area where there are large forests of the silver leaf ironbark tree *Eucalyptus melanoplhoia.*

Appearance

L. interrupta larvae are pale green or yellow (depending on time since molt) with longitudinal yellow stripes lateral to the back, and a thin black tail part. The most rostral part of the head is black, followed by an orange section with small white protuberances.

Circumstances of Poisoning

SLP occurs when grazing livestock consume sawfly larvae. SLP has been reported in cattle, sheep, and pigs in Australia. There has been a documented case of death of a puppy in Denmark, which has a sawfly that produces the same toxin as the Australian sawfly does. In Australia, most cases occur between July and October, although cases may occur in summer if rain dampens the dried-out remains of larvae. It appears that cattle develop a taste for sawfly larvae and will actively seek them out.

Toxicokinetics

Clinical signs develop within 3 days of experimental administration of larvae to calves.

Mode(s) of Action

The octapeptide lophyrotomin is the major toxin in the larvae of Australian sawflies.

Clinical Signs

Onset of clinical signs is acute, and cattle may be found dead, or may die within 24 hours of onset of clinical signs. Clinical signs in live cows are those of hepatotoxicosis and include depression, anorexia, diarrhea, ataxia, recumbency, tremors, paddling, and death. In cattle with a more protracted course of poisoning, clinical signs may include hemorrhagic diathesis, weight loss and illthrift, icterus, secondary photosensitivity, and/or signs of hepatic encephalopathy such as aggression and hyperexcitability.

Diagnostic Aids

Identification of larvae in leaf litter, and fragments of larvae in the rumen and reticulum of dead cattle.

Clinical chemistry is that of severe liver damage, i.e., elevated liver enzymes and bilirubin, decreased blood glucose, decreased clotting activity, but is not specific for this toxicosis.

Treatment

The remaining herd should be moved away from any silver leaf ironbark trees. Treatment is otherwise symptomatic and supportive. It has been suggested that silymarin may be beneficial.

Triage is appropriate, with euthanasia of severely affected animals and supportive treatment for less severely affected animals.

Prognosis

Prognosis depends on the severity of damage to the liver.

As with all hepatotoxicoses of livestock, it is appropriate to bear in mind that female animals may appear to be normal at the time of an acute outbreak but later succumb to the long-term effects of liver damage under the metabolic pressures of late pregnancy or early lactation.

Necropsy

Gross findings include ascites, swollen liver with accentuated lobular pattern, edema of the gall-bladder wall, and petechiae and ecchymosis over serosal surfaces in the thoracic and abdominal cavities. Sawfly larval body fragments and heads are typically present in the rumen, reticulum, and occasionally the abomasum of affected cattle.

Histopathology of the liver reveals of centrilobular to massive hepatocellular necrosis. Histopathology tends to be most severe in the right lobe of the liver. Mild to moderate lymphocyte necrosis may be present in lymphatic tissues.

Tubular degeneration may be present in the kidneys of cattle.

Prevention

Livestock should not be grazed where there are large numbers of silver leaf ironbark trees during the months July to October.

REDBACK SPIDERS, *LATRODECTUS HASSELTI*

Distribution

Redback spiders are widely distributed in Australia. They tend to live in close association to human habitation but prefer locations where they will not be disturbed, so they often occupy storage areas such as garages and tool-sheds. They are less common in deserts and are not found at the highest altitudes in Australia.

Redbacks have been inadvertently exported to New Zealand and to Japan, and have established self-sustaining colonies in New Zealand, but their distribution in New Zealand has not been fully defined.

Appearance

Female Redback Spiders are approximately 1 cm long, with a body about the size of a large pea, and slender legs. They are black (or, rarely, dark brown) with an obvious orange to red stripe, sometimes broken, on the dorsal abdomen, and an "hourglass" shaped red or orange spot on the ventral abdomen. Juvenile female redbacks have additional white markings on their abdomens.

The male is considerably smaller, averaging 3—4 mm, but similar general shape with slender legs. Males are light brown with dorsal stripe and ventral hourglass markings similar to, but often paler and less distinct than, those of the female. Males also retain white markings on the dorsal abdomen through adulthood.

Only female Redbacks build webs. The web is built in a dry sheltered site, and consists of a roughly funnel-shaped upper retreat area from which sticky catching threads run downward to ground attachments.

Circumstances of Poisoning

Both sexes synthesize venom but most bites of mammals, including humans, are from female Redbacks. Bites most often occur during the summer and in the late afternoon, when ambient temperature is high because this is when the spiders are most active. Redbacks can control the amount of venom they inject, and can deliver a "dry" bite (i.e., no venom is injected). In human beings, approximately 80% of bites have no clinical effect. However, a single Redback bite that injects venom can be sufficient to kill a small animal.

Toxicokinetics

Clinical signs begin almost immediately after the bite.

Mode(s) of Action

The major toxic element in the venom is α-latrotoxin, a presynaptic neurotoxin that causes release of neurotransmitters, including acetylcholine, adrenalin, and noradrenalin from presynaptic nerve terminals. Presynaptic neurotransmitter uptake is inhibited. Release of neurotransmitters occurs by both calcium-dependent and calcium-independent mechanisms. The toxin also acts to allow calcium influx into presynaptic nerve terminals.

Clinical Signs

Initial clinical signs in domestic pets include pain, ataxia, salivation, hyperpnea, and trembling. There may be vomiting and diarrhea. The spider bite is associated with intense local pain, but the site is not always evident.

Cats are not infrequently bitten when trying to eat a Redback, in which case the first sign of envenomation may be that the cat's tongue is protruding from its mouth.

Contraction and cramping of major muscle groups causes intense pain, muscle fasciculation, and muscle rigidity. There may be ascending motor paralysis, proceeding to fatal respiratory or cardiac failure.

Diagnostic Aids

Laboratory evaluation is that of nonspecific muscle damage and is not helpful.

Treatment

Calcium gluconate, in 10% solution, should be administered at a dose of 5–15 mL to cats and 10–30 mL for dogs, to treat muscle fasciculation and weakness.

A muscle relaxant, e.g., methocarbamol, may be administered to relieve muscle cramps.

Treat for shock and pain. Opioid or benzodiazepine pain relief is helpful in human patients.

There is an antivenom, which can be used in domestic animals, and should be used in feline patients. The antivenom can be diluted in saline (10–50 mL, depending on the size of the patient) and given by slow (15–20 minutes) intravenous infusion.

Respiratory and cardiac function must be monitored and supported as necessary.

Prognosis

Cats are particularly sensitive to *Latrodectus* venom, and suffer a high mortality rate. Guinea pigs are even more sensitive, but less likely to provoke a spider to bite them.

Necropsy

There are no distinctive lesions.

Public Health Considerations

Envenomation by Redback spider is unpleasant, but rarely lethal, in human beings.

Prevention

The risk of envenomation by a Redback is one of the many reasons why cats are safer as indoor-only pets, although this is not completely protective because Redbacks will come indoors.

TASMANIAN PARALYSIS TICK *IXODES CORNUATUS*

Clinical signs and treatment are as for Australian paralysis tick, *I. holocyclus* (q.v.), and APVMA-approved tick antiserum prepared for *I. holocyclus* envenomation should be administered.

FUNNEL-WEB SPIDERS (*ATRAX, HADRONYCHE, ILLAWARRA* SPP.) AND MOUSE SPIDERS (*MISSULENA* SPP.)

These species offer an interesting contrast to the situation with Australian tarantulas, in that their venoms are dangerously neurotoxic to primates, including human beings, but do not pose a significant risk to domestic animals. Funnel-web spiders may hold onto the victim and bite repeatedly with their large fangs, so domestic animals may suffer pain and distress, but they do not require therapy with antivenom.

FIDDLEBACK/HOBO SPIDERS (*LOXOSCELES* SPP.)

There are a small number of spiders of the genus *Loxosceles* in Australia, but the brown recluse, *Loxosceles reclusa* is not found in Australia, and the native Loxosceles spiders are not associated with the necrotic arachnism caused by *L. reclusa* bites.

SCORPIONS, CENTIPEDES, AND MILLIPEDES

Scorpions, centipedes, and millipedes in Australia are not particularly dangerous. The sting of a scorpion can cause burning pain that lasts for several hours. Centipedes in Australia can inflict a painful bite, and millipedes can squirt a venom that causes blistering, erythema, and swelling. Treatment is symptomatic.

Part 3: Venomous Terrestrial Invertebrates in New Zealand

In contrast to Australia, New Zealand has few venomous terrestrial animals, and no venomous vertebrates. Venomous invertebrates of significance are limited to the indigenous Katipo, *Latrodectus katipo*, the Australian redback spider *L. hasseltii*, which has been accidentally introduced, and various species of bee, bumblebee, or wasp.

Two species of Australian white-tailed spider, *Lampona cylindrata* and *Lampona murina*, have been introduced into New Zealand. Bites of *L. cylindrata* cause pain and some local erythema and pruritis, and have been claimed to lead to necrotic arachnidism. However, there is a lack of evidence that the spider venom, rather than possible secondary infection, is responsible for any necrotic effects.

The New Zealand tunnel web spider *Porrhothele antipodiana* is a large, rather alarming-looking spider that is sometimes mistaken for the deadly Sydney funnel-web spider, *Atrax robustus* (q.v.). However, although the bite of *P. antipodiana* is reported to be painful and may cause localized swelling, pruritis, or numbness, the venom does not appear to be dangerous.

KATIPO

Alternative Names

Black variants of the Katipo were previously thought to be a different species, *Latrodectus atritus*, but are now recognized as being members of the species *L. katipo*. The Katipo is so closely related to the Australian redback spider that it was formerly regarded as a subspecies with the Linnaean name *L. hasseltii katipo*, but is now recognized as a distinct species.

Distribution

Katipo are only found in coastal areas living among sand dunes, usually on the landward side. Their range includes both coasts the length of the North Island, and they are reported to be abundant on Great Barrier Island. In the

South Island, temperatures are too cold for Katipo eggs to survive south of Greymouth on the West Coast, but Katipo may be found as far south as Dunedin on the east coast. However, Katipo are declining in most areas and is considered to be endangered.

Katipo live close to the ground, because their prey is crawling insects. The disorganized webs are built in low-growing dune plants, under driftwood or stones, or under debris such as tin cans or bottles. Katipo do not thrive in plants that create a dense cover over sand, but prefer to spin their webs in plant cover that leaves patches of open sand.

Appearance

Katipo show a marked sexual dimorphism, with the female markedly larger than the male.

The mature female has a body size of 6—8 mm in length. The slender legs have a span up to 32 mm; the rounded abdomen is of similar size to a garden pea. In the "red Katipo," the abdomen is black with an orange or red stripe, bordered with white, running the length of it. The underside of the abdomen is black and very often has a red marking. The legs are usually black but may be brown on the extremities. In the "black Katipo" variant, which is found in the northern half of the North Island, there is no red stripe on the dorsal abdomen, the abdominal coloration may be lighter, and the marking on the underside of the abdomen is less distinct. There are variations in colors of individual Katipo. In some the base color of black is partially or wholly replaced with brown, and there may be cream spots on the dorsum.

Adult male Katipo, and juveniles, are about 1/6 the size of an adult female. Adult males retain the juvenile colors and markings, which are a brown carapace and with red or orange diamonds, bordered with black, running along the dorsum of the abdomen, which is otherwise white.

Circumstances of Poisoning

Most bites causing human envenomation have been adult female Katipo, although reports of envenomation from bites by males of the closely related *L. hasseltii* suggest that male Katipo should not be regarded as incapable of envenomation.

The Katipo, besides being endangered, is not an aggressive spider and generally tries to retreat from interference. Females may bite to defend their egg sac.

Envenomation by a spider of the genus *Latrodectus* is termed latrodectism, and clinical signs are similar between the various species of *Latrodectus* spider distributed worldwide. There is a lack of verified case reports of domestic animals being bitten by Katipo. However, there are veterinary reports of domestic pets suffering latrodectism as a result of *L. hasseltii* bites in Australia, or *Latrodectus mactans* (Black Widow) spiders in North America.

Toxicokinetics

There is a lack of specific information on the toxicokinetics of *Latrodectus* venom. Clinical signs usually commence almost immediately after the bite but may be delayed up to 8 hours. In a minority of cases, a *Latrodectus* bite is not envenomating.

Mode(s) of Action

Envenomation by a *Latrodectus* spider involves the injection of several biologically active proteins, of which the major component is α-Latrotoxin. The toxin binds to membrane receptors including neurexins and latrophilin/ calcium-independent receptor for α-latrotoxin. Through signal transduction pathway/s yet to be determined, this binding triggers a massive exocytosis in a variety of neurosecretory cells, with disruption of the acetylcholine, nor-adrenalin, dopamine, glutamate, and enkephalin systems.

A single bite from *L. mactans* is capable of delivering a lethal dose of venom to companion animals, although it is not known how *L. katipo* envenomation compares.

Clinical Signs

Cats often die as a result of *L. mactans* bite while dogs appear somewhat more resistant, although they suffer severe clinical signs.

Companion animals with latrodectism show evidence of severe pain. The release of acetylcholine stimulates contraction of major muscle groups and human victims report intensely painful muscle cramps. Companion animals typically exhibit salivation, muscular and abdominal rigidity, and ascending motor paralysis. Cats are particularly susceptible to paralysis. Death results from respiratory or cardiovascular failure.

Diagnostic Aids

There are no specific laboratory evaluations. There may be severe, life-threatening hypertension. Muscle spasms may lead to myoglobinuria.

Treatment

The most important therapeutic measure is intravenous administration of antivenin. Antivenin against the venom of *L. hasseltii* is effective in Katipo bite, and is held by some, but not all, hospitals. The response to the antivenin is usually apparent within 15−30 minutes of administration.

Other symptomatic measures, such as corticosteroids and fluids for shock, may be helpful but cannot substitute for the administration of antivenin. Methocarbamol has been suggested for relief of muscle spasms in animals, although human victims report that benzodiazepines are useful for this purpose. Human victims have reported that opioids relieve pain in latrodectism.

Prognosis

The animal must be closely monitored for myoglobinuria and consequent acute renal failure that may result from the muscle spasms in latrodectism. It may take several days for the animal to recover sufficiently for the practitioner to be confident of a favorable outcome. Complete recovery may take weeks. Severe myocarditis has been reported in one human victim of Katipo bite.

Necropsy

There are no distinctive findings on necropsy.

Public Health Considerations

Katipo are absolutely protected. However, their bite is dangerous to human beings who should be warned to leave the spiders undisturbed and preferably to avoid their habitats.

Prevention

Because of the protected status of Katipo, it is incumbent upon owners to control their animals to keep them away from Katipo, rather than seeking to eliminate the Katipo from the animal's environment.

REDBACK SPIDER

Alternative Names

Latrodectus hasselti.

Distribution

The redback spider was accidentally introduced into New Zealand from Australia and breeding colonies are now found in many parts of the country including Auckland, Tauranga, Coromandel, Gisborne, Hawke's Bay, Wanaka, and Queenstown.

Appearance

The adult female redback spider is approximately 10 mm in length, larger but similar in shape to the adult female Katipo, and is black or brown with a dorsal red or orange-red stripe on the round abdomen. White borders to this stripe are often less pronounced than those of the Katipo, and may be absent altogether. Juveniles and males are dull-colored.

Distinguishing redbacks from Katipo on physical characteristics requires specialist expertise. In any case the clinical signs and treatment of envenomation are the same regardless of which species is responsible.

Circumstances of Poisoning

The redback spider occupies a greater range of habitats than the Katipo and is more likely to be found in proximity to human habitation. Redbacks build their webs being built in dry, sheltered sites, such as among rocks, in logs, in junk-piles, and in sheds and outbuildings. They tend to seek shelter and warmth.

Toxicokinetics

As for Katipo. Human victims report that the bite is immediately painful.

Mode(s) of Action

As for Katipo.

Clinical Signs

As for Katipo.

Diagnostic Aids

As for Katipo.

Treatment

As for Katipo.

Prognosis

As for Katipo.

Necropsy

As for Katipo.

Public Health Considerations

The redback spider is not protected and poses a risk to the safety of human beings.

Prevention

Pest exterminators may be consulted to locate and remove redback spiders.

HYMENOPTERA

Alternate Names

The number and identity of species in the order Hymenoptera is poorly characterized in New Zealand, but well-known members with venomous stings include bees, bumblebees, and wasps. There are both native and introduced species of bee.

Distribution

Various, depending on species. Honey bees and bumblebees are most likely to be found in proximity to flowering plants. Queen wasps may hibernate in human habitation.

Appearance

Various, depending on species. The introduced stinging bees and wasps generally have yellow stripes on the abdomen, although feral bees are often black and have a reputation for aggression.

Circumstances of Poisoning

Honey bees generally only sting if provoked, and bumblebees only if severely provoked. An exception exists for sweaty horses, which may be attacked by multiple bees if they are ridden, tied, or allowed to stray near beehives. Dogs may snap at a hovering insect and sustain stings to the mouth as a result. Wasps are generally considered more aggressive than honey bees or bumblebees. All the common species of bee or wasp will attack if their hive or colony is disturbed.

Toxicokinetics

Localized pain is immediate and generalized hypersensitivity reactions, if they occur, generally follow rapidly. Hypersensitivity reactions appear to be less common in domestic animals than in human beings.

Mode(s) of Action

Venom in stings contains a wide range of substances of which some of the major ones, in terms of proportion and/or pathogenicity, are phospholipase A_2, acid phosphatase, hyaluronidase, melittin, histamine, dopamine, and noradrenaline.

Clinical Signs

Behavior consistent with acute pain. Swelling, erythema, and edema at the sting site/s. Urticarial wheals may develop, particularly if there are multiple stings. Vesicular lesions may develop on the skin. The pain associated with multiple stings has been reported to cause severe excitement in horses, with tachycardia and diarrhea developing.

If an animal is sting in or around the mouth or nostrils, local swelling may cause dyspnea.

Diagnostic Aids

No specific diagnostic aids.

Treatment

If the stinger is still present in the skin, remove it by scraping, taking care to avoid squeezing the venom sac. Apply a cold compress to minimize swelling. If signs of hypersensitivity reaction develop, treat with antihistamines or adrenaline as required. Airway patency must be maintained.

Prognosis

Prognosis depends on the number of stings, the site/s of stings and the presence or absence of hypersensitivity reaction.

Necropsy

No specific lesions.

Public Health Considerations

If the envenomation is the result of a domestic animal disturbing a wasp's nest, pest control services may be called to remove the nest for the protection of human beings.

Prevention

Puppies and kittens, in particular, should be observed to ensure that they do not try to eat or play with bees, wasps, or bumblebees. Horses, particularly when sweaty, should not be ridden, tied, or confined near beehives or colonies of wild stinging Hymenoptera. Commercial beehives should be fenced off with, at minimum, an electric wire or tape to keep livestock and horses away from them, for the protection of both the mammals and the bees.

Chapter 24

Poisonous Plants

Part 1: Toxicity of Introduced Plants

INTRODUCTION

Both Australia and New Zealand have numerous introduced plant species that have caused poisoning in animals. In this section, plants are categorized by the organ or system, which the most important target of toxicity. It should be noted that many plants cause some degree of gastrointestinal toxicity, but if the most important target of toxicity is an organ or system other than the gastrointestinal tract, the plant will be listed under that organ or system. Some plants that target several organs or systems are listed more than once, e.g., *Quercus* species.

For most plant poisonings, there is no specific antidote, and treatment is supportive. As a generalization, plant toxins are adsorbed by activated charcoal. The contraindications of using activated charcoal should be borne in mind. Ruminal emptying by rumenotomy may be indicated in the case of highly toxic material, if the value of the animal justifies it.

This chapter does not include details of the appearance of plants. There are high-quality photographs of most plants available on the internet, by searching in Google Images. When searching for information on the internet, the plant should always be searched by Linnaean name, because common names vary from region to region and the same common name may be used for different plants in different countries.

Details of distribution and identification, including photographs, are available for Australian readers in Dr. Ross McKenzie's authoritative work *Australia's Poisonous Plants, Fungi and Cyanobacteria* (CSIRO Press, 2012). Unfortunately, there is no reference book of comparable quality for poisonous plants in New Zealand. Those books that do exist are either poorly illustrated or far from comprehensive, or both.

It should be noted that a number of plants in this chapter have been introduced into Australia but not into New Zealand. New Zealand readers should not assume that any given species is present in New Zealand.

In those cases in which the toxicity associated with a given plant is due to a fungal infection, the toxicosis is covered in Chapter 21, Mycotoxins and Mushrooms, even if the fungus is an endophyte.

Examples include but are not limited to Ryegrass (*Lolium* spp.) staggers, *Phalaris* staggers, Tall Fescue toxicosis, *Paspalum* ergot, hemorrhagic diathesis associated with fungal infection of *Anthoxanthum odoratum* (sweet vernal grass) and pulmonary disease associated with moldy sweet potato (*Ipomea batatas*; kumara). The exception with regard to fungi is dihydroxycoumarin poisoning (see Subsection "Plants Associated With Clotting Defects" under Section "Plants With Toxic Effects on the Blood") because the plants synthesize the high levels of coumarol, which are converted by postharvest fungal action.

Categories in this section, are as follows:

- Neurotoxic plants
- Hepatotoxic plants
- Nephrotoxic plants
- Cardiotoxic plants
- Plants with toxic effects on the blood
- Plants with toxic effects on the gastrointestinal tract
- Plants with toxic effects on the respiratory system
- Plants with toxic effects on skin
- Plants with toxic effects on skeletal muscle
- Plants with toxic effects on the endocrine system and the mammary gland
- Plants with toxic effects on the immune system

With regard to reproductive effects, reference should also be made to Chapter 5, Vulnerable Patients.

NEUROTOXIC PLANTS

Introduced plants recognized to have neurotoxic effects in animals are listed and described in Table 24.1.

HEPATOTOXIC PLANTS

Plants Containing Pyrrolizidine Alkaloids

There are over 600 different pyrrolizidine alkaloids known, and they are produced by a wide variety of flowering plants. Pyrrolizidine alkaloids vary considerably in toxicity, but for most, the liver is the primary target of toxicity. A very small number are known to cause lung toxicity at lower doses than those at which they cause hepatotoxicity.

High doses of pyrrolizidine alkaloids cause liver necrosis, which is initially centrilobular in distribution. Low doses interfere with cell division in animals,

TABLE 24.1 Plants Introduced to Australia and/or New Zealand That Cause Neurotoxicity

Linnaean Name	Common Name	Type of Plant	Comments
Aesculus hippocastanum	Horse chestnut	Ornamental tree	Clinical toxicosis is most often reported in cattle and horses. The toxin principle, esculin, is a mixture of saponin glycosides. Clinical signs include incoordination, staggering, hypermetria, weakness, and collapse. Fatalities resulting from falling over cliffs or from drowning have been reported. Animals sometimes also show signs of gastroenteritis. The toxic effects are not permanent. Animals should be placed where they are safe from injuries resulting from falling.
Atropa belladonna	Deadly nightshade	Weed	The toxic principles are atropine, hyoscamine, and scopolamine. Poisoning is rare, but small animals occasionally eat the berries. Clinical signs include mydriasis, dry mouth, apparent hallucinations, ataxia, and hyperthermia. Seizures may occur in severe cases. The patient should be kept in a quiet dark place if possible. Diazepam or other benzodiazepine may be used for sedation. Physostigmine is helpful in severe cases.
Avena sativa	Oats	Crop	May cause "red tipped oats poisoning" in which dairy cows become hard to handle and highly sensitive to noise. They also exhibit ataxia and diarrhea. Up to 25% of a herd may be affected. Most recover within 5 days.
Beta vulgaris	Beet	Crop	May cause polioencephalomalacia in ruminants due to the presence of sulfur. Ruminants are susceptible if their total diet contains >0.5% sulfur. It is thought that ruminal microflora convert sulfur to hydrogen sulfide. Animals may be found dead. Others may exhibit depression, episodic excitement, apparent blindness, head-pressing, wandering, circling, and terminal convulsions. Mildly affected animals may respond to being moved from the offending pasture/crop and given 10–20 mg

(Continued)

TABLE 24.1 (Continued)

Linnaean Name	Common Name	Type of Plant	Comments
			thiamine/kg bodyweight, IV two to three times on the first day followed by the same dose IM b.i.d. for two or three more days. Valuable animals may be treated for cerebral edema. Mildly affected animals may survive and be productive despite mild brain damage.
Brassica spp.	Include rape, kale, cabbage, chou moellier, Brussels sprouts, kohlrabi, broccoli, turnips, and other vegetables	Crops	May cause polioencephalomalacia in ruminants due to the presence of sulfur (see entry for *B. vulgaris*).
			Other toxicoses associated with this large group of plants are nitrate poisoning, hemolysis, photosensitization, goiter.
Brugmansia spp.	Angel's trumpets	Ornamentals	Tropane alkaloids, as for *A. belladonna*, q.v.
Brunfelsia spp.	Francisia; Yesterday-today-and-tomorrow	Garden shrub	Toxicosis has been reported in dogs that eat the fruit of these plants. Clinical signs include muscle tremors and clonic/tonic convulsions as well as signs of gastroenteritis. The toxic principle is unknown and treatment is symptomatic.
Cannabis sativa	Cannabis, marijuana		See the section on illicit and recreational drugs.
Centaurea solstitialis	St Barnaby's thistle	Weed	Causes nigropallidal encephalomalacia in horses. Clinical signs include depression, drooped head, wandering, impaired grazing, protruding tongue with edges turned upward. Bilateral malacic lesions are present in the globus pallidus and substantia nigra. Most affected horses will require euthanasia although mildly affected horses may be able to adapt.

Chenopodium album	Fat hen	Weed	May cause polioencephalomalacia in ruminants due to sulfur content (see entry for *Beta vulgaris*, above). Also contains soluble oxalates and nitrates.
Conium maculatum	Poison hemlock	Weed	Poisoning due to poison hemlock is extremely rare because grazing animals find the plant unattractive. The toxic principles are coniine and related pyridine alkaloids. Clinical signs include muscle tremors, weakness, convulsions, and coma. There may also be gastrointestinal signs of vomiting and diarrhea. Pyridine alkaloids have also been shown experimentally to be teratogenic in cattle and pigs.
Datura stramonium	Thorn apple; Angel's Trumpet	Garden ornamental	Toxic principles include atropine, hyoscamine, and hyoscine. Clinical signs and treatment are as for *A. belladonna* (q.v.).
Delphinium	Delphinium, larkspur	Garden ornamental	The toxic principles are polycyclic diterpene alkaloids, which act as neuromuscular blocking agents on cholinergic and nicotinic receptors. Toxicosis has been reported in ruminants and horses. Clinical signs include excitability, disorientation, muscle tremors, stiff movement and paresis, progressing to prostration and seizures. The clinical course is rapid. Poisoning resembles hypomagnesemia. Ruminants may develop bloat which must be relieved. Physostigmine, 0.6 mg/kg IV, should be administered to relieve the neuromuscular blockade.
Duranta erecta	Duranta	Garden shrub	The toxin is unknown. Toxicosis has been observed in a variety of domestic species as well as in human beings. Clinical signs are predominantly nervous, including depression, drowsiness, ptosis, bradycardia, tremors, and convulsions, but vomiting and diarrhea may also occur.
Gelsemium sempervirens	Carolina jessamine, night-blooming jessamine	Ornamental vine	Toxins are indole alkaloids that may be found in all parts of the plant. Clinical signs and symptoms in human beings include muscle weakness, mydriasis, biplopia, headache, trembling of limbs, falling of the jaw, bilateral ptosis, dyspnea, paralysis, and death. Some people experience spasms of the limbs and/or general rigidity.

(Continued)

TABLE 24.1 (Continued)

Linnaean Name	Common Name	Type of Plant	Comments
Gomphrena celpsioides	Gomphrena weed	Weed	Causes a disease of horses called "coastal staggers" or "Bundaberg horse disease." Onset is delayed for >3 weeks after horses begin grazing pasture heavily contaminated with this plant. Clinical signs include incoordination, ataxia, inappetence. Mild cases will recover fully if removed from the pasture containing the weed.
Hyoscyamus niger	Henbane	Weed	Poisoning is extremely rare because the plant is not palatable to livestock. Toxic principles include hyosyamine and scopolamine. Clinical signs and treatment are the same as for *A. belladonna* (q.v.).
Hypochaeris radicata	Cat's ear	Weed	Associated with stringhalt in horses. Horses have uncontrolled flexion of the hocks, are unable to back, and have muscle atrophy over the hind legs. Horses may also develop laryngeal hemiplegia. Most horses recover. Phenytoin may be helpful.
Ipomea spp.	Morning Glory	Ornamental vine	Toxic principles include lysergic acid and related indole alkaloids, and are most concentrated in the seeds. Poisoning in dogs has been reported. Clinical signs include mydriasis, bizarre behavior, and apparent hallucinations. Dogs may develop diarrhea and may be hypotensive. Sedation may be indicated but hypotensive sedatives such as acetyl promazine should be used with caution.
Laburnum anaglyroides	Laburnum	Ornamental tree	The toxic principle is cytisine. Clinical signs include emesis, drowsiness, weakness, ataxia, mydriasis, and tachycardia.

Lamium amplexicaule	Henbit	Weed	Staggers due to this plant are reported in New South Wales, but not in New Zealand. Affected animals are ruminants and horses. Staggers occur when animals are forced to move. Animals have hindleg stiffness and will move only a short distance before stopping and exhibiting tremors in the legs. Animals may collapse and die if forced to continue moving. Henbit staggers may be shown for some time after animals are removed from access to henbit, but eventually resolve. The toxic principle is unknown.
Lantana camara	Lantana	Weed	The toxin is unknown. Consumption of milk from dams that have grazed this plant causes "scrub ataxia" in calves. Clinical signs include posterior ataxia, high head carriage, dermal damage on the forelimbs, partial or complete blindness, dry crusty facial and dorsal skin, diarrhea, urinary incontinence, epiphora. Most calves will recover after being weaned.
Lantana montevidensis	Creeping lantana	Weed	
Macadamia	Macadamia	Nut-bearing tree	Toxicosis due to ingestion of macadamia nuts has been reported in dogs. Clinical signs of muscular weakness are transient and recovery is generally complete within 24 hours. The toxic principle is unknown, but is not destroyed by roasting.
Malva parviflora	Small-flowered mallow	Weed	Staggers due to ingestion of this plant are reported in Australia but not in New Zealand. Sheep are most often affected and exhibit weakness, trembling, tachycardia, and increased respiration when forced to move. Sheep may die if hard-pressed to move. *M. parviflora* is also known to cause nitrite poisoning and skeletal muscle necrosis.
Modiola caroliniana	Creeping mallow	Weed	Creeping mallow has been suspected of causing staggers in Australia and in the US. It also grows in New Zealand but has not been reported to cause staggers.

(Continued)

TABLE 24.1 (Continued)

Linnaean Name	Common Name	Type of Plant	Comments
Nicotiana spp.		Garden shrubs or weeds	Introduced species in this genus include *N. glauca* (tree tobacco), *N. tabacum* (tobacco), and *N. rustica* (wild tobacco). The toxic principle in *N. glauca* is anabasine, which is pharmacologically similar to, but more potent than, nicotine, whereas nicotine predominates in the other species. Clinical signs include ataxia, tremors, tachycardia, clonic convulsions, and prostration. Death is due to asphyxia.
Phalaris spp.		Pasture grasses or weeds	"Phalaris staggers" affect ruminants and are caused by Indole alkaloids Clinical signs include hyperexcitability, muscle tremors, and paresis. Toxicosis may be prevented by administering cobalt by slow-release intraruminal "bullet," commencing prior to exposure to *Phalaris*.
R. raphanistrum	Wild radish	Weed	May cause polioencephalomalacia in ruminants due to the presence of sulfur (see entry for *Beta vulgaris*, above).
R. rugosum	Turnip weed	Weed	Although better known as a goitrogen, this weed may cause hemolysis and/or polioencephalomalacia in ruminants that ingest it (see entry for *Beta vulgaris*, above). The hemolysis is attributed to the presence of S-methylcysteine sulfoxide and the polioencephalomalacia to the presence of sulfur.
Romulea spp.	Onion grass	Weed	Associated with staggers in sheep, particularly in the autumn, although it is not clear whether the toxin is synthesized by the plant itself or by fungi infecting the plant.
Sisymbrium irio	London rocket	Weed	Sulfur in this plant may cause polioencephalomalacia in ruminants (see entry for *Beta vulgaris*, above). Also contains nitrate.

Stachys arvensis	Staggerweed	Weed	An unidentified toxin causes staggers in ruminants and horses that ingest this weed. Staggers generally resolve when access is halted.
Solanaceae family	Nightshade family	Tomato, potato, some ornamentals, some weeds	The toxic principles are solanine and solanidine. The clinical course is rapid with animals either succumbing or recovering within 48 hours. Clinical signs include depression, ataxia, tremors, posterior weakness, and prostration. There may also be gastrointestinal signs such as vomiting and diarrhea, and large doses may cause intestinal atony. Potatoes (*Solanum tuberosum*) should never be eaten if partially green. Both the potato plant and the tomato plant (*Lycopersicon* spp.) are toxic.
Trachyandra divaricata	Branched onion weed	Weed	An unknown toxin causes CNS degeneration in horses and sheep that graze this weed. Clinical signs are ataxia and recumbency, and postmortem histopathology shows intense lipofuscinosis of neurons. There is no treatment.
Tribulus terrestris	Puncture vine	Weed	ß-Carboline alkaloids cause progressive, irreversible posterior ataxia in sheep.

leading to hepatomegalocytosis featuring giant multinucleate hepatocytes. The latter phenomenon is not seen in human toxicosis. Pyrrolizidine alkaloid hepatotoxicity is cumulative in effect, so liver failure is the end result, whether poisoning is acute or chronic. Toxicosis in livestock is most frequently chronic, because animals find the plants unpalatable and will avoid eating them if they can. However, many weeds containing pyrrolizidine alkaloids are relatively drought-resistant and may be the only grazing available in dry conditions.

Sheep are relatively resistant to toxicosis, when compared to horses and cattle. Pyrrolizidine alkaloid concentrations are reduced but not eliminated by drying associated with haymaking. Pigs have been poisoned by eating *Crotalaria retusa* seeds in contaminated feed grain.

Clinical signs of chronic pyrrolizidine alkaloid toxicosis are icterus, depression, anorexia, and failure to thrive. Hepatic encephalopathy may develop, particularly in horses. Signs of hepatic encephalopathy include aimless wandering, head-pressing, and disoriented behavior. Animals may suffer secondary photosensitization, particularly on skin unprotected by hair, wool, or melanin. Lesions in the liver include megalocytosis, hepatocellular

TABLE 24.2 Introduced Plants That Contain Pyrrolizidine Alkaloids

Linnaean Name	Common Name
Amsinckia calycina	Ironweed
Amsinckia intermedia	Ironweed
Amsinckia lycosoides	Ironweed
Crotalaria species	Rattlepod
Delairea odorata	*Senecio mikanioides*, German ivy, Cape ivy
Echium vulgare	Alpine borage, Viper's Bugloss
Echium plantagineum	Paterson's curse, Salvation Jane
Heliotropium amplexicaule	Blue heliotrope
Heliotropium europaeum	Common heliotrope
Heliotropium ovalifolium	
Senecio bipinnatisectus	Fireweed
Senecio jacobaea	Ragwort, tansy ragwort
Senecio madagascariensis	Fireweed
Senecio quadridentatus	Cotton fireweed
Senecio vulgaris	Groundsel
Symphytum officinale	Comfrey
Symphytum x uplandicum	Russian comfrey, blue comfrey

necrosis, biliary hyperplasia, nodular hyperplasia, and extensive fibrosis. Treatment is usually futile by the time toxicosis is diagnosed.

Introduced plants in Australia and/or New Zealand that have been associated with pyrrolizidine alkaloid poisoning are listed in Table 24.2. It should be noted that some indigenous plants in both countries also produce pyrrolizidine alkaloids.

Plants within the genus *Crotalaria* may contain the pyrrolizidine alkaloids monocrotaline or fulvine, both of which may cause pulmonary disease at doses lower than that required to produce hepatic toxicosis. Pulmonary toxicosis has been reported in horses and in sheep.

Plants that produce hepatotoxicity by toxic principles other than pyrrolizidine alkaloids are presented in Table 24.3.

TABLE 24.3 Plants Introduced to Australia and/or New Zealand That Cause Hepatotoxicity by Toxic Principles Other Than Pyrrolizidine Alkaloids

Linnaean Name	Common Name	Type of Plant	Comments
Brachiaria spp.	Signal grass, para grass	Grass	The toxic principles are steroidal saponins. Disease is most often manifested as secondary photosensitization although other clinical signs may include hemoglobinuria, dependent subcutaneous edema and hepatic encephalopathy. Ruminants and horses are affected. *Brachiaria* species also contain oxalates that cause secondary hyperparathyroidism in horses.
Cestrum parqui	Green cestrum	Garden plant	Diterpenoid glycosides parquin and carboxyparquin cause acute necrosis of hepatocytes in ruminants. Animals are often found dead but may survive long enough to develop hepatic encephalopathy.
Cycas revoluta	Sago palm	Garden plant	Dogs eating seeds of cultivated specimens of *C. revoluta* have suffered liver necrosis. The toxic principle is methylazoxymethanol.
Lythrum hyssopifolia	Lesser loosestrife	Weed	Sheep grazing this plant have developed heaptic necrosis as well as renal tubular necrosis. The toxic principle is unknown.
Panicum spp.		Grass	Steroidal saponins cause hepatogenous photosensitization in ruminants. These

(Continued)

TABLE 24.3 (Continued)

Linnaean Name	Common Name	Type of Plant	Comments
			plants also contain oxalates that may cause secondary hyperparathyroidism in horses.
Quercus spp.	Oak	Trees	Acorns are poisonous to ruminants although generally well-tolerated by pigs. The toxic principle is gallotannin. Affected ruminants exhibit depression, anorexia, and ruminal atony, and are usually constipated although hemorrhagic scouring has been reported. Icterus, hematuria, polyuria, and hyposthenuria may be present. Necropsy findings include severe hepatitis and centrilobular necrosis in acute cases. Gastroenteritis and nephritis are also evident and perirenal edema is characteristic.
Salvia reflexa	Mint weed	Weed	Appears to contain an unidentified hepatotoxin in addition to nitrate.
Xanthium occidentale	Noogoora burr	Weed	A carboxyatractyloside causes acute necrosis of hepatocytes in pigs and ruminants that eat the burrs. Animals are often found dead but may survive long enough to develop hepatic encephalopathy.

NEPHROTOXIC PLANTS

Plants Containing Soluble Oxalates

A wide range of plants cause nephrotoxicity because they contain soluble oxalates. Once ingested and absorbed into the body, soluble oxalates react with serum calcium to form calcium oxalate. In the concentrating environment of the renal tubules, calcium oxalate can crystallize to form distinctive rosette-shaped crystals that can be observed using a polarizing filter. The precipitation of calcium oxalate crystals leads to renal tubular necrosis and death from renal failure.

The formation of calcium oxalate in the circulation also leads to depletion of calcium ions and functional hypocalcemia, which can cause muscle twitching, mild seizures, recumbency, and death, particularly if animals are forced to move. In addition the hypocalcemia caused by ingesting soluble oxalates may lead to secondary hyperparathyroidism in horses.

Hypocalcemia may be treated with calcium borogluconate IV, as for a cow with postparturient hypocalcemia.

Clinical signs of renal failure in animals as a result of ingesting soluble oxalates include depression, azotemia, and oliguria later changing to polyuria and hyposthenuria. Animals may die of hyperkalemic heart failure.

The calcium oxalate crystals will eventually dissolve if the animal can be kept alive and renal throughput maintained, but renal function may be permanently reduced. Horses with secondary hyper parathyroidism should be removed from the pasture and supplemented for at least 6 months with 2 kg/week of a mineral supplement containing a Ca:P ratio of 2:1, in order to remineralize the bones.

Introduced plants that contain soluble oxalates are listed in Table 24.4. It should be noted that some indigenous Australian plants also contain toxic

TABLE 24.4 Plants Introduced to Australia and/or New Zealand That Cause Nephrotoxicity Due to Soluble Oxalates

Linnaean Name	Common Name	Comments
Acetosa vesicaria	Ruby dock	
Acetosella vulgaris	Sheep sorrel	Also known as *Rumex acetosella*.
Amaranthus retroflexus	Redroot pigweed	*Amaranthus* spp. also appear to have nephrotoxic actions by means of unidentified toxin/s.
Averrhoa carambola	Carambola	
Beta vulgaris	Beet	Also contains sulfur and nitrate.
Brachiaria spp.	Signal grass, para grass	See Table 24.3.
C. ciliaris	Buffel grass	
C. album	Fat hen	
Emex australis	Spiny emex	
Mesembryanthemum spp.	Ice plants	
Oxalis corniculata		
Oxalis pes-caprae	Bermuda buttercup, soursob	
Portulaca spp.	Pigweed	
Rheum x cultorum	Rhubarb	
Rumex spp.	Docks	
Salsola australis	Soft roly-poly	
S. sphacelata		
Trianthema spp.	Black pigweed, red spinach	

levels of soluble oxalates. All the plants in Table 24.4 are found in both Australia and New Zealand, although in some cases toxicity has only been observed in Australia. This difference may reflect different gene pools and/ or different growing conditions.

Anagallis arvensis

Anagallis arvensis or Scarlet Pimpernel has caused severe renal tubular necrosis in sheep in Australia. It may also cause gastrointestinal toxicosis.

Aristolochia spp.

There are both introduced and native Australian species of *Aristolochia*. Their common name is birthwort. They contain aristolochic acid that is a potent nephrotoxin. Acute renal failure has occurred in horses, sheep, and human beings consuming these plants. Consumption of aristolochic acid is also associated with neoplasia of the urinary tract in human beings.

Hemerocallis spp. Daylilies

AND

Lilium spp. Lilies

An unknown toxin in these ornamentals causes renal failure in cats. All parts of the plants are toxic. Clinical signs develop within 2 hours of cats eating the plants. Initial clinical signs are vomiting, hypersalivation, and depression. There may be tremors or seizures if *Hemerocallis* spp. have been consumed. After 12–30 hours, cats develop polyuria, with progression to anuria. Unless treatment is prompt and aggressive, cats usually die within 5 days. Prognosis is grave to hopeless if the cat is anuric. If consumption is recent, activated charcoal may be helpful. Intravenous fluid therapy should be established early in order to maintain urinary throughput at approximately twice the normal level.

Lythrum hyssopifolia, Lesser loosetrife

The toxic principle in this weed is unknown. Poisoning is most often reported when sheep have grazed on crop stubbles in which the plant is present. Necropsy findings are those of renal tubular necrosis as well as necrosis of hepatocytes. This plant is present in both Australia and New Zealand but poisoning cases have not been reported in New Zealand.

Quercus Species, Oaks

The gallotannins in *Quercus* species (oaks) are toxic to the kidney as well as the liver and gastrointestinal tract. Refer to Table 24.3.

Vitis *Species, Grape Vine*

Acute renal tubular necrosis has been reported in dogs following ingestion of grapes or raisins. However, many dogs have been recorded to have eaten large quantities of grapes or raisins with no ill-effects, and there is no clear dose–response relationship evident from case reports. The toxin may be a mycotoxin, or may be a toxin synthesized by the grape plant itself (*Vitis* spp.) but only produced under some conditions. Cases of grape or raisin poisoning have been reported from the US, Europe, and South Korea, and have been associated with both seeded and seedless grapes, homegrown and purchased grapes, and with grape pressings from wineries. Hemorrhagic gastroenteritis, fibrinous peritonitis, and cardiac myositis have also been found in some affected dogs on necropsy, and metastatic calcification may be present in multiple organs in chronic or recovered cases. In some cases, brownish crystals have been observed in the renal pelvis. Clinical signs including vomiting, diarrhea, depression, anorexia, ataxia, and oliguria develop within 6–24 hours of ingestion. It is estimated that the toxic dose of raisins is 2.8 mg/kg, and as few as four to five grapes may be fatal in a small dog. Affected dogs should be treated vigorously with supportive therapy for renal failure, and renal throughput maintained. Activated charcoal may be helpful for gastrointestinal decontamination. Grape/raisin poison has not been confirmed in cats.

Cattle have suffered toxicosis from consumption of large quantities of grapes. Clinical signs include anorexia, bruxism, ruminal stasis, pyrexia, tachycardia, dyspnea, and ruminal tympany. The mechanism appears to be ruminal acidosis. Prognosis is poor and ruminal emptying should be considered for valuable animals.

CARDIOTOXIC PLANTS

Plants Containing Grayanotoxins

Plants introduced into Australia and New Zealand that synthesize cardiotoxic grayanotoxins (also sometimes called andromedotoxins) include *Rhododendron* species, which include rhododendrons and azaleas, Kalmia species and *Pieris japonica*, also known as Japanese pieris or lily-of-the-valley tree. All of these plants are attractive ornamental trees or shrubs. Grayanotoxins are water-soluble diterpenoid compounds found in leaves and nectar, which bind to and modify the sodium channels of cell membranes, leading to prolonged depolarization and excitation. In the heart, this results in a strong inotropic effect. Poisoning has been reported in horses and ruminants, and may occur when the animals have unaccustomed access to the plants because prunings are thrown into a paddock. Goats have been known to become poisoned by voluntarily browsing the plants. It has been estimated that a mass of leaves as little as 0.2% of the animal's bodyweight is sufficient to cause lethal toxicosis. The plants cause some hypersalivation and apparent oral discomfort on ingestion. Clinical signs develop rapidly and include diarrhea, muscular weakness, dyspnea, depression, and collapse. Hypotension develops as a result of vasodilation, and auscultation reveals bradycardia and atrioventricular block. Bradycardia may respond to atropine and isoproterenol or sodium channel blockers may be useful.

Introduced plants causing cardiotoxicity due to toxic principles other than grayanotoxins are listed in Table 24.5.

TABLE 24.5 Plants Introduced to Australia and/or New Zealand That Cause Cardiotoxicity Other Than Grayanotoxicosis

Linnaean Name	Common Name	Type of Plant	Comments
Acokanthera oblongifolia	Bushman's poison	Ornamental	Toxic principles are cardiac glycosides (see preamble).
Aconitum napellum	Monkshood, aconite	Garden plant	The toxic principles, aconitine and related compounds, are found throughout the plant. Clinical signs include oral inflammation, hypersalivation, hypotension, cardiac arrhythmia, and weakness.
Adonis microcarpa	Pheasant's eye, red chamomole	Weed	This species is not known in New Zealand and is designated as an "unwanted organism." In Australia it has caused poisoning of ruminants, horses, and pigs due to the presence of cardiac glycosides (see preamble).
Araujia sericifera	White moth plant	Weed	The toxic principles are unknown, but are thought to be cardiac glycosides.
Argemone spp.	Mexican poppy	Weed	Poisonings have occurred in poultry and ruminants following ingestion of seeds or the dried plant in hay. The toxic principles are isoquinoline alkaloids which cause cardiomyopathy. Clinical signs include those of pulmonary and subcutaneous edema.
Asclepias curassavica	Red-head cotton-bush, Red cotton	Weed, may be grown to support Monarch butterflies	Toxic principles are cardiac glycosides (see preamble).

(Continued)

TABLE 24.5 (Continued)

Linnaean Name	Common Name	Type of Plant	Comments
Calotropis procera	Calotrope	Weed	Toxic principles are cardiac glycosides (see text). In addition, the sap is irritant to skin and eyes of human beings.
P. americana	Avocado	Tree, cultivated for fruit	Leaves, and the skin or pit of the fruit, have been reported to be toxic to domestic pets, birds and horses. The toxic principle is persin, which causes gastrointestinal irritation and also induces myocardial degeneration and necrosis, and pericardial effusion. Ingestion of avocado leaves may also cause severe sterile mastitis.
Bryophyllum spp.	Kalanchoe, mother-of-millions	Garden plant or garden-escaped weed	Flowering plants are the most toxic. The toxic principles are cardiac glycosides (see text).
Cascabela thevetia	Yellow oleander, *Thevetia peruviana*		The toxic principles are cardiac glycosides (see text).
Convallaria majalis	Lily-of-the-valley		The toxic principles are cardiac glycosides (see text).
Corchorus olitorius	Jute	Weed	The toxic principles are cardiac glycosides (see text).
Cryptostegia grandiflora	Rubber vine	Weed	The toxic principles are cardiac glycosides (see text).
Digitalis purpurea	Foxglove	Weed, sometimes grown as garden plant	The toxic principles are cardiac glycosides (see text).
Gomphocarpus spp.	Balloon cotton, swan plant	Garden plant or weed	The toxic principles are cardiac glycosides (see text).
Gossypium spp.	Cotton	Crop	See Gossypol Toxicity in Chapter 19, Agricultural and Feed-Related Toxicants.

(Continued)

TABLE 24.5 (Continued)

Linnaean Name	Common Name	Type of Plant	Comments
Helleborus spp.	Christmas rose	Garden plant	Cardiac glycosides including hellebrin, helleborin, helleborein. Gastroenteric clinical signs predominate but arrhythmia and hypotension may develop in severe poisonings (see text).
Homeria flaccida	One-leaf Cape tulip	Weeds	The toxic principles are cardiac glycosides (see text).
Homeria miniata	Two-leaf Cape tulip		
Iris spp.	Iris	Ornamentals and weeds	The toxins are unidentified.
Melianthus major	Cape honey flower	Ornamental or escaped weed	The toxic principles are cardiac glycosides (see text). Necropsy findings include hemorrhage and edema of the lungs, pericardial hemorrhage, general cyanosis and congestion of the liver and kidney. However, palatability is low so poisoning occurs only if animals are extremely hungry.
Moraea setifolia	Thread iris	Weed	The toxic principles are cardiac glycosides (see text).
Nerium oleander	Oleander	Ornamental shrubs	Extremely toxic to all domestic species. The toxic principles are cardiac glycosides (see text).
Ornithogallum umbellatum	Star of Bethlehem	Weed	The toxic principles are cardiac glycosides (see text).
Taxus baccata	English yew	Tree	The taxine alkaloids are highly toxic to herbivores. Cattle and horses are often found dead. Clinical signs include trembling, muscle weakness, dyspnea, and collapse. Auscultation reveals arrhythmia and bradycardia. Diastolic heart block is the cause of death.

For many of the species listed in Table 24.5, the toxic principles are *cardiotoxic glycosides*. These substances disrupt electrical conductivity in the myocardium, leading to conduction block and eventual asystole. Cardiotoxic glycosides are generally readily absorbed from the gastrointestinal tract, and may undergo enterohepatic cycling. Initial clinical signs are usually gastroenteric and include vomiting, signs of abdominal pain, and diarrhea which may be bloodstained. Signs of acute cardiotoxicity ensue and include weakness, depression, dyspnea, recumbency, coma, and death. Findings on auscultation include arrhythmia, ventricular premature systole, paroxysmal tachycardia, and asystole. As a generalization, cardiac glycosides are adsorbed by activated charcoal. Phenytoin may assist atrioventricular conduction. Atropine and propanolol have also been suggested to alleviate arrhythmia. Serum potassium should be monitored and hyperkalemia corrected as necessary.

PLANTS WITH TOXIC EFFECTS ON THE BLOOD

Plants Containing Nitrates

A number of plants contain, at least under some growing conditions, high levels of nitrates in their stalks and/or leaves. Nitrate levels tend to increase by high soil moisture, acid soil, rapid growth, use of phenoxy herbicides, and frosts. Forage nitrates exceeding 1% on a dry-weight basis may cause acute nitrate/nitrite toxicosis. The LD_{50} for dietary nitrate in ruminants is in the range of $0.5-1$ g/kg bodyweight. Nitrates may be converted to nitrites prior to ingestion by heating, such as when hay becomes damp, but more often nitrate/nitrite toxicosis is the result of conversion of nitrates to nitrites in the rumen. Nitrite ions absorbed into the bloodstream oxidize iron in hemoglobin from the ferrous to the ferric state, resulting in formation of methemoglobin which cannot transport oxygen. Clinical signs become apparent when methemoglobin levels reach 30%−40%, and death ensues when they reach 80%− 90%. The clinical course is rapid with clinical signs developing within 4 hours of ingestion. Clinical signs are anxiety, rapid respiration, dyspnea and rapid, weak pulse. Animals may be weak and intolerant of exercise, but should be removed from the source forage immediately. Mucous membranes are "muddy" or have a bluish cast. In many cases animals are found dead. On necropsy, chocolate-brown blood is a distinctive finding although it will change to dark red with exposure to air. Postmortem samples are generally unstable although ocular fluid may be useful. Analysis of forage, hay, and water for nitrate levels is generally more rewarding. The recommended reducing agent is methylene blue 1%, administered intravenously at $4-15$ mg/kg. Because the rumen continues to produce nitrites, methylene blue administration may need to be repeated at 6 hour intervals. Unfortunately methylene blue is not approved by the APVMA for use in food-producing animals.

Introduced plants that may contain toxic levels of nitrates are listed in Table 24.6. This list may not be comprehensive. It should be noted that some Australian native plants may also contain toxic levels of nitrates.

TABLE 24.6 Introduced Plants That May Contain Toxic Levels of Nitrates

Linnaean Name	Common Name	Type of Plant
Acacia spp.	Acacias, wattles	Trees
Amaranthus spp.	Amaranth	Weed
Apium graveolens	Celery	Garden vegetable
Avena sativa	Oat	Crop
Beta vulgaris	Mangels, fodder beet, sugar beet	Crop
Brassica spp.	For example, rape, turnip	Crop
Chenopodium album	Fat hen	Weed
Crypostemma calendula	Cape weed, *Arctotheca calendula*	Weed
Glycine max	Soybean	Crop
Hordeum vulgare	Barley	Crop
Ipomoea batatas	Sweet potato	Crop
Malva parviflora	Marsh mallow, Egyptian mallow, little mallow	Weed
Medicago sativa	Lucerne	Crop
Raphanus raphanistrum	Wild radish	Weed
Salvia reflexa	Mint weed, narrow-leaf sage	Weed
Secale cereale	Rye	Crop
Silybum marianum	Variegated thistle	Weed
Sisymbrium irio	London rocket	Weed
Stellaria media	Chickweed	Weed
Sorghum spp. and hybrids	Sorghum, Sudan grass	Crops
Trianthema spp.		Weed
Tribulus terrestris	Puncture vine	Weed
Triticum spp.	Wheat	Crop
Urochloa panicoides	Liverseed grass	Grass
Zea mays	Maize	Crop

Plants Containing Cyanogenic Glycosides

Cyanogenic glycosides have been found in more than 800 plants, from at least 80 plant families. There are a variety of introduced plants that contain cyanogenic glycosides, which yield hydrogen cyanide upon hydrolysis. Ruminants are particularly susceptible to toxicosis from these plants, because the rumen flora produces large amounts of β-glucosidase, which hydrolyses the glycosides to hydrogen cyanide (HCN). Toxicosis is most likely if the animal eats large amounts of the cyanogenic glycosides in a short time, which overwhelms the natural detoxification pathway catalyzed by the enzyme rhodanese. HCN reacts with the iron in cytochrome oxidase, preventing electron transfer and blocking cellular respiration. Toxic levels of cyanogenic glycosides are highest in actively growing parts of the plant and are increased under conditions of stress, high soil nitrogen, and low soil phosphorus. The clinical course is rapid with clinical signs becoming evident within 30 minutes of ingestion of a toxic dose. Animals exhibit excitement, tremors, rapid respiration, tachycardia, dyspnea, collapse, terminal convulsions, coma, and death. Blood and tissues are a characteristic cherry-red because the hemoglobin is oxygenated but calls cannot take up the oxygen. The blood clots slowly or not at all. Hemorrhages are often present under the epicardium and endocardium. There may be a bitter almond smell to the ruminal contents, but not all people can detect this odor. Ruminal content should be frozen if later analysis is desired. Urine may be frozen for later thiocyanate analysis. The recommended therapeutic regimen for large animals is 10−20 mg/kg sodium nitrite administered IV as a 20% solution, together with up to 600 mg/kg of sodium thiosulfate as a 20% solution. The sodium nitrite induces formation of cyanmethemoglobin, which dissociates cyanide from cytochrome oxidase. The thiosulfate is required as a substrate for the detoxifying activity of rhodanese.

Some introduced plants that are significant sources of cyanogenic glycosides are listed in Table 24.7. In addition to those listed in Table 24.7, various legumes including clovers and vetches may contain cyanogenic glycosides.

Plants Causing Hemolysis

Plants that may induce intravascular hemolysis include:

- *Acer* spp.; maples
- *Allium* spp.; including onions and garlic
- *Brassica* spp.; including rape (*Brassica napus*) and the various forms of *Brassica oleraceae* that include cabbage, cauliflower, kale, broccoli, Brussels sprouts, etc.
- *Raphanus raphanistrum*, wild radish
- *Rapistrum rugosum*, turnip weed

TABLE 24.7 Introduced Plants That May Contain Toxic Levels of Cyanogenic Glycosides

Linnaean Name	Common Name	Type of Plant
Euphorbia spp.	Spurges	Weed
Glyceria maxima	Reed sweet grass	Grass
Linum spp.	Flax	Crop or weed
Manihot esculenta	Cassava	Shrub
Osteospermum ecklonis	African daisy, South African daisy, Cape daisy	Garden ornamental or weed
Prunus spp.	Includes peaches, apricots, cherries, almonds and *Prunus laurocestus*, the cherry laurel	Fruit trees and ornamentals
Sambucus nigra	Elder, elderberry	Tree
Sorghum spp. and hybrids	Sorghum, Sudan grass	Crop
Zea mays	Maize	Crop

The toxic principle in *maples* is unknown. Horses are most often affected and may be poisoned by as little as 0.3% of their bodyweight in leaves. Toxicity is not lost on wilting or drying. The hemolytic principle in *Allium* spp. is *N*-propyl disulfide, which is present in the edible bulb. Toxicosis has been reported in ruminants, dogs, horses, and rabbits. The toxic principle in *Brassica* and *R. raphanistrum* and *R. rugosum* is *S*-methyl cysteine sulfoxide. Poisoning has been most often reported in ruminants.

Clinical signs of poisoning with any of these plants include depression, icterus, anemia, hemoglobinemia, and hemoglobinuria (redwater). Anemia leads to tachycardia and polypnea. Blood transfusion may be required to sustain life. Forced diuresis by aggressive fluid therapy reduces the risk of hemoglobin nephrosis.

Plants Associated With Clotting Defects

Introduced plants associated with clotting defects are *Anthoxanthum odoratum* (perennial sweet vernal grass) and *Melilotus albus* (white sweet clover). Both of these plants produce coumarol. The action of unspecified fungi postharvest converts coumarol to dihydroxycoumarin, which has the same toxic mechanism as anticoagulant rodenticides (q.v.). Clinical signs and treatment are as for anticoagulant rodenticides.

PLANTS WITH TOXIC EFFECTS ON THE GASTROINTESTINAL TRACT

Plants Containing Insoluble Oxalates

Insoluble calcium oxalate crystals in a number of plants form needle-like raphides that penetrate the oral and pharyngeal mucosa, causing inflammation, hypersalivation, and edema that may be sufficient to cause choking or to significantly inhibit respiration. Cooling liquids or demulcents may be helpful. Antihistamines should be administered, and respiration maintained, by tracheostomy if necessary. Effects may last for hours. Introduced plants associated with significant toxicity due to insoluble oxalates are listed in Table 24.8.

Plants Containing Protoanemonin (Ranunculin)

Protoanemonin is an irritant oil glycoside that is not readily absorbed from the gastrointestinal tract or metabolized in it, with the result that irritation is likely to occur in the oral cavity and throughout the gastrointestinal tract. The toxin is most abundant in the roots, which may be eaten by grazing animals that inadvertently pull up the whole plant when

TABLE 24.8 Introduced Plants That May Contain Toxic Levels of Insoluble Oxalates

Linnaean Name	Common Name	Type of Plant
Alocasia macrorrhiza	Elephant's ear, giant taro	Ornamental garden plant
Anthurium spp.	Flamingo flowers	Ornamental garden plant
Arisaema spp.	Jack-in-the-pulpit, cobra lily	Ornamental garden plant
Arum italicum	Italium arum, Italian lords-and-ladies	Ornamental garden plant
Colocasia esculenta	Taro	Grown for edible corms
Dieffenbachia spp.	Dumbcane	Ornamental garden or house plant
Philodendron spp.		Ornamental house or garden vines
Zantedeschia aethiopica	Arum lily, calla lily	Ornamental garden plant

soil is soft. Clinical signs include oral irritation, hypersalivation, diarrhea, depression, and irritated skin of the muzzle. Introduced plants known to contain significant levels of protoanemonin include *Ranunculus* spp. (buttercups), *Anemone* spp. (anemones), *Helleborus* spp. (hellebores), and *Clematis vitalba* (Old Man's Beard; Traveller's Joy).

Plants causing gastrointestinal toxicity due to toxic principles other than insoluble oxalates or protoanemonin are listed in Table 24.9. It should be noted that hemorrhagic gastroenteritis is a common clinical sign when plants containing cardiac glycosides are ingested (see Table 24.5 and preamble to that table).

TABLE 24.9 Plants Introduced to Australia and/or New Zealand That Cause Gastrointestinal Toxicosis Due to Toxic Principles Other Than Insoluble Oxalates or Protoanemonin

Linnaean Name	Common Name	Type of Plant	Comments
Anagallis arvensis	Scarlet Pimpernel	Weed	Also causes nephrotoxicity. Low palatability means that toxicosis is unlikely unless animals are starved. Contains saponins but it is not clear what the toxic principle is.
Aleurites fordii	Tung	Tree	All parts of the tree are poisonous but the seeds are the most toxic. Ingestions of one seed is sufficient to kill a human being.
Buxus sempervirens	Box	Shrub, used for hedges	The leaves and stems are poisonous. Toxicity to horses is estimated to be 0.15% (green-weight basis) of bodyweight. Deaths have also occurred in cattle and sheep.
Cestrum spp.	Cestrum	Garden plant or escape	Belongs to the Solanaceae family. All parts of the plant are poisonous, causing hemorrhagic gastroenteritis.
Citrullus spp.	Colocynth, Pie melons	Vine	Toxic principles are cucurbitacins that cause gastrointestinal irritation and rapid death. Ripe fruits are the most toxic part of the plants. Cattle are most often affected.

(Continued)

TABLE 24.9 (Continued)

Linnaean Name	Common Name	Type of Plant	Comments
Colchicum autumnale	Autumn crocus, naked lady	Garden plant	Toxic principle is colchicine, an antimitotic agent. All parts are toxic, especially the bulb and seeds. Leaves are toxic at about 0.1% of an animal's weight. Poison is not destroyed by haymaking or ensiling. Kidney failure, hepatic necrosis, dyspnea, coagulopathy, bone narrow suppression, and heart failure are among reported effects, but the predominant clinical signs are usually those of the gastrointestinal tract.
Cucumis spp.	Paddy melons	Vine	Toxic principles are cucurbitacins; toxicity as for *Citrullus* spp.
Daphne spp.	Daphne	Garden shrub	Toxic principles are daphnetoxin and mezerein. Not palatable to animals but poisoning have occurred. Causes severe hemorrhagic gastroenteritis.
Dittrichia graveolens	Stinkwort	Weed	Strictly speaking, this plant exerts its effects by a physical rather than a toxic mechanism. The bristles in the seed-heads become embedded in the intestinal mucosa of sheep. Sheep develop anorexia and diarrhea. Most sheep will recover following removal of the flock from the affected pasture.
Euonymus europaeus	Spindle tree	Ornamental shrub or tree	Poisoning has been reported in horses and ruminants, but is rare because palatability is low.
Euphorbia spp.	Milkweeds, spurges	Weed	Clinical signs include mucosal vesicles, hypersalivation, and

(Continued)

TABLE 24.9 (Continued)

Linnaean Name	Common Name	Type of Plant	Comments
			diarrhea. Dermatitis and/or ocular irritation may also occur. Toxic principles are complex diterpene or phorbol esters. Ingestion of plant material in excess of approximately 1% of bodyweight is sufficient to cause toxicosis.
Gloriosa superba	Flame lily, climbing lily, creeping lily, glory lily, tiger claw, fire lily	Ornamental	Contains colchicine and related compounds; toxicity as for *C. autumnale*.
Hedera helix	English ivy	Vine	Toxic principles are hederagenin and falcarinol. Poisoning is rare but may occur if prunings are dumped in pastures.
Iris	Iris	Garden ornamentals or weeds	Toxic principle is iridin.
Jatropha spp.	Physic nut	Garden ornamentals or weeds	Flowering plants in the spurge family, *Euphorbiaceae*, and with similar toxic properties to *Euphorbia* spp. Western Australia has identified *J. gossypiifolia* as an invasive, highly toxic weed.
			Jatropha curcas contains curcin, a toxalbumin similar in action to, although less toxic than, ricin (see *Ricinus communis* below).
Ligustrum	Privet	Shrub used for hedges	The toxic principle is unknown. Poisoning has been reported in horses, sheep, and cattle.

(Continued)

TABLE 24.9 (Continued)

Linnaean Name	Common Name	Type of Plant	Comments
Mercurialis annua	Mercury	Weed	Toxic principle is mercurialine. Hematuria in sheep, and agalactia in cattle, have also been reported in addition to gastrointestinal toxicity.
Narcissus	Daffodils	Garden ornamental or escapes	The toxic principles are lycorine and related alkaloids that have an irritant effect. The highest concentration is in the bulbs and less than one bulb can be toxic to small animals. In addition to gastrointestinal clinical signs, hypotension, tremors, and seizures have been reported.
Papaver nudicaule	Iceland poppy	Garden ornamentals	Toxic principles include amurine, nudaurine, and protopine. Gastrointestinal toxicity may be complicated by the presence of cyanogenic glycosides.
Pennisetum clandestinum	Kikuyu grass	Grass	The toxic principle is unidentified, and the grass appears to be toxic only under some conditions. Most poisoning cases have affected cattle and sheep appear to be relatively resistant. Clinical signs include depression, hypersalivation, sham drinking, dehydration, and ruminal distension. Inflammation and necrosis of the mucosa of the forestomachs are found on necropsy.
Phytolacca octandra	Inkweed	Shrub	The toxic principle in this species of *Phytolacca* is unknown. Occasional losses

(Continued)

TABLE 24.9 (Continued)

Linnaean Name	Common Name	Type of Plant	Comments
			have occurred in cattle and pigs.
Quercus spp.	Oaks	Trees	See entry in Table 24.3.
Ricinus communis	Castor oil plant	Shrub	The toxic principle is ricin, a toxalbumin that is one of the most toxic substances, on a per bodyweight basis, known. One seed can kill a dog, particularly if chewed. Clinical signs in animals are those of hemorrhagic gastroenteritis, ataxia, convulsions, coma, and death. Hemolytic anemia and kidney failure have been reported in human beings. The latent period between ingestion and onset of clinical signs may be up to 24 hours.
Robinia pseudoacacia	Black locust	Tree	The toxic principle is robin, a toxalbumin similar in action to, although less toxic than, ricin (see *Ricinus communis*, above).
Romulea spp.	Onion grass	Weed	Ruminants and horses consuming these weeds may develop phytobezoars.
Sambucus nigra (*elderberry*)	Elder, elderberry	Shrub or tree	Low palatability means that poisoning is rare. This plant also contains cyanogenic glycosides but some reported cases or poisoning are of gastrointestinal toxicity rather than cyanide poisoning, and are attributed to an unknown alkaloid or alkaloids.

PLANTS WITH TOXIC EFFECTS ON THE RESPIRATORY SYSTEM

Plants with toxic effects on the respiratory system are listed in Table 24.10.

TABLE 24.10 Plants Introduced to Australia and/or New Zealand That Cause Toxicosis of the Respiratory System

Linnaean Name	Common Name	Type of Plant	Comments
Crotalaria spp.	Crotalaria	Weed	Crotalaria contain pyrrolizidine alkaloids, best known for hepatotoxicity. However, a major pyrrolizidine alkaloid in Crotalaria is monocrotaline, one of a small number of pyrrolizidine alkaloids that cause pulmonary toxicosis at doses lower than those required to cause hepatotoxicity. Early changes are congestion, alveolar hemorrhage, and chronic effects pulmonary fibrosis and Clara cell proliferation. The primary lesion is pulmonary hypertension following hypertrophy of the tunica media of pulmonary arterioles. Most cases have been reported in horses.
Eupatorium (or *Ageratina*) *adenophorum*	Crofton weed, Mexican devil	Weed	Chronic pulmonary inflammation and fibrosis in horses. The toxic principle is unknown. Clinical signs include coughing, exercise intolerance, and dyspnea, and horses may die of cardiac failure. The disease is called Crofton weed poisoning, Numinbah Horse Sickness, or Tallebudgera Horse Disease.
Eupatorium riparium	Mist flower	Weed	As for *E. adenophorum*.
Galega officinalis	Goat's rue	Weed	The toxic principles are alkaloids of which galegine and peganine are the most abundant. The plant has low palatability but hungry animals may be poisoned. Most cases of poisoning have occurred in sheep, which develop dsypnea with shallow, rapid respiration, and frothy exudate from the nares. On necropsy the distinctive finding is a large volume (up to 2 or 3 L) of pleural exudate in the thoracic cavity. This straw-colored fluid is high in protein and solidifies into a gel on cooling to room

(Continued)

TABLE 24.10 (Continued)

Linnaean Name	Common Name	Type of Plant	Comments
			temperature. Other findings are abundant frothy fluid in the airways and pulmonary congestion and edema of the lungs. The lungs often do not collapse when the chest is opened, and have an abnormally high number of rib impressions on them. There may be subendocardial hemorrhage.
Persea americana	Avocado	Tree cultivated for fruit	Toxic effects on the respiratory system include pulmonary edema secondary to the cardiomyopathy (see Table 24.5) and edema of the neck, which has been reported in horses, rabbits, and goats and which may impair respiration, particularly in horses.
Verbesina encelioides	Crownbeard	Weed	Like *G. officinalis*, this weed contains galegine and similarly causes acute respiratory distress, edema, and cardiac failure.

PLANTS WITH TOXIC EFFECTS ON SKIN

The most common toxic effect on skin observed in veterinary practice is photosensitivity, which particularly affects unpigmented areas of dorsal or lateral skin, and areas where skin is thin such as muzzle, periocular areas, ears, udder, and escutcheon. Photosensitivity may be primary or secondary. Primary photosensitization occurs when the toxic principle or its metabolite is photodynamic and reacts when exposed to sunlight. Secondary photosensitization occurs when the toxic principle impairs liver function, with the result that conjugation and excretion of phylloerythrin, a photodynamic metabolite of chlorophyll, is reduced. Photosensitization is first manifested as erythema and edema, followed by pruritis, hyperesthesia, and vesiculation and ulceration of the skin. Animals are typically photophobic and, if severely affected, are likely to be depressed. If the muzzle or lips are affected, feed intake may greatly decrease. Animals may stop feeding their young because of udder and teat pain, and breeding may also be impaired. Affected animals should be provided with abundant shade. Inert sunblocks may be helpful.

Other mechanisms of toxicity include direct irritant effects, direct trauma, and induction of allergic dermatitis.

Plants known to cause dermal toxicity are listed in Table 24.11, categorized by mechanism.

TABLE 24.11 Introduced Plants That May Cause Photosensitivity Reactions

Linnaean Name	Common Name	Comments
Plants Causing Primary Photosensitization		
Ammi majus	Bishop's weed	Photodynamic agents are furanocoumarins
Apium graveolens	Celery	Photodynamic agents are furanocoumarins
Avena sativa	Oat	Unknown photosensitising agent
Heracleum mantegazzianum	Cow parsnip	Photodynamic agents are furanocoumarins
Hypericum perforatum	St. John's Wort	Hypericin, the toxic principle, is also found in other members of the genus *Hypericum*
Medicago spp.	Medic, lucerne	Unknown photosensitising agent
Persicaria spp.	Smartweed	Unknown photosensitising agent
Trifolium hybridum	Alsike clover	Unknown photosensitising agent
Trifolium pratense	Red clover	Unknown photosensitising agent
Trifolium repens	White clover	Unknown photosensitising agent
Echinochloa utilis	Japanese millet	Unknown photosensitising agent
Erodium cicutarium	Storksbill	Unknown photosensitising agent
Erodium moschatum	Musky storksbill	Unknown photosensitising agent
Pastinaca sativa	parsnip	Photodynamic agents are furanocoumarins
Petroselinum crispum	Parsley	Photodynamic agents are furanocoumarins
Polygonum spp.	Willow weeds	Unknown photosensitising agent
Plants Causing Secondary (Hepatogenous) Photosensitization		
Brachiaria spp.	Signal grass, para grass	Toxic principles are steroidal saponins
Crotalaria spp.	Crotalaria	Pyrrolizidine alkaloids; see Table 24.2
Delairea odorata		Pyrrolizidine alkaloids; see Table 24.2
Echium spp.	See Table 24.2	See Table Pyrrolizidine alkaloids; see Table 24.2
Heliotropium spp.	Heliotropes	Pyrrolizidine alkaloids; see Table 24.2

(Continued)

TABLE 24.11 (Continued)

Linnaean Name	Common Name	Comments
Lantana camara	Lantana	
Panicum spp.		Toxic principles are steroidal saponins
Senecio spp.	Ragworts and groundsels	Pyrrolizidine alkaloids; see Table 24.2
Tribulus terrestris	Calthrop, puncture vine	Toxic principles are steroidal saponins
Plants Having a Direct Irritant Effect		
E. cicutarium	Storksbill	Penetrating awns
Euphorbia spp.	Milkweeds, spurges	
Ranunculus spp.	Buttercups	Protoanemonin
Synadenium grantii	African milk bush	Diterpenoid esters
Toxicodendron radicans	Poison ivy	The irritant principle is urushiol
Urtica spp.	Nettles	As for *Urtica ferox* (q.v.) but introduced nettles inject much less toxin
Polygonum spp.	Willow weeds	Unknown irritant
Plants Causing Allergic Dermatitis		
Beta napus	Rape	
Raphanus raphanistrum	Wild radish	
Raphanus sativus	Fodder radish	
Tradescantia spp.	Wandering jew	
Plants Causing Direct Trauma		
Tribulus terrestris	Puncture vine	
Plants Causing Hair Loss		
Leucaena leucocephala		Mimosine and related chemicals are the toxic principles

PLANTS WITH TOXIC EFFECTS ON SKELETAL MUSCLE

Malva parviflora, the small-flowered mallow, has been listed previously in this chapter because it causes staggers and may contain toxic levels of nitrates. In addition, this weed contains an unknown toxic principle that causes skeletal muscle necrosis.

Two *Senna* species, *Senna occidentalis* (Coffee senna) and *Senna obtusifolia* (sickle pod) have become naturalized in parts of Australia. These plants contain an unidentified toxic principle that causes degeneration and necrosis of striated muscle, with myoglobinuria. The most toxic parts of the plants are the seeds and seed pods.

PLANTS WITH TOXIC EFFECTS ON THE ENDOCRINE SYSTEM AND THE MAMMARY GLAND

Plants Affecting the Thyroid Gland

A number of plants produce goitrogens, including:

- *Brassica* spp.
- *Leucaena leucocephala*
- *R. rugosum*

Goiter is usually self-correcting with time if animals are removed from the toxic pasture, but poisoning may have serious effects on fertility and production.

Plants Causing Secondary (Nutritional) Hyperparathyroidism

This response may be seen in horses following prolonged ingestion of any of the following plants:

- *Brachiaria* spp.
- *Cenchrus ciliaris*
- *Megathyrsus maximus*
- *Panicum* spp.
- *Pennisetum clandestinum*
- *Setaria sphacelata*

Clinical signs include lameness, weight loss, and characteristic enlargement of the facial bones. Horses should be removed from the pasture and fed a corrective mineral supplement containing a Ca:P ratio of 2:1, at a rate of 2 kg/week for at least 6 months.

Plants Containing Phytoestrogens

Trifolium subterraneum, subterranean clover, may contain physiologically significant concentrations of phytooestrogens that impair fertility, particularly in sheep. Lactation has occurred in wethers as a result of grazing *Trifolium pratense*; red clover. The phytoestrogens in clovers are genistein, formononetin, and biochanin A. Genistein and formononentin are also found in soya bean, *Glycine max.*

Plants Causing Agalactia

Persea americana, the avocado, is known to cause severe sterile mastitis, best described in goats. Mastitis occurs within 24 hours of ingestion, and milk production drops sharply. That milk which is produced is watery and curdled. Microscopically, the secretory epithelium shows degeneration and necrosis, and there is interstitial edema and hemorrhage. Analgesics and anti-inflammatories may be helpful.

Plants Causing Spontaneous Abortion

Consumption of *Cupressus macrocarpa*, the Monterey cypress, a tree commonly used for windbreaks, may cause abortion, particularly in the third trimester, or premature calving in cattle. No effective treatment is known. The toxic principle may be isocupressic acid, but this is uncertain. Cows may exhibit profound depression prior to aborting. Retention of fetal membranes is a common complication of macrocarpa abortion, and cattle that abort close to term typically have greatly reduced or absent lactation.

Plants Causing Infertility

Species of *Romulea* (onion grass) are associated with infertility, abortion, vulvitis, and testicular atrophy in sheep, although it is not clear whether the toxin responsible is synthesized by the plants themselves or by fungi infecting the plants.

For toxicity of *Gossypium* spp., see the description of gossypol poisoning in Chapter 19, Agricultural and Feed-Related Toxicants.

PLANTS WITH TOXIC EFFECTS ON THE IMMUNE SYSTEM

Vicia spp., woolly-pod vetch (*Vicia villosa* ssp. *dasycarpa*) and popany vetch (*Vicia benghalensis*), are leguminous weeds that cause systemic granulomatous disease in cattle and occasionally in horses. Clinical signs include severe pruritic dermatitis with self-trauma, and illthrift. Cattle are typically anorexic and other reported clinical signs include conjunctivitis and/or nasal discharge, hyperexcitability, diarrhea, pyrexia, and stiffness. The disease may be fatal. On necropsy, granulomas are found in many organs. Commonly affected organs include the skin, kidney, liver, heart, adrenal glands, and lymph nodes. Granulomas feature eosinophils, macrophages, plasma cells, and lymphocytes. Macrophages may include multinucleate giant cells. Herd morbidity tends to be less than 10%, but mortality is high among affected animals. The disease appears to be a Type IV hypersensitivity response to one or more absorbed components of vetch that act as haptens or complete antigens. Prognosis is poor, but some animals may be saved if removed from the pasture immediately, particularly if they are only mildly affected, and treated with corticosteroids. Convalescence is prolonged, and exposure of recovered animals to *Vicia* species must be avoided.

Part 2: Poisonous Native Plants of Australia

INTRODUCTION

There are a large number of poisonous plants of Australia. Details of distribution, identifying characteristics and color photographs, are thoroughly covered in Dr. Ross McKenzie's recent book *Australia's Poisonous Plants, Fungi and Cyanobacteria* (CSIRO Publishing, 2012). There appears to be no value in attempting to replicate that level of coverage in this book. Therefore this chapter is composed with a view to being a "ready reference" only, and the reader is referred to Dr. McKenzie's authoritative work for further details and for illustrations of the plants.

In this chapter, as in the chapter on introduced plants, plants are categorized by the organ or system that is the most important target of toxicity. It should be noted that many plants cause some degree of gastrointestinal toxicity, but if the most important target of toxicity is an organ or system other than the gastrointestinal tract, the plant will be listed under that organ or system. A few plants that target several organs or systems are listed more than once.

For most plant poisonings, there is no specific antidote, and treatment is supportive. As a generalization, plant toxins are adsorbed by activated charcoal. The contraindications of using activated charcoal should be borne in mind. Ruminal emptying by rumenotomy may be indicated in the case of highly toxic material, if the value of the animal justifies it.

This chapter does not include details of the appearance of plants, because there are high-quality photographs of most plants available in Dr. McKenzie's book, and also on the internet, by searching in Google Images. When searching for information on the internet, the plant should always be searched by Linnaean name, because common names vary from region to region and the same common name may be used for different plants in different countries.

In those cases in which the toxicity associated with a given plant is due to a fungal infection, the toxicosis is covered in Chapter 21, Mycotoxins and Mushrooms, even if the fungus is an endophyte.

Categories in this chapter are as follows:

- Neurotoxic plants
- Hepatotoxic plants
- Nephrotoxic plants
- Cardiotoxic plants
- Plants with toxic effects on the blood
- Plants with toxic effects on the gastrointestinal tract
- Plants with toxic effects on the respiratory system
- Plants with toxic effects on skin
- Plants with toxic effects on skeletal muscle
- Plants with toxic effects on the skeleton
- Plants with toxic effects on the reproductive system
- Plants that contain high levels of selenium

NEUROTOXIC PLANTS

Corynetoxin Poisoning and Associated Plants

Corynetoxicosis is not strictly a plant poisoning. Corynetoxins are synthesized by bacteria of thes species *Rathayibacter toxicus* when they are infected with a bacteriophage. The toxigenic bacteria are carried on the skin of nematode worms of the species *Anguina agrostis* and *Anguina paludicola*. These nematodes invade grass seeds, resulting in the formation of galls. The toxin persists indefinitely in hay made from the affected grass.

Sheep are most commonly affected by corynetoxicosis. The toxic dose is in the range of 3–5 mg/kg. The toxins inhibit the production of glycoproteins essential to the normal structure of cell membranes. The brain is the organ most severely affected. Poisoning usually occurs from November to January, and is associated with sheep grazing grass with mature seed-heads. Onset of poisoning can occur in as little as 4 days, but may take weeks to develop. Forced exercise, high ambient temperature and cobalt deficiency all exacerbate this toxicosis. Clinical signs include gait abnormalities, nodding or swaying of the head, muscle spasms, collapse, nystagmus, and tetanic seizures. If left undisturbed, animals may recover from these seizures and regain their feet. Deaths may occur within hours of onset of clinical signs, or the course of the toxicosis may take days. Subclinical toxicosis is associated with decreased wool growth. Control involves feeding pasture before the seed-heads mature, mowing to remove seed-heads, and if necessary destroying infected pasture and resowing affected areas.

Polypogon monspeiensis (annual beard grass; introduced)
Lachnagrostis filiformis (blow-away grass; native)
Lolium rigidum (annual ryegrass; introduced)

Fluoroacetate Poisoning and Associated Plants

The vertebrate pesticide fluoroacetate (1080) occurs naturally in a number of Australian native plants. Fluoroacetate poisoning is described in Chapter 10, Vertebrate Pesticides, and only details relevant to fluoroacetate in plants are covered here.

The most toxic parts of the plants are flowers, seed pods, and new leaves. The plants that synthesize fluoroacetate are quite palatable to grazing animals. Secondary toxicosis can occur if dogs, dingos, or pigs consume the bodies of grazing animals that have died from eating these plants. While dogs and pigs show predominantly nervous signs such as running fits and convulsions, herbivores most commonly die of heart failure. There is no treatment available for poisoned livestock.

Australian native plants that contain fluoroacetate include:

Acacia georginae	Georgina gidyea
Gastrolobium calycinum	York Road poison
Gastrolobium floribundum	Wodjil poison
Gastrolobium laytonii	Kite-leaf poison
Gastrolobium parviflorum	Box poison
Gastrolobium polystachyum	Horned poison
Gastrolobium racemosum	Net-leaf poison
Gastrolobium spinosum	Prickly poison
Gastrolobium villosum	Crinkle-leaf poison
Gastrolobium tetragonophyllum	Brother-brother
Gastrolobium bennettsianum	Cluster poison
Gastrolobium bilobum	Heart-leaf poison of Western Australia
Gastrolobium crassifolium	Thick-leaf poison
Gastrolobium cuneatum	River poison
Gastrolobium microcarpum	Sandplain poison
Gastrolobium oxyloboides	Champion Bay poison
Gastrolobium parvifolium	Berry poison
Gastrolobium velutinum	Stirling Range poison
Gastrolobium grandiflorum	Wallflower poison, heart-leaf poison bush, desert poison bush

Nicotine and Related Alkaloid Poisoning

There are 22 species of *Nicotiana* native to Australia, of which *N. megalosiphon*, *N. suaveolens*, *N. velutina*, and *N. glauca* (tree tobacco) are associated with poisoning, most commonly of cattle or sheep. *Duboisia hopwoodii* (pituri) also contains nicotine and related alkaloids.

Poisoning most often occurs in cattle and sheep, but cases have been recorded in horses and cattle. Although dried plant material is less toxic than fresh, poisoning has occurred in livestock fed hay in which there were suckers of *D. hopwoodii*. Clinical signs of poisoning include incoordination, muscle tremors, mydriasis, weakness, recumbency, paddling, and paralysis.

There may be diarrhea and signs of abdominal pain. In severe poisoning, there may be sudden death. There is no specific treatment.

Anabasine, one of the alkaloids related to nicotine, is teratogenic.

Swainsonine and Calystegine Poisoning and Associated Plants

Plants native to Australia that contain swainsonine and/calystegine include numerous members of the genus *Swainsona* (*S. brachycarpa*, *S. canescens*, *S. galegifolia*, *S. greyana*, *S. luteola*, *S. procumbens*, *S. swainsonioides*) as well as the vines *Ipomoea muelleri* (poison morning glory) and *Ipomoea polpha* subsp. *weirana* (Weir vine).

Swainsonine inhibits the enzyme α-mannosidase, leading to build-up of mannose-rich sidechains of glycoproteins in lysosomes. Calystegines inhibit other enzymes involved in breakdown of sugar sidechains of molecules, such as β-glucosidase and α-galactosidase, leading to build-up of these sugars in cells. Abnormal storage of these products can be demonstrated in many tissues but the clinical signs are principally related to the brain. Animals appear to develop a taste for plants containing these toxins. Horses need to eat these plants for 2 weeks or more, and ruminants need to eat them for 4 weeks or more, before clinical signs develop. Clinical signs include weight loss, lethargy, "star-gazing," head shaking, tremor, head-pressing, incoordination, abortion, and inability to feed normally. Horses in particular may become excitable and dangerous to handle. There is no effective treatment. Animals may recover if moved away from the plants early in the course of the toxicosis.

Tropane Alkaloid Poisoning and Associated Plants

Native plants of Australia that contain tropane alkaloids include the corkwoods, *Duboisia leichhardtii* and *Duboisia myoporoides*; hybrids of the two *Duboisia* species; and two *Solanum* species, *Solanum quadriloculatum* (wild tomato) and *Solanum sturtianum* (Sturt's nightshade). The latter two plants generally cause only gastroenteric toxicity.

Tropane alkaloids include atropine, scopolamine, hyoscyamine, hyoscine, and related alkaloids. These alkaloids have anticholinergic effects. Clinical signs include mydriasis, dry mouth, apparent hallucinations, ataxia, and hyperthermia. Seizures may occur in severe cases. The patient should be kept in a quiet dark place if possible. Diazepam or other benzodiazepine may be used for sedation. Opiates are contraindicated. Physostigmine is helpful in severe cases.

There is mnemonic for the clinical signs of tropane alkaloid poisoning: "hot as hare, blind as a bat, dry as a bone, red as a beet, and mad as a hatter," representing hyperthermia, mydriasis, dry mouth, flushed skin, and mucous membranes, delirium.

Zamia Staggers and Associated Plants

The plants associated with Zamia staggers are the cycads, of which there are a number of native species in Australia, as well as some introduced species of the genus *Cycas*. Species of native Australian plant associated with Zamia staggers include *Bowenia serrulata*, *Bowenia spectabilis*, *Cycas* species, *Lepidozamia peroffskyana*, and *Macrozamia* species. Methazoxymethanol (MAM) is one of the toxic principles in the cycads, causing hepatotoxicity, but other unidentified toxin/s are responsible for Zamia staggers. It is possible that the neurotoxin is a metabolite of MAM, produced by the action of ruminal microflora. Poisoning is most often observed in cattle. Cattle develop Zamia staggers after consuming the plants for weeks or months. Zamia staggers most often occur when there has been good summer rain but then a dry autumn and winter, leading to decreased pasture growth in association with abundant seeds on the cycads. Clinical signs most often develop in winter. Cattle develop stiffness of the hind legs, knuckling-over at the hind fetlocks, wasting of the muscles of the hindquarters and finally paralysis of the hindquarters. There is no treatment for Zamia staggers.

Australian plants recognized to have neurotoxic effects in animals by mechanisms other than those described above are listed Table 24.12:

TABLE 24.12 Native Australian Plants That Cause Neurotoxicity by Mechanisms Other Than Corynetoxicosis, Fluoroacetate Poisoning, Swainsonine/Calystegine Poisoning, or Zamia Staggers

Linnaean Name	Common Name	Type of Plant	Comments
Alstonia constricta	Bitter bark	Tree	Toxins are indole alkaloids with strychnine-like activity. Clinical signs include diarrhea, muscle tremors, ataxia, inducible tetanic seizures, and death from asphyxia.
Atalaya hemiglauca	Whitewood	Tree	An unidentified toxin causes lethargy, staggering, stiffness, and apparent blindness in cattle. Horses may also show trembling, staggering, and weakness but this appears to be the result of cardiotoxicity in this species.
Cheilanthes sieberi	Mulga fern	Fern	Toxic action of thiaminase may cause staggers in horses, sheep, or pigs following consumption for days or weeks. Treat with
Cheilanthes distans	Wooly cloak fern	Fern	

(Continued)

TABLE 24.12 (Continued)

Linnaean Name	Common Name	Type of Plant	Comments
			thiamine, IV to horses, IV or SC to pigs or sheep.
Hoya australis subsp. *australis*	Wax flower	Vine	The toxin is unknown. Poisoning is most often seen in cattle although sheep are susceptible. Clinical signs include incoordination, muscle tremor, knuckling-over of fetlocks, nystagmus, and inducible seizures. Prognosis is poor once animals are unable to stand.
Indigofera linnaei	Birdsville indigo	Herb	An unidentified toxin causes Birdsville horse disease. Horses exhibit inappetence, lethargy, incoordination, hindlimb weakness, and dragging of the toes. Horses have difficulty turning. Ocular discharge, stomatitis, and abortion have also been reported. Mild cases may recover if denied access to the plant.
Lomandra longifolia	Spiny-headed mat-rush	Grass-like perennial	One of the species associated with "wamps," a syndrome of posterior ataxia, urinary incontinence and weight loss in sheep and cattle. The toxic principle is unknown. Prolonged grazing appears to be required. Wallerian degeneration may be evident microscopically, but wamps is reversible with nursing.
Macadamia spp.	Macadamia	Nut-bearing trees	Toxicosis has only been reported in dogs, following consumption of the nuts. Dogs develop lethargy, hindlimb weakness, muscle tremors, and recumbency. The leg joints may be painful and swollen. Emesis and hyperthermia are sometimes present. Dogs usually recover fully in 12–24 hours. Ingestion of the nuts has also been associated with gastrointestinal obstruction in dogs.

(Continued)

TABLE 24.12 (Continued)

Linnaean Name	Common Name	Type of Plant	Comments
Marsilea drummondii	Common nardoo	Fern	Toxic action of thiaminase may cause staggers in horses, sheep, or pigs following consumption for days or weeks. Treat with thiamine, IV to horses, IV or SC to pigs or sheep.
Melia azedarach	White cedar	Tree	Native to Australia but also occurs in Asia and Africa. Nervous signs include drowsiness, incoordination, muscle tremors and spasms, coma. Nervous signs typically accompanied by signs of severe gastroenteritis.
Pteridium esculentum	Austral bracken	Fern	Toxic action of thiaminase may cause staggers in horses, sheep, or pigs following consumption for days or weeks. Treat with thiamine, IV to horses, IV or SC to pigs or sheep.
Pteridium revolutum	Hairy bracken	Fern	
Rhodomyrtus macrocarpa	Finger cherry	Shrub or small tree	Ingestion of the fruit has caused sudden onset of permanent blindness in human beings.
Sarcostemma brevipedicellatum	Pencil caustic	Vine	Pregnane glycoside poisoning affecting sheep, cattle, swine, and horses. Clinical signs include restlessless, staggering, muscle tremors, nystagmus, and inducible seizures.
Sarcostemma viminale subsp. *australe*	Pencil caustic	Vine	
Stypandra glauca	Blind grass, Candyup poison, nodding blue lily	Perennial herb with blue/purple flowers	Toxic principle is stypandrol. Toxicosis is most common is sheep and goats but has also occurred in horses and poultry. Affects the brain, particularly the optic nerves. Clinical signs include blindness, incoordination, and death. Survivors may be permanently blind.
Terminalia oblongata	Yellow-wood	Tree	Transient inducible seizures. Plant may also cause liver and kidney damage.

(*Continued*)

TABLE 24.12 (Continued)

Linnaean Name	Common Name	Type of Plant	Comments
Tribulus microccocus	Yellow vine	Ground-hugging herb	May cause a distinctive staggers in sheep, with hocks flexed, legs swung outward when walking, and with knuckling-over at the fetlocks. The hindquarters may be dragged. Occasionally the front legs may be affected. Sheep will recover if further exposure to *T. microccocus* is prevented.
Tribulus terrestris[a]	Caltrop	Ground-hugging herb	Causes Coonabarabran staggers in sheep. Sheep cannot walk in a straight line but consistently deviate to the left or right. Hind legs are weak and one side is affected more than the other. Eventually the weakness spreads to the forelegs, sheep have difficulty standing and starve to death. There is no treatment.
Solanum quadriloculatum	Wild tomato	Shrub	Severe poisoning may feature delirium visual disturbances, drowsiness, and coma, but veterinary cases are usually limited to gastroenteric irritation.
Solanum sturtianum	Sturt's nightshade	Shrub	
Xanthorrhea spp.	Grass-trees, yacca	Large grass-like pants	Several of these species are associated with "wamps," a syndrome of posterior ataxia, urinary incontinence and weight loss in cattle, and all species are probably poisonous. The toxic principle is unknown. Prolonged grazing appears to be required. Wallerian degeneration may be evident microscopically, but wamps is reversible with nursing.

[a] *This species also occurs in other countries. It is not clear whether* T. terrestris *in Australia is native or introduced.*

HEPATOTOXIC PLANTS

Methylazoxymethanol Poisoning and Associated Plants

MAM poisoning is one of the toxic effects of the cycads, of which there are a number of native species in Australia, as well as some introduced species of the genus *Cycas*. Species of native Australian plant associated with MAM poisoning include *B. serrulata*, *B. spectabilis*, *Cycas* species, *L. peroffskyana*, and *Macrozamia* species. Poisoning has also been reported in human beings, dogs, and sheep, and all cycads should be regarded as toxic to human beings and domestic animals. It appears that MAM is metabolized in the liver to a hepatoxic metabolite. Acutely, MAM causes acute liver necrosis, and may also cause severe gastroenteritis with bloody diarrhea in dogs. Chronic toxicosis, with progressive hepatic fibrosis and hepatic megaocytosis is also reported. Chronic toxicosis resembles that of pyrrolizidine alkaloids. There are no specific treatments for either acute or chronic toxicosis.

Pyrrolizidine Alkaloids and Associated Plants

High doses of pyrrolizidine alkaloids cause liver necrosis, which is initially centrilobular in distribution. Low doses interfere with cell division in animals, leading to hepatomegalocytosis featuring giant multinucleate hepatocytes. Pyrrolizidine alkaloid hepatoxicity is cumulative in effect, so liver failure is the end result, whether poisoning is acute or chronic. Toxicosis in livestock is most frequently chronic, because animals find the plants unpalatable and will avoid eating them if they can. However, many weeds containing pyrrolizidine alkaloids are relatively drought-resistant and may be the only grazing available in dry conditions.

Sheep are relatively resistant to toxicosis, when compared to horses and cattle. Pyrrolizidine alkaloid concentrations are reduced but not eliminated by drying associated with haymaking.

Clinical signs of chronic pyrrolizidine alkaloid toxicosis are icterus, depression, anorexia, and failure to thrive. Hepatic encephalopathy may develop, particularly in horses. Signs of hepatic encephalopathy include aimless wandering, head-pressing, and disoriented behavior. Animals may suffer secondary photosensitization, particularly on skin unprotected by hair, wool, or melanin. Lesions in the liver include megalocytosis, hepatocellular necrosis, biliary hyperplasia, nodular hyperplasia, and extensive fibrosis. Treatment is usually futile by the time toxicosis is diagnosed.

Native Australian plants in Australia that have been associated with pyrrolizidine alkaloid poisoning are listed in Table 24.13.

Plants within the genus *Crotalaria* may contain the pyrrolizidine alkaloids monocrotaline or fulvine, both of which may cause pulmonary disease at doses lower than that required to produce hepatic toxicosis. Pulmonary toxicosis has been reported in horses and in sheep.

Plants that produce hepatotoxicity by toxic principles other than pyrrolizidine alkaloids are presented in Table 24.14.

TABLE 24.13 Australian Native Plants That Contain Pyrrolizidine Alkaloids

Linnaean Name	Common Name
Crotalaria crispata	Kimberly horse poison
Crotalaria dissitiflora	Gray rattlepod
Crotalaria eremaea subsp. *eremaea*	Bluebush pea
Crotalaria medicaginea var. *neglecta*[a]	Trefoil rattlepod
Crotalaria mitchelli	Yellow rattlepod
Crotalaria novae-hollandiae	New Holland rattlepod
Crotalaria ramosissima	Kimberly horse poison
Crotalaria retusa	Wedge-leaf rattlepod
H. ovalifolium	
Senecio brigalowensis	Brigalow fireweed
Senecio linearifolius	fireweed
Senecio magnificus	Perennial yellowtop
Senecio quadridentatus	Cotton fireweed
Trichodesma zeylanicum	Camel bush

[a]More commonly associated with Chillagoe horse disease.

NEPHROTOXIC PLANTS AND PLANTS AFFECTING THE URINARY TRACT

Plants Containing Soluble Oxalates

A wide range of plants, some native to Australia and others introduced, cause nephrotoxicity because they contain soluble oxalates. Once ingested and absorbed into the body, soluble oxalates react with serum calcium to form calcium oxalate. In the concentrating environment of the renal tubules, calcium oxalate can crystallize to form distinctive rosette-shaped crystals that can be observed using a polarizing filter. The precipitation of calcium oxalate crystals leads to renal tubular necrosis and death from renal failure.

The formation of calcium oxalate in the circulation also leads to depletion of calcium ions and functional hypocalcemia, which can cause muscle twitching, mild seizures, recumbency, and death, particularly if animals are forced to move. In addition the hypocalcemia caused by ingesting soluble oxalates may lead to secondary hyperparathyroidism in horses.

Hypocalcemia may be treated with calcium borogluconate IV, as for a cow with postparturient hypocalcemia.

TABLE 24.14 Native Australian Plants Cause Hepatotoxicity by Toxic Principles Other Than Methylazoxymethanol or Pyrrolizidine Alkaloids

Linnaean Name	Common Name	Type of Plant	Comments
Argentipallium blandowskianum	Woolly everlasting	Herb with daisy-like flowers	Causes acute lliver necrosis. Toxin is unknown
Eremophila deserti	Ellangowan poison bush, turkey bush	Shrub	Toxins are furanosesquiterpenes
Indigofera linnaei	Birdsville indigo	Herb	Chronic liver disease in dogs fed the meat of horses or camels that have been grazing on the plant
Lythrum hyssopifolia	Lesser loosestrife	Herb	Toxin is unknown, but damages hepatocytes first, followed by renal tubular cells
Myoporum montanum	Boobialla	Shrub	Toxins are furanosesquiterpenes
Panicum decompositum	Native millet	Grass	Toxicosis usually manifested as secondary photosensitization
Terminalia oblongata	Yellow-wood	Tree	Also causes kidney damage and seizures
Trema tomentosa	Poison peach	Tree	Toxin is trematoxin, which causes acute liver necrosis. Cattle are most often affected
Wedelia asperrima	Sunflower daisy	Herb with yellow flowers	Toxin is wedeloside, which causes acute liver necrosis

Clinical signs of renal failure in animals as a result of ingesting soluble oxalates include depression, azotemia, and oliguria later changing to polyuria and hyposthenuria. Animals may die of hyperkalemic heart failure.

The calcium oxalate crystals will eventually dissolve if the animal can be kept alive and renal throughput maintained, but renal function may be permanently reduced. Horses with secondary nutritional parathyroidism should be removed from the pasture and supplemented for at least 6 months with 2 kg/week of a mineral supplement containing a Ca:P ratio of 2:1, in order to remineralize the bones.

Native Australian plants that contain soluble oxalates are listed in Table 24.15.

TABLE 24.15 Australian Plants That Cause Nephrotoxicity Due to Soluble Oxalates

Linnaean Name	Common Name	Comments
Atriplex muelleri	Annual saltbush, Mueller's saltbush	
Averrhoa carambola	Carambola	
Enchylaena tomentosa	Ruby saltbush	
Neobassia proceriflora	Soda bush	
Portulaca spp.	Pigweeds	
Rumex brownii	Swamp dock, hooked dock, slender dock	Introduced docks also contain soluble oxalates
Sclerolaena calcarata	Red burr	
Trianthema spp.	Pigweeds	

Aristolochic Acid Poisoning

There are both native Australian and introduced species of *Aristolochia* spp. (birthworts) in Australia. These plants contain aristolochic acid that is a potent nephrotoxin and can also cause cancers of the urinary tract. Acute renal failure from consumption of these plants has been observed in sheep and horses in Australia.

Iforrestine Poisoning

A number of species of *Isotropis* in Australia, notably *Isotropis cuneifolia* (lamb poison) and *Isotropis atropurpurea* (poison sage) may contain the nephrotoxin iforrestine. The plants appear to be readily palatable to livestock. Clinical signs include inappetence, lethargy, diarrhea, and oliguria progressing to anuria. Although large doses can kill within an hour, most animals take 2−7 days to die. On necropsy there is perirenal edema around pale, swollen kidneys. Microscopically there is necrosis of the proximal renal tubules. Other gross findings are congestion of the epithelium of abomasum and intestines, edema of the abomasal wall, and excessive fluid in the abdominal cavity. Necrosis of hepatocytes and cardiac myocytes has also been reported, as well as pulmonary edema. There is no effective treatment.

Toxic Ferns

Native ferns of toxicological importance include the bracken ferns *Pteridium esculentum* and *Pteridium revolutum*, as well as the mulga fern *Cheilanthes sieberi* and the woolly cloak fern *Cheilanthes distans*.

The toxins in ferns are norsesquiterpene glycosides, notably ptaquiloside, and also thiaminase. Prolonged consumption of norsesquiterpene glycosides may lead to bovine enzootic hematuria, which is a clinical manifestation of neoplasia of the urinary bladder. The toxicity of these toxins is covered in detail the chapter on poisonous plants of New Zealand, under Rarauhe (bracken fern).

CARDIOTOXIC PLANTS

Simplexin Poisoning and Plants Containing Simplexin

Plants that contain simplexin include *Pimelea simplex* (desert rice flower), *Pimelea elongata*, *Pimelea latifolia* subsp. *altior*, *Pimelea neo-anglica*, and *Pimelea trichostachya*.

Simplexin poisoning is also known as St George disease or Marree disease. Simplexin poisoning is most often seen in cattle. Grazing of *Pimelea* plants for ≥12 days causes constriction of pulmonary venules, which in turn causes right-sided cardiac insufficiency. The jugular veins become distended and there is marked edema of the chest, brisket, and head. The toxin is also irritant to the gastrointestinal tract, and may cause diarrhea. Anemia also develops, although the mechanism is unclear. Grazing animals other than cattle may develop diarrhea, and horses may develop the full syndrome. Necropsy findings in affected cattle include distended left ventricle of the heart, hydrothorax, and severely congested liver. There is no specific treatment. Cattle will recover fully if moved away from *Pimelea* early in the course of the disease. *Pimelea* species are unpalatable and will only be grazed by animals as a last resort.

Australian plants causing cardiotoxicity due to toxic principles other than simplexin are listed in Table 24.16.

PLANTS WITH TOXIC EFFECTS ON THE BLOOD

Plants Containing Nitrates

A number of plants contain, at least under some growing conditions, high levels of nitrates in their stalks and/or leaves. Nitrate levels tend to increase by high soil moisture, acid soil, rapid growth, use of phenoxy herbicides, and frosts. Forage nitrates exceeding 1% on a dry-weight basis may cause acute nitrate/nitrite toxicosis. The LD_{50} for dietary nitrate in ruminants is in the range 0.5−1 g/kg bodyweight. Nitrates may be converted to nitrites prior

TABLE 24.16 Native Australian Plants That Cause Cardiotoxicity Other Than Simplexin Poisoning

Linnaean Name	Common Name	Type of Plant	Comments
Atalaya hemiglauca	Whitewood	Tree	An unidentified toxin causes degeneration and necrosis of heart muscles, skeletal muscles, liver and kidneys in horses. Clinical signs include muscle weakness, staggering, fluid build-up under the skin of the head, myoglobinuria.
Diplarrena moraea	Butterfly flag, white iris, native lily, white lily	Perennial herb with white iris-like flowers	Toxic principles are cardiac glycosides.
Erythrophleum chlorostachys	Ironwood	Tree	Toxic principles are diterpenoid alkaloids. Clinical signs include anorexia, arrhythmia, diarrhea, dyspnea, and collapse.
Trachymene glaucifolia, T. ochracea, and *T. cyanantha*	Wild parsnips	Annual or biennial herbs	Diarrhea and heart failure have occurred in young ruminants exercised after grazing on large amounts of these plants.
Triunia spp.	Spice bushes	Shrubs or small trees	The toxin is unidentified. Poisoning only reported in human beings. Symptoms and clinical signs include nausea, diaphoresis, bradycardia, hypotension, headache, miosis, and diarrhea.

to ingestion by heating, such as when hay becomes damp, but more often nitrate/nitrite toxicosis is the result of conversion of nitrates to nitrites in the rumen. Nitrite ions absorbed into the bloodstream oxidize iron in hemoglobin from the ferrous to the ferric state, resulting in formation of methemoglobin which cannot transport oxygen. Clinical signs become apparent when methemoglobin levels reach 30%–40%, and death ensues when they reach 80%–90%. The clinical course is rapid with clinical signs developing within 4 hours of ingestion. Clinical signs are anxiety, rapid respiration, dyspnea, and rapid, weak pulse. Animals may be weak and intolerant of exercise, but

TABLE 24.17 Native Australian Plants That May Contain Toxic Levels of Nitrates

Linnaean Name	Common Name	Type of Plant
Atriplex muelleri	Annual saltbush, Mueller's saltbush	Herb
Dactyloctenium radulans	Button grass	Grass
Dysphania spp.	Crumbweeds, goosefoots	Herb
Rumex brownii	Swamp dock, hooked dock, slender dock	Herb
Tribulus terrestris	Caltrop	Herb

should be removed from the source forage immediately. Mucous membranes are "muddy" or have a bluish cast. In many cases animals are found dead. On necropsy, chocolate-brown blood is a distinctive finding although it will change to dark red with exposure to air. Postmortem samples are generally unstable although ocular fluid may be useful. Analysis of forage, hay, and water for nitrate levels is generally more rewarding. The recommended reducing agent is methylene blue 1%, administered intravenously at 4−15 mg/kg. Because the rumen continues to produce nitrites, methylene blue administration may need to be repeated at 6 hour intervals. Unfortunately methylene blue is not approved by the APVMA for use in food-producing animals.

Native Australian plants that may contain toxic levels of nitrates are listed in Table 24.17.

Cyanogenic Glycosides and Associated Plants

Cyanogenic glycosides have been found in more than 800 plants, from at least 80 plant families. There are a variety of native and introduced plants in Australia that contain cyanogenic glycosides, which yield hydrogen cyanide upon hydrolysis. Ruminants are particularly susceptible to toxicosis from these plants, because the rumen flora produces large amounts of β-glucosidase, which hydrolyses the glycosides to HCN. Toxicosis is most likely if the animal eats large amounts of the cyanogenic glycosides in a short time, which overwhelms the natural detoxification pathway catalyzed by the enzyme rhodanese. HCN reacts with the iron in cytochrome oxidase, preventing electron transfer and blocking cellular respiration. Toxic levels of cyanogenic glycosides are highest in actively growing parts of the plant and are increased under conditions of stress, high soil nitrogen, and low soil

TABLE 24.18 Native Australian Plants That May Contain Toxic Levels of Cyanogenic Glycosides

Linnaean Name	Common Name	Type of Plant
Alectryon oleifolius	Boonaree	Tree
Brachyachne convergens	Native couch	Grass
Chamaesyce spp.(?)	Caustic weeds	Herb
Dysphania spp.	Crumbweeds, goosefoots	Herb
Eremophila maculata	Fuchsia bush	Shrub
Eucalyptus cladocalyx	Sugar gum	Tree
Euphorbia boophthona (?)	Gascoyne spurge	Herb
Goodia lotifolia	Golden tip	Shrub
Leptopus decaisnei	Andrachne	Herb
Lotus australis	Native bird's-foot trefoil	Herb

phosphorus. The clinical course is rapid with clinical signs becoming evident within 30 minutes of ingestion of a toxic dose. Animals exhibit excitement, tremors, rapid respiration, tachycardia, dyspnea, collapse, terminal convulsions, coma, and death. Blood and tissues are a characteristic cherry-red because the hemoglobin is oxygenated but calls cannot take up the oxygen. The blood clots slowly or not at all. Hemorrhages are often present under the epicardium and endocardium. There may be a bitter almond smell to the ruminal contents, but not all people can detect this odor. Ruminal content should be frozen if later analysis is desired. Urine may be frozen for later thiocyanate analysis. The recommended therapeutic regimen for large animals is 10–20 mg/kg sodium nitrite administered IV as a 20% solution, together with up to 600 mg/kg of sodium thiosulfate as a 20% solution. The sodium nitrite induces formation of cyanmethemoglobin that dissociates cyanide from cytochrome oxidase. The thiosulfate is required as a substrate for the detoxifying activity of rhodanese.

Native Australian plants that are significant sources of cyanogenic glycosides are listed in Table 24.18.

PLANTS WITH TOXIC EFFECTS ON THE GASTROINTESTINAL TRACT

Native Australian plants causing gastrointestinal toxicity are listed in Table 24.19.

TABLE 24.19 Native Australian Plants That Cause Gastrointestinal Toxicosis

Linnaean Name	Common Name	Type of Plant	Comments
Abrus precatorius	Gidee-gidee, rosary pea, jequirity bean	Vine	The toxin is abrin. Clinical signs are usually delayed for hours after ingestion, but include severe abdominal pain, severe diarrhea or dysentery, vomiting, weakness, shock, and collapse. Hemolytic anemia and renal failure have been reported in human cases. On necropsy, in addition to severe gastroenteritis, there may be hepatic and renal degeneration/necrosis, enlarged lymph nodes and spleen, and hemorrhagic lesions throughout the body.
Alocasia brisbanensis	Cunjevoi, spoonlily, elephant's ear	Large herbaceous plant	Contains insoluble calcium oxalate crystals that form needle-like raphides that penetrate the oral and pharyngeal mucosa, causing inflammation, hypersalivation, and edema that may be sufficient to cause choking or to significantly inhibit respiration. Cooling liquids or demulcents may be helpful. Antihistamines should be administered, and respiration maintained, by tracheostomy if necessary. Effects may last for hours.
Castanospermum australe	Black bean, Moreton Bay chestnut	Tree	The toxic principle is unidentified. Toxicosis is usually due to cattle eating the seeds. Clinical signs include severe diarrhea, oliguria, and dehydration. Postmortem lesions include hemaorrhagic gastroenteritis, myocardial necrosis, nephrosis, and cytoplasmic vacuolation of up to 5% of circulating lymphocytes.

(Continued)

TABLE 24.19 (Continued)

Linnaean Name	Common Name	Type of Plant	Comments
Crotalaria aridicola subsp. *aridicola*	Chillagoe horse poison	Shrub	Cause "Chillagoe horse disease," in which horses develop severe ulceration of the esophagus and cardiac part of the stomach. The ulceration leads to partial or complete esophageal obstruction. Horses exhibit bruxism, coughing, halitosis, and drooling, and are hungry and thirsty but have great difficulty swallowing and may regurgitate ingesta through the nose. Horses can die of dehydration and/or starvation. Horses may be saved with intensive nursing, including administering water and feed through a nasogastric tube, and providing food that is easily swallowed such as molasses. Toxicosis develops after horses have been eating the plants for at least 2 weeks, but may be delayed up to 4 weeks after horses are moved from access to the plants. Horses may develop a liking for the plants and seek them out.
C. medicaginea var. *neglecta.*	Trefoil rattlepod	Shrub	
Cucumis melo supsp. *agrestis*	Ulcardo melon	Vine	Cucurbitacins cause extremely severe gastrointestinal irritation and may also affect cardiac function.
Melia azedarach	White cedar	Tree	Severe diarrhea, vomiting, and colic. Also causes nervous signs.
Phaleria clerodendron	Rosy apple	Shrub or small tree	Toxins are irritant diterpenoids.

(Continued)

TABLE 24.19 (Continued)

Linnaean Name	Common Name	Type of Plant	Comments
Pimelea decora	Flinders poppy	Herb or shrub	Toxins are irritant diterpenoids or phorbol esters. These plants also contain simplexin; see Section "Cardiotoxic Plants." Species other than cattle usually exhibit gastrointestinal toxicity (diarrhea) rather than cardiotoxicity.
P. elongata			
Pimelea haematostachya	Pimelea poppy		
P. latifolia subsp. *altior*			
P. neo-anglica	Poison pimelea		
P. simplex	Desert rice flower		
P. trichostachya	Flax-weed		
Ranunculus inundatus			Contain protoanemonin, an irritant oil glycoside that is not readily absorbed from the gastrointestinal tract or metabolized in it, with the result that irritation is likely to occur in the oral cavity and throughout the gastrointestinal tract. The toxin is most abundant in the roots, which may be eaten by grazing animals that inadvertently pull up the whole plant when soil is soft. Clinical signs include oral irritation, hypersalivation, diarrhea, depression, and irritated skin of the muzzle.
Ranunculus undosus			
Wikstroemia indica	Tie bush		Toxins are irritant diterpenoids.

PLANTS WITH TOXIC EFFECTS ON THE RESPIRATORY SYSTEM

Plants with toxic effects on the respiratory system are listed in Table 24.20.

PLANTS WITH TOXIC EFFECTS ON SKIN

Plants known to cause dermal toxicity are listed in Table 24.21, categorized by mechanism.

TABLE 24.20 Native Australian Plants That Cause Toxicosis of the Respiratory System

Linnaean Name	Common Name	Type of Plant	Comments
Dendrocnide spp.	Stingers	Trees	Although the most severe toxic effect of these trees is the pain of their stings (see Section on plants toxic to the skin) inhalation of fine particles in their vicinity can be associated with severe nose and throat irritation.
Schoenus asperocarpus	Poison sedge	Grass-like herb	Toxin is galegine, which causes acute pulmonary edema and pleural effusion, with proteinaceous exudate that sets on cooling. Sheep are most commonly affected. There is no treatment.
Zieria arborescens	Stinkwood	Tall shrub or tree	Pulmonary edema, emphysema, and damage to pulmonary arterioles in cattle, due to an unidentified toxin.

PLANTS WITH TOXIC EFFECTS ON SKELETAL MUSCLE

Leiocarpa brevicompta (flat billy buttons) is a low-growing annual with yellow flowers that grows mainly on the floodplains of the Darling River, particularly after flooding. Poisoning most often occurs in sheep, and occurs after they consume the seeds as more than 50% of their diet, for 14 days or more. The toxidrome is called "summer staggers" or "tiring syndrome." The primary lesion is a skeletal and cardiac myopathy, but in addition to muscle pallor, particularly of the hindlimbs, gross lesions also include pulmonary edema, hepatic degeneration, renal degeneration, and cerebral edema. The usual toxidrome is weakness and exercise intolerance, with irregular heartbeat, tachypnea, and hyperthermia. Some animals show apparent nervous signs; when disturbed, they run until they collapse and die suddenly. Clinical pathology reveals marked increases in creatine kinase and AST. Animals may recover with nursing. Cattle are relatively although not wholly resistant to toxicosis, and can be used to graze the plants. If sheep are moved away from the toxic pasture when clinical signs are first noticed, some sheep will die as a result of being moved but there will be no further deaths after 7–10 days.

Atalaya hemiglauca causes degeneration and necrosis of skeletal muscle as well as heart muscle, liver, and kidney in horses. See entry in Table 24.16.

PLANTS WITH TOXIC EFFECTS ON THE SKELETON

For plants associated with "Big Head" in horses, see Section "Plants Containing Soluble Oxalates".

TABLE 24.21 Native Australian Plants That May Cause Dermal Effects

Linnaean Name	Common Name	Comments
Plants Causing Primary Photosensitization		
Cullen spp.	Scurf-peas	The toxins are furanocoumarins. Horses may develop corneal edema
Plants Causing Secondary Photosensitization		
Panicum decompositum	Native millet	Toxins are steroidal or lithogenic saponins
Panicum effusum	Hairy panic	
Persicaria lapathifolia	Smartweed, pale knotweed, pink knotweed	It is not clear whether photosensitization is primary or secondary, but liver damage has been reported in some cases
Persicaria orientalis	Oriental smartweed, oriental knotweed, princes feathers	
Also see the Section "Hepatotoxic Plants"—any plant that causes chronic hepatic damage can cause secondary photosensitization in grazing animals		
Plants Having a Direct Irritant Effect		
Dendrocnide corallodesme	Mango-leaved stinger	These plants, which are shrubs or small trees all belong to the nettle family, and have stinging hairs on leaves and small stems. They are found along the Eastern coast of Australia. The stings are excruciatingly painful and horses in particular may scream and throw themselves about violently, with great risk of injury to themselves or their handlers. Human beings, cattle, and dogs have also been stung. Humans stung by *D. moroides*, *D. cordata*, or *D. corallodesme* have reported pain lasting for up to 3 months. Euthanasia may be required for animals stung by *Dendrocnide* spp.
Dendrocnide cordata	Stinger	
Dendrocnide excelsa	Giant stinger	
Dendrocnide moroides	Gimpi-gimpi	
Dendrocnide photinophylla	Shining-leaved stinger	
Grevillea spp.	Caustic bushes	The toxicants are urushiols, which cause blistering

Bent-Leg in Lambs

This condition occurs when pregnant ewes graze the mature fruits of *Trachymene glaucifolia*, *Trachymene ochracea*, or *Trachymene cyanantha*.

These plants have common names including wild parsnip, wild carrot, and blue parsnip. Lambs are born normal, but subsequently develop lateral or medial deviation of the carpus. The effect may be apparent within days of birth but may develop later, even after weaning. A proportion of affected lambs will recover over time. The defect is in the epiphyseal plates. Usually only the forelimbs are affected, but occasionally lambs may be born missing their distal hindlimbs, or with micrognathia or hydrocephalus.

PLANTS WITH TOXIC EFFECTS ON THE REPRODUCTIVE SYSTEM

Plants Causing Infertility

Consumption of *Trachymene* spp. is associated with infertility in ewes, possibly due to early embryonic loss. The mechanism is unknown.

Plants Causing Teratogenic Effects

The plants that cause nicotine and related alkaloid poisoning (see under neurotoxic plants, above) may contain the nicotine-like alkaloid anabasine, that may case teratogenic effects including cleft palate, scoliosis, and arthrogryposis.

PLANTS THAT CONTAIN HIGH LEVELS OF SELENIUM

Selenium poisoning is covered elsewhere in this book. Native Australian plants that can cause selenium poisoning due to storage of high concentrations of selenium include *Neptunia amplexicaulis* (selenium weed) and *Morinda reticulata* (mapoon).

Part 3: Poisonous Native Plants of New Zealand

In this section, plants that are known or suspected to be poisonous are listed in alphabetical order using their Maori names. While not all these species are unique to New Zealand, they are included in this chapter if they were not introduced by human colonization. Toxicity, or suspected toxicity, of the following plants is described in this section:

Maori Name	Common Name	Linnaean Name
Kakariki	Rock fern	*Cheilanthes sieberi*
Karaka	Karaka	*Corynocarpus laevigatus*
Kowhai	Kowhai	*Sophora* species
Ngaio	Ngaio	*Myoporum laetum*
Ongaonga	Tree Nettle	*Urtica ferox*

(*Continued*)

(Continued)

Maori Name	Common Name	Linnaean Name
Pinatoro	Pinatoro	*Pimelea prostrata*
Poroporo	Poroporo	*Solanum aviculare, Solanum laciniatum*
Porokaiwhiri	Pigeonwood	*Hedycarya arborea*
Pukatea	Pukatea	*Laurelia novae-zelandiae*
Rangiora	Rangiora	*Brachyglottis repanda*
Rarauhe	Bracken	*Pteridium esculentum*
Titoki	Titoki	*Alectryon excelsus*
Turutu	New Zealand blueberry	*Dianella nigra*
Tutu	Tutu	*Coriaria* species
Waoriki	Waoriki	*Ranunculus amphitrichus*
Whauwhaupaku	Five-finger	*Pseudopanax arboreum*

KAKARIKI *CHEILANTHES SIEBERI*

Alternative Names

Rock fern, Poison rock fern, Mulga fern.

Distribution

This fern is found in rocky coastal to sunny montane habitats, and is endemic to New Zealand, Australia, and New Caledonia. It prefers damp locations, but is drought-tolerant in that although it dies back in drought, it regenerates rapidly after the drought breaks.

Appearance

Kakariki is a small upright fern, usually reaching not more than 30 cm.

Circumstances of Poisoning

Kakariki is usually eaten only when other grazing is scarce. It is rapidly growing and is often one of the first plants to regenerate after drought, when it may be the only feed available to hungry stock. Poisoning has been recorded most frequently in Australia.

Absorption, Distribution, Metabolism, and Excretion

There is a lack of information on the toxicokinetics of the toxic principle/s in Kakariki, ptaquiloside and thiaminase I, the same toxic principles as in Rarauhe (bracken fern; q.v.); however, the effects of consumption tend to become apparent after prolonged exposure (1—3 months).

Mode(s) of Action

Ptaquiloside and thiaminase I, the same toxic principles as those responsible for toxicosis due to Rarauhe (bracken fern; q.v.) are also responsible for toxicoses due to Kakarike.

Clinical Signs

Clinical signs are as for the more common and better-known toxicoses caused by Rarauhe (bracken fern; q.v.); hemorrhagic syndrome, enzootic hematuria, and polioencephalomalacia.

Diagnostic Aids

These are the same as for the more common and better-known toxicoses caused by Rarauhe (bracken fern; q.v.).

Treatment

These are the same as for the more common and better-known toxicoses caused by Rarauhe (bracken fern; q.v.).

Prognosis

These are the same as for the more common and better-known toxicoses caused by Rarauhe (bracken fern; q.v.).

Necropsy

These are the same as for the more common and better-known toxicoses caused by Rarauhe (bracken fern; q.v.).

Public Health Considerations

People should not consume any part of this plant because of the risk of carcinogenesis.

Prevention

Stock find this species unpalatable and generally eat it only when other feed is not available, so provision of safer and more palatable feed is preventative. Inclusion of Kakariki in hay should be avoided.

KARAKA *CORYNOCARPUS LAEVIGATUS*

Alternative Names

New Zealand Laurel; Kopi (on the Chatham Islands, Kopi being the Moriori name).

Distribution

This tree is common on the two main islands and is also found on some outlying islands. It is most commonly found in coastal habitats. It is popular as an ornamental tree, although seedlings and saplings are frost-tender.

Appearance

The Karaka tree grows up to 15 m in height and has large, glossy leaves up to 200 mm in length. It produces erect panicles of small cream flowers between August and November. The ovoid fruit are produced between January and April, and ripen from green to orange. "Karaka" is the Maori word for the color orange.

Circumstances of Poisoning

Dogs are susceptible to Karaka poisoning, and some dogs will voluntarily eat the Karaka fruit. Neurotoxic effects have been reported in kiwi (*Apteryx* species) as a result of ingestion of Karaka fruit.

Cattle, sheep, and pigs appear to be able to ingest Karaka with impunity, although diarrhea and depression in goats has been attributed to Karaka. The toxicity of Karaka to horses is unclear.

Toxicokinetics

There is no robust information on the toxicokinetics of karakin or the other toxic principles that may be present in Karaka. Case reports suggest that clinical signs are often delayed for 2 hours or more after ingestion.

Mode(s) of Action

The kernels of the fruit are toxic, containing the alkaloid karakin. Other toxic principles may be present.

Karakin has the empirical formula $C15H21O15N3$, and the chemical name 1:4: ß-tris-(-nitropropionyl) D-glucopyranose. Unpollinated Karaka fruit do not contain nuts and are not considered to be toxic, although they are bitter.

Clinical Signs

Clinical signs of karaka poisoning in the dog include vomiting, dyspnea, weakness, paralysis, and convulsions.

Clinical signs observed in kiwi have included weakness, ataxia, leg paralysis, and convulsions.

Clinical signs in human beings may include severe tonic convulsions. The Maori recognized that survivors could be left with limbs permanently fixed in contorted positions, and it was tradition to bury poisoned children up to their neck until the convulsions had passed, in order to prevent this outcome.

Diagnostic Aids

There are no characteristic findings on clinical pathology or radiology, and no standard test for karakin or other putative toxic principles that can be applied to biological samples from the live animal.

Treatment

There is no specific antidote or treatment for Karaka poisoning. The animal should be stabilized to maintain vital functions and convulsions controlled, by general anesthesia if necessary.

Given the delayed onset of toxicosis in reported cases, decontamination is extremely unlikely to be effective once clinical signs are evident. However, prophylactic gastric decontamination may have some value if performed within 15 minutes of ingestion.

Prognosis

Anecdotal evidence suggests that if a dog survives for more than 24 hours after onset of toxicosis, it is likely to survive, although convalescence may be prolonged.

Necropsy

There is no standard test for karakin or other putative toxic principles, and no characteristic lesions of Karaka poisoning. Whole or macerated parts of Karaka kernels in the gastrointestinal tract may support the diagnosis.

Public Health Considerations

Poisoning from ingestion of Karaka fruit has occurred in humans, particularly children. Karaka was a traditional food crop of Maori, following careful processing of the kernels.

Prevention

Karakin is reported to be heat-labile and unstable in storage over time, but there is no established, reliable method to make Karaka kernels nontoxic. Even among Maori for whom it was a staple of the diet, human poisoning cases occurred. Prevention of access to Karaka fruit is the only reliable preventative measure.

KOWHAI *SOPHORA* SPECIES

Alternative Names

Kohai
Eight species: *Sophora chathamica, Sophora fulvida, Sophora godleyi, Sophora longicarinata, Sophora microphylla, Sophora molloyi, Sophora prostrata,* and *Sophora tetraptera.*

Distribution

Kowhai are found throughout New Zealand, usually on the edge of forest or in open areas, and are often planted as an ornamental tree and to attract native songbirds such as the bellbird and tui.

Appearance

The Kowhai is usually a small tree up to 12 m in height, with fairly smooth bark and a somewhat weeping form. It has small greyish-green leaves and may be deciduous or semi-deciduous. The racemes of yellow flowers are produced from July to November. The hard yellow seeds are produced in 4-winged segmented pods.

Circumstances of Poisoning

All parts of Kowhai are considered poisonous, and the seeds are alleged to be particularly toxic. However, there is a lack of evidence, in the form of case reports, that voluntary ingestion of Kowhai has caused serious toxicity in any species. The seeds, although often shed in abundance, are very hard and are bitter if chewed, so clinical poisoning is considered to be unlikely.

The alleged toxicity of Kowhai may be largely an extrapolation from the well-established toxicity of Texas Mountain Laurel, *Sophora secundiflora,* which is found in North America and contains the neurotoxic quinolizidine alkaloids, cytisine, and sparteine.

Extracts from the seeds of Kowhai have been reported to be toxic to mice. The nectar of the Kowhai causes narcosis in honey bees.

Absorption, Distribution, Metabolism, and Excretion

There is no information on the toxicokinetic profile of ingested Kowhai *per se*.

In experimental animals, the C_{max} of ingested cytisine may be reached at 35 minutes, and the half-life is less than an hour. These values may be moderately increased if cytisine-containing plant material, rather than purified cytisine, is ingested.

In human beings, onset of poisoning in human beings by the related species *S. secundiflora* is reported to be rapid, occurring within 30 minutes of ingestion.

Mode(s) of Action

The toxic principle in Kowhai is cytisine, an alkaloid with both nicotinic and muscarinic effects.

Clinical Signs

Chewing on Kowhai seeds has been reported to cause a burning sensation in the mouth, and gastric distress, in human beings.

Poisoning due to the related species *S. secundiflora* causes stiff gait, exercise intolerance and ataxia in ruminants, and exercise intolerance, muscle rigidity and periodic weakness or syncope in dogs. Recovery is reported to be rapid in dogs.

Toxic effects of *S. secundiflora* ingestion in human beings include nausea, emesis, mydriasis, delirium, parasthesias, loss of muscle tone, drowsiness, and occasionally convulsions. Cytisine has the potential to paralyze respiratory muscles.

Diagnostic Aids

There are no characteristic findings on clinical pathology or radiology. Testing for cytisine is not commercially available and would not be useful, given the short half-life.

Treatment

Treatment is symptomatic and supportive. Seizures should be controlled and respiratory support provided if necessary.

Gastric decontamination is highly unlikely to be useful because of the rapid absorption and excretion of cytisine, and may be hazardous because cytisine is an emetic. Likewise, the rapid absorption of cytisine means that activated charcoal is unlikely to be beneficial.

Prognosis

Prognosis is excellent.

Necropsy

There is no standard test for cytisine or sparteine, and no characteristic lesions of Kowhai poisoning. Parts of Kowhai in the gastrointestinal tract may support the diagnosis.

Public Health Considerations

Because of the lack of evidence that Kowhai is a significant source of poisoning to human beings or domestic animals in New Zealand, there is no justification for removing Kowhai as a public health measure.

Prevention

Toxic exposure is unlikely and therefore preventative measures are not required. Kowhai may be found growing undisturbed in paddocks and does not appear to be attractive to livestock. The related toxic species *S. secundiflora* is unpalatable to ruminants, and toxicosis of livestock in North America generally only occurs if the animals do not have alternative plants to graze.

NGAIO *MYOPORUM LAETUM*

Alternative Names

Mousehole tree.
Note: Australian Ngaio, *Myoporum insulare*, has similar toxic properties.

Distribution

Coastal or lowland forests.

Appearance

Ngaio grow as shrubs or spreading trees, up to 1−0 m in height. They have glossy yellow-green to dark green leaves. The leaves contain oil glands that can be seen as small see-through spots if leaves are held up to the light. New shoots on the Ngaio are dark and have a sticky feel. The bark is gray to brown, thick, rough, and furrowed. Ngaio flower from October to January. The flowers are small and white with purple spots. The fruits are purple and ripen from December to June.

Circumstances of Poisoning

The leaves of Ngaio contain the toxic principle, Ngaione. Ngaio is generally unpalatable to livestock although cattle, in particular, may eat it if there is no other feed available, or out of curiosity if fallen or trimmed branches are available. Toxicosis has also been reported in sheep and pigs, and there has been a possible case reported in a horse.

Absorption, Distribution, Metabolism, and Excretion

Ngaione requires metabolic activation. The toxicokinetics of ngaione are otherwise unknown.

Clinical signs in cattle developed 24–72 hours after a single experimental ingestion, and the duration of clinical poisoning was up to 7 days.

Mode(s) of Action

Ngaione, the hepatotoxic principle in Ngaio, is a furanoid sesquiterpene ketone and constitutes 70%–80% of the oil in Ngaio.

Clinical Signs

Clinical signs include anorexia, colic, ruminal stasis, constipation, depression, serous ocular and nasal discharge, icterus, photosensitivity, and mucosal petechiation. Lactating animals may develop mammary edema and agalactia, and pregnant animals may abort. Tenesmus and tooth grinding have been reported in sheep.

Diagnostic Aids

Serum levels of AST, GGT, and bilirubin are elevated.
Liver biopsy may confirm hepatotoxicity in surviving animals.

Treatment

Treatment is supportive. Shade must be provided to minimize photosensitivity. If possible, animals should be housed during the day. Skin lesions should be treated with wound management techniques, and secondary infections or myiasis prevented. A soap-and-water enema may be helpful to relieve constipation.

Prognosis

Prognosis is variable, depending on the severity of liver damage. Livestock that are severely affected but which survive may not return to full production. Female ruminants that suffer severe liver damage and survive, may succumb to ketosis under the metabolic pressures of late pregnancy or lactation.

Necropsy

Macerated pieces of Ngaio may be present in the rumen or gastrointestinal tract.

Gross findings include abomasitis, a pale mottled liver, widespread petechiae and ecchymoses, subcutaneous edema, generalized icterus, excessive fluid in serous cavities, and hemorrhage within the epicardium and endocardium.

Hepatic degeneration and necrosis is usually periportal but may also be midzonal. Portal fibrosis and bile ductule proliferation, and hypertrophy of surviving hepatocytes, are observed in livers of recovering animals.

Public Health Considerations

There is no evidence of risk to public health. Children should not be allowed to eat Ngaio fruits.

Prevention

Livestock should not be grazed in areas with access to Ngaio. Ngaio trimmings should not be dumped where livestock have access to them, and branches of Ngaio that fall into grazing areas should be promptly removed.

ONGAONGA *URTICA FEROX*

Alternative Names

Tree Nettle; Giant Tree Nettle; Native Stinging Nettle.

Distribution

Ongaonga is found throughout the main islands of New Zealand, as far south as Otago.

It grows at less than 600 m in altitude is mainly found in coastal and lowland areas. It tends to grown on the margins of forests or in scrub, and may form thickets. It is frost-hardy to −8°C.

Appearance

Ongaonga grows up to 3 m tall and, unusually for a member of the genus *Urtica*, has woody stems. The leaves are coarsely toothed and have numerous white stinging hairs (trichomes) up to 6 mm in length. Trichomes are also found on young stalks and on leaf veins.

The flowers and fruit are insignificant.

Circumstances of Poisoning

Poisoning of horses, dogs, or human beings have occurred when the victim makes physical contact with Ongaonga. Poisoning of other species has not been recorded. Goats and deer have been recorded to browse on Ongaonga.

Absorption, Distribution, Metabolism, and Excretion

There is no experimental information on the toxicokinetics of the combination of toxins released by Ongaonga. Pain at the site is immediate. Systemic clinical signs usually commence within 15−30 minutes and reach their greatest intensity within 60−90 minutes. Severe systemic effects may persist for 3 days. A prolonged peripheral neuropathy has been reported in humans and replicated experimentally in rats.

Mode(s) of Action

When a trichome on Ongaonga is touched, the sharp tip pierces the skin and then breaks off. The trichome is hollow, and the toxic principles are released into the skin and subcutis. Toxicants include acetylcholine, serotonin, and histamine. Delayed effects of Ongaonga toxicosis are attributed to unidentified neurotoxin(s).

Clinical Signs

Reported clinical signs in dogs include hypersalivation, weakness, ataxia, dyspnea, tremors, and seizures. There may be vomiting and/or diarrhea.

Horses have also been fatally stung by Ongaonga, and may die within hours if severely stung. Clinical signs include dyspnea, collapse, and seizures.

Human victims of Ongaonga stings report that the local pain is intense and accompanied by pruritis. The stung area becomes inflamed and blisters may develop. Local effects may last for 36 hours or more. Depending on the number of stings, systemic effects may also develop, typically within 30 minutes. These may include abdominal pain, hypersalivation, visual blurring or loss of vision, numbness or paresthesia, muscle weakness, incoordination, paralysis, and dyspnea. A human fatality occurred in 1961.

A prolonged peripheral neuropathy occurs occasionally in human victims of Ongaonga stings. This neuropathy has been replicated experimentally in rats, and neurophysiological and pathological features of axonopathy were observed.

Diagnostic Aids

Diagnosis is made on the basis of history and clinical signs, and there are no specific diagnostic aids.

Treatment

Immediate washing of the sting site with water has been recommended as a decontamination measure in animals, although since the trichomes inject the toxins into or through the skin it is not clear why this would alter the absorption of the toxins, and no testing has been conducted to determine whether it alters clinical outcome in severe toxicosis. However, in human cases, cooling of the affected skin is reported to reduce local pain and pruritis.

Mild cases of Ongaonga toxicosis are self-limiting, and there are anecdotal accounts of dog owners successfully controlling toxicosis by administering oral antihistamines.

However, if systemic clinical signs are evident, the animal should be treated with atropine, parenteral antihistamine, parenteral short-acting corticosteroids, and fluid therapy. Respiratory dunction should be closely monitored, and Intubation and respiratory support provided if required. Adrenalin may be required to control anaphylactic/anaphylactoid response.

Prognosis

Life-threatening respiratory compromise generally responds rapidly to treatment, but neurological signs such as muscle weakness and ataxia may persist for a few weeks.

Necropsy

Internal findings are nonspecific. Pulmonary congestion, abundant foam in the trachea and abundant saliva in the stomach support the diagnosis. Specimens of the site/s of stings may be fixed for histopathology.

Public Health Considerations

Because of the risk of human toxicosis by Ongaonga, local authorities should be notified of the location of the plants responsible for veterinary cases.

Prevention

Owners should be informed of the dangers of walking a dog, or riding a horse, in areas where Ongaonga grows, and also informed of the risks to themselves or other people.

Removal of plants by local authorities may be appropriate in some locations, but it should be borne in mind that Ongaonga is an important source of food and protection for the caterpillars of the Red Admiral (*Brassaris gonerilla*; *Vanessa gonerilla*; kahukura) butterfly, which is native to New Zealand, and the Yellow Admiral (*Vanessa itea*; kahukowhai) butterfly, which is native to Australia and New Zealand.

PINATORO *PIMELEA PROSTRATA*

Alternative Names

Pimelea, Strathmore weed, New Zealand daphne.

Not that there are multiple species of the genus *Pimelea* in New Zealand, and the use of the name Pinatoro for them varies depending on source. Poisoning of horses and cattle has been specifically attributed to *Pimelea prostrata* or to *Pimelea urvilleana*, which was thought to be a subspecies of *P. prostrata* but has been reclassified. The toxicity of other species of *Pimelea* in New Zealand is unclear, but it seems likely that they would contain similar toxic principles. A comprehensive list of *Pimelea* species in New Zealand, together with their distributions, can be found at http://www.nzpcn.org.nz.

Distribution

P. prostrata and other members of the genus, that are likely to contain the same or similar toxins, are found in grassland, shrubland, on river terraces and on rocky or graveled areas on both main islands and many offshore islands, to an altitude of 1500 m.

Appearance

Most *Pimelea* in New Zealand are small to medium sized shrubs with prostrate habit, flexible stems and small leaves. Flowers are small, white and often hairy, and produced between September and May, with some species variation. Fruits are produced from October to July, again with some species variation, and are small, fleshy and usually white, although some species may produce red fruit.

Circumstances of Poisoning

Pinatoro is poisonous to horses and cattle that graze on it, but sheep appear to be tolerant of it.

Absorption, Distribution, Metabolism, and Excretion

There is no information on the toxicokinetics of prostratin.

Mode(s) of Action

The toxic principle is prostratin, which is chemically similar to the toxins in Daphne and *Euphorbia* species.

Clinical Signs

Cattle develop inflammation of the mucous membranes and the abomasum.

Cattle poisoned by related *Pimelea* species in Australia develop depression, diarrhea, ventral edema, and exercise intolerance. The toxic principle responsible for Pimelea poisoning in Australia is simplexin, which is in the same chemical class as prostratin.

Clinical signs of Pinatoro poisoning observed in horses include marked depression, severe stomatitis and glossitis, colic, abundant watery diarrhea, and icterus. Eyelids may be edematous.

Diagnostic Aids

There is a lack of information on the clinical pathology of Pinatoro poisoning in New Zealand, but hypoproteinemia, anemia, leucopenia, and elevation of liver enzymes have been reported in bovine *Pimelea* poisoning in Australia, which is caused by a chemically related toxin.

Treatment

Treatment is symptomatic and supportive.

Prognosis

Prognosis is moderate, depending on severity of clinical signs. Functional reserve of the liver may be reduced in survivors.

Necropsy

Stomatitis, glossitis, esophagitis, gastritis, and hyperemia of the intestinal mucosa have been reported in horses with Pinatoro poisoning. Similar lesions would be expected in cattle. Mucosal inflammation may include bullae and/or ulceration.

Liver lesions of *Pimelea* poisoning in Australia are reported to include disruption of the sinusoidal architecture with development of large blood-filled spaces.

Public Health Considerations

Pinatoro does not appear to pose any risk to human beings.

Prevention

Horses and cattle should be restricted from access to Pinatoro, and should be provided with sufficient grazing of nontoxic plants.

POROPORO *SOLANUM AVICULARE, SOLANUM LACINIATUM*

Alternative Names

Kangaroo Apple (*S. aviculare*).

Distribution

S. aviculare is native to both Australia and New Zealand. It is uncertain whether *S. aviculare* and *S. laciniatum* are two different species, or one. Plants are found on both main islands of New Zealand and the Chatham islands, in coastal and lowland forest margins and shrubland, but the lighter-flowered plant, *S. aviculare* is found in the northern part of the North Island of New Zealand, while the plant found south of Auckland has darker purple flowers and may be a separate species, *S. laciniatum*.

Appearance

Poroporo can grow up to 4 m tall. The leaves are 8−30 cm long. Flowers range in color from white through mauve to blue-violet, and are 25−40 mm wide. The fruit are 10−15 mm wide and range in color from orange-red to scarlet.

Circumstances of Poisoning

All green parts of Poroporo, and the unripe fruit, contain toxic Solanum alkaloids. However, there is a lack of well-documented evidence of Poroporo poisoning in New Zealand, and reports of poisonings of sheep and cattle appear to be anecdotal or at best circumstantial. As a generalization the presence of Solanum alkaloids makes plants of the genus unpalatable to livestock.

Absorption, Distribution, Metabolism, and Excretion

Poisoning with solasodine or related alkaloids generally has a rapid clinical course, although clearance of tritiated solasodine from the liver has been shown to be protracted. Limited toxicokinetic data suggest that solasodine in the circulation is predominantly bound to erythrocytes, and that more solasodine is excreted by the fecal route than by the renal route.

Mode(s) of Action

The leaves and unripe fruit of *S. aviculare* contain the alkaloid solasodine and related alkaloids, which are also produced by a number of other plants within the genus *Solanum*. Clinical signs would be expected to be similar as those for related glycoalkaloids produced by plants of the *Solanum* genus.

Clinical Signs

Gastrointestinal signs of Solanum alkaloid poisoning include colic, diarrhea, and in those species that can easily vomit, emesis. In severe cases, there may be partial or complete intestinal atony, and constipation. Clinical findings also include mydriasis, dry mucous membranes, tachycardia, hypotension, and arrhythmia. Neurological effects include agitation, ataxia, paralysis, convulsions, and coma. There may be behavioral evidence of delirium, which is reported in human patients with solasodine poisoning. Human patients also report headache. Human beings who have tasted unripe fruits of Poroporo report a burning sensation in the mouth.

In laboratory rodents, solasodine has been shown to be teratogenic, toxic to the testes, and to inhibit lymphocyte proliferation.

Diagnostic Aids

There are no specific diagnostic aids.

Treatment

Treatment is symptomatic and supportive.
If a breeding female is affected, the owner should be warned that solasodine may be teratogenic. If a breeding male is affected, the owner should be warned that fertility may be adversely affected.

Prognosis

The clinical course of Solanum alkaloid poisoning is generally rapid with animals either succumbing or recovering in 24—48 hours.

Necropsy

Lesions are nonspecific or absent. There may be gastroenteritis.
Plant material in the gastrointestinal tract may be sufficiently intact to permit identification.

Public Health Considerations

Solanum aviculare is an attractive plant and may be planted in gardens for this reason. The unripe fruit are toxic to human beings and may be attractive to children. However, the burning sensation reported by people who have tasted unripe fruit would be a deterrent.

Prevention

Prevent grazing and browsing animals from access to Poroporo, and provide them with sufficient nontoxic grazing.

POROKAIWHIRI *HEDYCARYA ARBOREA*

Alternative Names

Pigeonwood.

Distribution

This tree is found in the North and South Islands as well as the Three Kings islands. On the eastern side of the South island, it is uncommon south of Kaikoura and not found south of Banks Peninsula, but on the western side it is found as far south as Fiordland. It is common in coastal and lowland forest, and may extend into montane areas in the warmer parts of the North Island.

Appearance

Porokaiwhiri is a small upright fragrant tree that grows to a maximum height of 12 m. It has ascending branches with a trunk with smooth, dark gray or brown-gray bark up to 50 cm in diameter. The leaves are bright green, thick, and leathery with saw toothed margins and distinct veins. It flowers in

Spring. Flowers on male plants are 10 mm across and those on female plants, 6 mm across.

Berries are bright orange to red.

Circumstances of Poisoning

Porokaiwhiri has been suspected of causing poisoning in cattle, but there is little information and no recent information.

Absorption, Distribution, Metabolism, and Excretion

No information.

Mode(s) of Action

No information. Alkaloids have been shown to be present in the foliage, bark, and berries. However, possums (*Trichosurus vulpecula*) eat the berries with impunity. Kereru (wood pigeons; *Hemiphaga novaeseelandiae*) also eat the berries with impunity. The tree was given its common name because it was thought that the berries were a favorite food of kereru, but there is recent evidence that suggests that kereru eat the berries only when other food is in short supply.

Clinical Signs

No information.

Diagnostic Aids

No information.

Treatment

No information.

Prognosis

No information.

Necropsy

No information.

Public Health Considerations

No information. Because the male flowers in particular are fragrant, porokai-whiri may be grown as a garden tree, but no human poisonings have been reported.

Prevention

No information.

PUKATEA *LAURELIA NOVAE-ZELANDIAE*

Alternative Names

None.

Distribution

Pukatea is found throughout the North Island and in the northern third of the south Island. It is found in lowland forest, usually where there is plenty of moisture, such as in gullies and on the edges of streams. It does best in a temperate to warm subtropical climate with only very slight winter frosts not below −4°C, and with high summer heat. The tree prefers well-drained, slightly acidic soil rich in organic matter.

Appearance

Pukatea is a tall forest tree that can grow to a height of 40 m. It is unusual in being the only New Zealand native tree developing large plank-buttresses in maturity. Plank-buttresses are thin triangular flanges extend up to the trunk and along the roots, and in this species they are believed to help to support the heavy crown. The trunk is straight and up to 2 m in diameter. The bark is pale. The thick leathery leaves are bright green, glossy on top and pale underneath, and have serrated margins. Green flowers, 6 mm in diameter, are borne on stalks during October to November. It then develops urn-shaped seed cases up to 2.5 cm long, which split and release hair-covered seeds, which are dispersed by the wind.

Circumstances of Poisoning

There is a lack of information on Pukatea poisoning, beyond a 1909 report that pukateine caused strychnine-like convulsions in rabbits, and muscle contraction in frogs.

Absorption, Distribution, Metabolism, and Excretion

There is no information on the toxicokinetics of pukateine.

Mode(s) of Action

The Maori used a bark extract as an analgesic for toothache. Pukateine, an alkaloid extracted from the bark, is similar in structure to glaucine and tetrahdropalmatine that are found in Chinese medicinal herbs used as analgesics. Pukateine acts as an agonist at the D_2 dopamine receptor and an antagonist at the $\alpha 1$ adrenergic receptor.

There have been some claims that pukateine has morphine-like effects, but people who have tried Pukatea bark preparations as a recreational drug have reported little effect other than a numb tongue.

Clinical Signs

Strychnine-like convulsions in rabbits experimentally administered pukateine.

Diagnostic Aids

No information.

Treatment

No information.

Prognosis

No information.

Necropsy

No information.

Public Health Considerations

No information.

Prevention

No information.

RANGIORA *BRACHYGLOTTIS REPANDA*

Alternative names

Pukapuka, Wharangi, Bushman's Friend, Bushman's toilet paper.

Distribution

Rangiora is common in scrub and forest throughout the North Island and upper South Island.

Appearance

It is a bushy shrub with large leaves, which are dull green on the upper surface. The undersides of the leaves are white with a soft furry underside. It has small, fragrant creamy flowers that are abundant in spring.

Circumstances of Poisoning

Rangiora is reputed to cause staggers in cattle and horses, but clinical cases appear to be very rare.

Absorption, Distribution, Metabolism, and Excretion

No information.

Mode(s) of Action

Maori used the plant for a number of medicinal uses. The leaves appeared to have some antiseptic quality and were used for wounds and old ulcerated sores to keep dust and flies away. The bark and tips of the branches on the west side of the bush were cut and the gum that exuded was chewed (but not swallowed) for halitosis. The leaves were bruised, mixed with olive oil and applied to boils as a poultice. The antiseptic principle responsible for these effects has not been identified.

Rangiora contains senkirkine, a pyrrolizidine alkaloid. Pyrrolizidine alkaloids are hepatotoxic and it is possible that the "staggers" reported in cattle and horses may be the result of hepatic encephalopathy. Alternatively, it is possible that Rangiora contains some unidentified neurotoxin.

Clinical Signs

No information.

Diagnostic Aids

No information.

Treatment

No information.

Prognosis

No information.

Necropsy

No information.

Public Health Considerations

No information.

Prevention

Rangiora is not palatable to livestock and likely to be eaten only if more palatable grazing is not available.

RARAUHE *PTERIDIUM ESCULENTUM*

Alternative Names

Austral bracken, Bracken, Bracken fern. Alternative Maori names are rahurahu or rarahu.

Distribution

Rarauhe is found throughout New Zealand, and, under other names, in most states of Australia, Malaysia, Polynesia, and New Caledonia.

Appearance

Rarauhe grows from creeping rhizomes, which are covered with dull reddish-brown or orange-brown hair. Large, stiff, roughly triangular fronds, which grow to up to 3 m tall, arise from the rhizomes.

Circumstances of Poisoning

Poisoning has been reported in cattle, horses, and pigs, and has been induced experimentally in sheep. There have been few reports of field poisoning in sheep. Clinical toxicosis is most commonly reported in cattle.

Young fronds and the underground rhizomes are more toxic than mature fronds.

Absorption, Distribution, Metabolism, and Excretion

There is a lack of information on the toxicokinetics of the toxic principles in Rarauhe. However, the clinical conditions in horses and cattle generally occur after 4−6 weeks of continuous exposure by grazing. Suckling calves may be poisoned through milk.

Mode(s) of Action

The toxic principles responsible for bone marrow suppression in cattle are ptaquiloside and related norsesquiterpene glycosides. It is assumed that these are also the cause of hemorrhagic diasthesis observed in experimental poisoning in sheep.

Horses have not been reported to develop bone marrow suppression, but are susceptible to the toxic effects of thiaminase I in Rarauhe. This enzyme inactivates thiamine (vitamin B_1), with polioencephalomalacia and clinical signs of neurological abnormality resulting. A similar condition has occasionally been reported in pigs. Ruminants may also be affected by this form of poisoning.

The toxic principle responsible for the retinal degeneration which occurs sometimes as part of Rarauhe poisoning in sheep is unknown.

Rarauhe also contains carcinogenic and mutagenic principles including, but not limited to, shikimic acid. The presence of the cyanogenic glycoside prunasin has also been detected but clinical poisoning consistent with this toxin has not been reported.

Clinical Signs

Poisoning in ruminants may present as an acute hemorrhagic disease or a chronic disease with urinary bladder neoplasia (enzootic hematuria).

Clinical signs in ruminants include pyrexia, failure to thrive, anorexia, and depression. On the examination, there is evidence of hemorrhagic diathesis, including anemia, hematuria, and ventral edema. Mucous membranes are pallid and often show petechiae and/or ecchymoses. Epistaxis and melaena have been observed. Calves tend to present with dyspnea.

Sheep are susceptible to "bright blindness" as part of Rarauhe poisoning. This is an irreversible blindness with tapetal hyperreflectivity, and affected sheep tend to be nervous and hyperalert.

Clinical signs of polioencephalomalacia in ruminants include depression, head-pressing, and incoordination. However, ruminants are more likely to exhibit signs of hemorrhagic diathesis and bone marrow suppression.

Horses are relatively resistant to the effects of ptaquiloside and to instead succumb to the toxic effects of thiaminase I. The clinical signs in horses are loss of condition, weakness, tremors, wandering, chronic ataxia and, in advanced cases, convulsions. A crouching stance is characteristic. Horses tend to become nervous and may lie down and be unable to rise.

Diagnostic Aids

Hematology in cattle shows nonregenerative anemia, granulocytopenia, and thrombocytopenia. Clotting time is prolonged.

Treatment

Animals should be removed from pasture containing Rarauhe, and provided with a high-quality diet. Blood transfusion may be beneficial in severely affected ruminants with acute hemorrhagic syndrome if their value justifies this measure. Horses may respond to intravenous thiamine injections if they are mildly affected.

Although many older textbooks recommend the use of DL batyl alcohol, this has been found to be of little value.

Prognosis

Prognosis is guarded to poor.

Necropsy

On necropsy, ruminants have thin watery blood, serosal petechiae and/or ecchymoses, and pale bone marrow, and hematuric urine in the urinary bladder. There may be neoplasia in the urinary bladder in the more chronic cases. Bone marrow should be submitted for histopathology to support the diagnosis.

There are no specific necropsy findings in monogastric animals.

In addition to bladder tumors, adenocarcinomas and pulmonary adenomas have been induced experimentally in laboratory animals.

The neurological syndrome of thiamine deficiency is due to polioencephalomalacia. This may show as fluorescence when a sliced brain is examined with a Wood's lamp, but the absence of fluorescence does not preclude the presence of polioencephalomalacia on microscopic examination.

On histopathology, bright blindness in sheep has lesions of severe atrophy of the retinal rods, cones, and outer nuclear layer, most pronounced in the tapetal portion of the retina.

Public Health Considerations

People should not eat any part of the plant, particularly the "fiddleheads," raw, because of the risk of carcinogenesis. Although the rhizomes were an important carbohydrate source for pre-European Maori, they were soaked and roasted according to a traditional procedure which minimized or removed the carcinogenic principles.

Prevention

Animals, particularly cattle, should not be grazed on pasture infested with Rarauhe. The palatability of the plant is generally low, so alternative safe feed should be provided if exposure cannot be avoided. Inclusion of Rarauhe in hay should be avoided.

TITOKI *ALECTRYON EXCELSUS*

Alternative Names

New Zealand Ash, New Zealand Oak.

Distribution

Titoki grow in coastal and lowland forests, and are also often planted as a specimen tree or shade tree in gardens. Although frost-tender when young, the Titoki is found throughout most of the North Island and from Banks Peninsula to central Westland in the South Island.

Appearance

Titoki can grow up to 18 m in height. It has smooth dark bark and glossy dark green leaves, and forms a spreading canopy. Titoki produce small, inconspicuous purple flowers, which have a pleasant fragrance, in spring. The seeds develop in hairy, woody capsules that split open to reveal bright red fruit that somewhat resemble raspberries. The fruit contains a shiny black seed. The fruit can take up to a year to mature, so a tree may simultaneously bear flowers and fruit.

Circumstances of Poisoning

There appears to be only one case of unconfirmed Titoki poisoning of live-stock. The tree is generally inaccessible to grazing animals.

Absorption, Distribution, Metabolism, and Excretion

No information. Likely to be similar to other plants containing cyanogenic compounds (q.v.).

Mode(s) of Action

Titoki belongs to the family *Sapindaceae*. Many members of this family synthesize cyanolipids, from which HCN is liberated. The presence of cyanolipids has not been confirmed in Titoki, but the plant does liberate HCN and theoretically at least, could be a cause of cyanide poisoning (q.v.).

Clinical Signs

See cyanide poisoning.

There have been no confirmed cases of titoki poisoning in animals in New Zealand. The seeds are reputed to be poisonous. The toxicity of the fruit is a matter of debate. The fruit is eaten by native birds such as kereru with no ill-effects.

Diagnostic Aids

See cyanide poisoning.

Treatment

See cyanide poisoning.

Prognosis

See cyanide poisoning.

Necropsy

See cyanide poisoning.

Public Health Considerations

The toxicity of Titoki appears to be theoretical, but given the grave prognosis of cyanide poisoning, consumption of the fruits or seeds is probably ill-advised.

Prevention

Because no cases of Titoki poisoning have been recorded, despite anecdotal accounts of cattle grazing on Titoki seedlings, there is no indication for preventative measures.

TURUTU *DIANELLA NIGRA*

Alternative Names

New Zealand blueberry, Inkberry, Flaxlily.

Distribution

Turutu colonises a wide range of habitats throughout both main islands of New Zealand and is commonly observed on the forest floor, on banks and along the sides of tracks.

Appearance

Turutu is an evergreen herb which forms diffuse, tussock-like clumps. The elaves are grass-like. It produces white star-shaped flowers in May. The berries are approximately 7 mm long and range in color from gray-white to deep violet-blue.

Circumstances of Poisoning

There is only one case of supposed Turutu poisoning recorded, that of a toddler who died in 1891 after eating several berries. The death may have been unrelated to the consumption of Turutu berries.

Absorption, Distribution, Metabolism, and Excretion

No information.

Mode(s) of Action

No information.

Clinical Signs

No information.

Diagnostic Aids

No information.

Treatment

No information.

Prognosis

No information.

Necropsy

No information.

Public Health Considerations

No information.

Prevention

No information.

TUTU *CORIARIA* SPECIES

Alternative Names

None.
There are six species of Coriaria in New Zealand, all known as Tutu:

Coriaria angustissima	*Coriaria arborea*
Coriaria lurida	*Coriaria plumosa*
Coriaria pteridoides	*Coriaria sarmentosa*

Distribution

Toxic species of Tutu are widely distributed throughout New Zealand and are commonly found along stream banks, in regenerating native forest and on broken ground such as the banks of rural roads.

Appearance

Most species of Tutu are shrubs of 1 m or less in height, although the tree tutu, *Coriaria arborea*, may form a small tree up to 6 m in height. Tutu has a straggling growth pattern. The glossy green leaves grow opposite on long, flexible stems. The small green flowers are produced in drooping racemes. The fruit are black or purple.

Circumstances of Poisoning

Veterinary cases of Tutu poisoning have been reported in cattle, sheep, and elephants. Horses do not seem to find Tutu palatable. Poisoning has been produced experimentally in pigs. All parts of the plants, except the flesh of the fruits, contain the toxic principle, tutin.

A form of relay toxicosis has been reported, in that dogs that ate the rumen contents of a poisoned lamb developed clinical signs.

Absorption, Distribution, Metabolism, and Excretion

There is a lack of information on the toxicokinetics of tutin. In a recent case report of human poisonings, it was observed that clinical signs may not commence until 6 hours after ingestion of the fruits. Onset of clinical signs from consumption of Tutu plants may be delayed for as long as 48 hours in cattle.

Delirium has been reported to last for several days in a human case.

Mode(s) of Action

Tutin inhibits glycine receptors in spinal neurons. Glycine acts as an inhibitory neurotransmitter, so the action of tutin results in enhanced neuronal excitability.

Clinical Signs

Clinical signs include hypersalivation, agitation, seizures, exhaustion, coma, and respiratory distress. Cattle may become aggressive, and/or may develop ruminal tympany. Death generally results from asphyxiation during seizures.

In human cases, patients reported that the neurological signs were preceded by nausea, and patients have also reported blurred vision and, during convalescence, memory deficits. Pyrexia and tachycardia have been observed in human patients during the clinical phase.

Diagnostic Aids

There are no specific diagnostic aids.

Treatment

There is no specific antidote. Seizures must be controlled with diazepam or, if necessary, barbiturate anesthesia. Respiratory function must be maintained.

Prognosis

Prognosis is good if seizures are controlled, and respiratory function is maintained.

Necropsy

Pulmonary congestion is likely, and mucous membranes may also be congested. Plant material in the gastrointestinal tract may be sufficiently intact to permit identification.

Public Health Considerations

Most recent cases of tutin toxicity in human beings have occurred as a result of tutin contamination of honey. People should be warned not to eat the berries of Tutu.

Prevention

Tutu remains an important toxicant to grazing ruminants in New Zealand. Access to tutu should be prevented.

WAORIKI *RANUNCULUS AMPHITRICHUS*

Alternative Names

New Zealand oxygen plant; Water buttercup; *Ranunculus rivularis*.

Distribution

This indigenous buttercup is found in the North, South, and Chatham Islands of New Zealand, and is also indigenous to Australia.

In New Zealand, Waoriki is found from coastal to montane altitudes. It is often partially submerged in shallow water, wet grassland, and at the margins of lakes, ponds, or tarns. It is sometimes found in moist clearings within forest or tussock grassland. It is easily propagated and may be grown around ornamental ponds.

Appearance

Waoriki is a perennial herb with small, lace-like, green scalloped leaves, and tiny yellow flowers.

Circumstances of Poisoning

As for other buttercups, Waoriki is not palatable to livestock but they may ingest it if there is heavy invasion of grazing or if it is the only feed available.

Absorption, Distribution, Metabolism, and Excretion

Protoanemonin is not readily absorbed from the gastrointestinal tract, with the result that effects are seen in the oral cavity and gastrointestinal mucosa. The toxin is most abundant in the roots, but these may be pulled up by grazing animals because Waoriki grows in soft, wet soil.

Mode(s) of Action

Protoanemonin is an irritant oil glycoside.

Clinical Signs

Clinical signs include oral irritation, hypersalivation, diarrhea, depression, and irritated skin of the muzzle.

Diagnostic Aids

None.

Treatment

Treatment is supportive. Remove the animals from grazing containing Waoriki, or provide alternative palatable feed.

Prognosis

Prognosis is favorable provided exposure is halted.

Necropsy

Lesions on necropsy are those of inflammation of the oral cavity, esophagus, and gastrointestinal tract.

Public Health Considerations

None.

Prevention

Avoid grazing that is heavily infested with Waoriki, and provide adequate alternative feed.

WHAUWHAUPAKU *PSEUDOPANAX ARBOREUS*

Alternative Names

Five-finger, Puahou.

Distribution

Whauwhaupaku is common throughout New Zealand in lowland forests and open scrub. It may be epiphytic.

Appearance

Whauwhaupaku, or Five-finger, is a small tree growing up to 8 m in heights. It has large, glossy light green leaves divided into five to seven leaflets with serrated edges. It produces pink or white flowers from June to August and small purple or black fruits from August to February.

Circumstances of Poisoning

Although it is much eaten by brushtail possums (*T. vulpecula*), Whauwhaupaku is theorized to be toxic because it is related to ivy (*Hedera helix*, q.v.).

Absorption, Distribution, Metabolism, and Excretion

No information.

Mode(s) of Action

No information.

Clinical Signs

Presumably similar to ivy, *H. helix*, q.v.

Diagnostic Aids

No information.

Treatment

Presumably similar to ivy, *H. helix*, q.v.

Prognosis

No information.

Necropsy

No information.

Public Health Considerations

No information.

Prevention

No information.

Index

Printed in the United States
By Bookmasters